PHARMACOTHERAPY APPROACHES TOWARD ENDOCRINE AND METABOLIC DISEASES

PHARMACOTHERAPY APPROACHES TOWARD ENDOCRINE AND METABOLIC DISEASES

Thakur Gurjeet Singh, PhD

Sanjana Mehta, PhD

Editors

AAP | APPLE ACADEMIC PRESS

First edition published 2026

Apple Academic Press Inc.
1265 Goldenrod Circle, NE,
Palm Bay, FL 32905 USA

760 Laurentian Drive, Unit 19,
Burlington, ON L7N 0A4, Canada

CRC Press
2385 NW Executive Center Drive,
Suite 320, Boca Raton FL 33431

4 Park Square, Milton Park,
Abingdon, Oxon, OX14 4RN, UK

Library and Archives Canada Cataloguing in Publication

CIP data on file with Canada Library and Archives

Library of Congress Cataloging-in-Publication Data

CIP data on file with US Library of Congress

ISBN: 978-1-779640-14-7 (hbk)
ISBN: 978-1-779640-15-4 (ebk)
DOI: 10.1201/9781779640154

About the Editors

Prof. (Dr.) Thakur Gurjeet Singh
M. Pharm (Pharmaceutical Sciences—Pharmacology),
PDCR (Clinical Research & PCPV (Pharmacovigilance)),
PhD (Pharmaceutical Sciences)

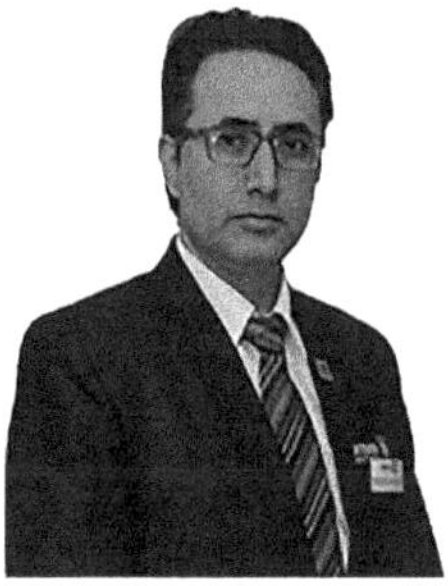

Thakur Gurjeet Singh, PhD, brings to the forefront a wealth of expertise and leadership cultivated through his role as Dean at Chitkara College of Pharmacy, Chitkara University, Punjab, India. Dr. Singh is globally recognized researcher consecutively for the last three years as one of the top 2% of scientists, an honor bestowed by Stanford University.

Spanning over 16 years, his academic and industrial experience is distinguished by more than 250 published papers, accruing an impressive 3950 citations, reflecting his significant scholarly impact, characterized by an H-Index surpassing 33 and an i10 Index of 104. Notably, his contributions are underscored by an Impact Factor of 890.5 and an RG score of 1598.

With a doctoral specialization in pharmacology and a prolific career focused on neuropharmacology, substance dependence, pharmacological preconditioning, and drug discovery, Dr. Singh has mentored more than 20 PhD scholars and over 90 postgraduate research candidates, contributing significantly to translational science in neurodegenerative and metabolic disorders. His expertise spans both preclinical and clinical research, with deep insights into animal modeling, behavioral pharmacology, and experimental therapeutics.

Under his visionary leadership, Chitkara College of Pharmacy became the first institute in Punjab to establish the IPA-SF (Indian Pharmaceutical Association-Student Forum) Punjab State Chapter, fostering professional engagement and national-level visibility for student pharmacists. He also serve as a Faculty Advisor at the ISPOR (Professional Society for Health Economics and Outcomes Research) Student Chapter at Chitkara College of Pharmacy, empowering students to explore health economics, outcomes research, and value-based healthcare practices.

An editorial board member and Editor of the *Journal of Pharmaceutical Technology, Research and Management*, Dr. Singh is a recognized contributor to scholarly publishing. His academic footprint includes numerous book chapters published by global leaders such as Elsevier, Springer Nature, Taylor & Francis, and Apple Academic Press, in areas ranging from nanotechnology and diabetes management to pharmacoeconomics and clinical therapeutics.

He has received multiple prestigious awards, including the Outstanding Researcher Award, Teacher's Excellence Awards, and accolades for innovation, patent filings, and research consultancy. Dr. Singh's enduring commitment to academic excellence, scientific inquiry, and institutional growth continues to elevate Chitkara College of Pharmacy as a hub of innovation, regulatory alignment, and interdisciplinary research in India's pharmaceutical landscape.

ORCID ID: 0000-0003-2979-1590,
Scopus ID: 27667828700,
Google Scholar ID: puCyockAAAAJ&hl,
Vidwan ID: 383169

Sanjana Mehta
PharmD, PhD
Pharmaceutical Sciences—Pharmacy Practice
Researcher, Educator, Innovation Catalyst, Clinical Pharmacology Expert

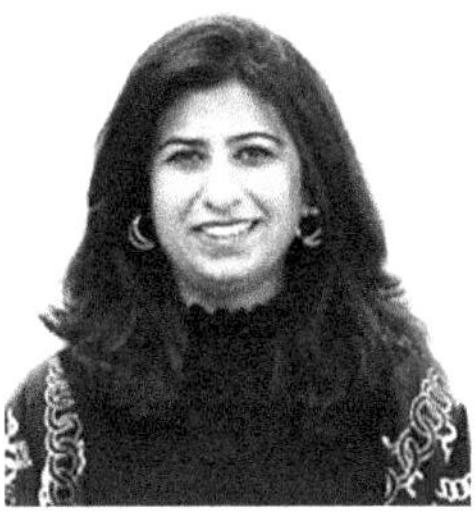

Sanjana Mehta, PharmD, PhD, is a dedicated academician, researcher, and innovation mentor with PharmD and PhD in Pharmaceutical Sciences. Currently serving as Assistant Professor at Chitkara College of Pharmacy, Chitkara University (Punjab), she brings over five years of experience in academic leadership, clinical pharmacology, and translational research.

She actively coordinates the Institutional Innovation Cell (IIC) where she fosters a vibrant ecosystem for student-led innovation, start-up incubation, and interdisciplinary research. In her roles as Education Officer of the ISPOR (Professional Society for Health Economics and Outcomes Research) Student Chapter and Faculty Coordinator for IPA-SF (Indian Pharmaceutical Association-Students' Forum) Punjab State Chapter, Dr. Mehta empowers students to engage with global trends in pharmacoeconomics, public health policy, and community pharmacy practice.

Beyond research, she is a trained professional in vaccine administration and basic life support (BLS) under the prestigious IPA-FIP (Indian Pharmaceutical Association-International Pharmaceutical Federation) collaborative "Train the Trainer" program, equipped with hands-on expertise in vaccine delivery, CPR, AED use, and ethical emergency response protocols. This training further enhances her role in healthcare education and community outreach.

She continues to mentor PharmD, MPharm, and PhD scholars in innovative, patient-centered research. Her research focus lies in advanced pharmacotherapeutics, metabolic disorders, and patient-centric innovations, with several patents and funded projects to her credit.

She also has a registered copyright (L-110308/2022) to her credit, the DN-22 QoL Questionnaire (Diabetic Neuropathy Quality of Life Questionnaire).

Recognized with awards including the Best PhD Award, Dr. Mehta is known for her academic rigor, mentoring excellence, and commitment to public health advancement.

ORCID ID: 0000-0002-5517-4273
Scopus ID: 57213267102
Google Scholar ID: V3hUwOgAAAAJ
Vidwan ID: 381413

Contents

Contributors

Deepankar Akoliya
Faculty of Medical and Health Sciences, Pharmacy, University of Auckland, New Zealand

Venkata Sita Rama Raju Allam
Department of Medical Biochemistry and Microbiology, Biomedical Centre (BMC), Uppsala University, Uppsala, Sweden

Geetansh Allawadhi
Chitkara College of Pharmacy, Chitkara University, Chandigarh, Punjab, India

Somasundaram Arumugam
Department of Pharmacology and Toxicology, National Institute of Pharmaceutical Education and Research (NIPER), Kolkata, West Bengal, India

Hema Arya
School of Pharmacy, Sharda University, Greater Noida, Uttar Pradesh, India

Shubham Singh Bartwal
National Institute of Pharmaceutical Education and Research (NIPER), Hyderabad, Telangana, India

Ruby Bhatia
Maharishi Markandeshwar Institute of Medical Science and Research (MMIMSR), Mullana, Ambala, Haryana, India

Indrajit Bhattacharya
Department of Pharmacology and Toxicology, National Institute of Pharmaceutical Education and Research (NIPER), Kolkata, West Bengal, India

Teeshyo Bhattacharya
Department of Pharmacology and Toxicology, National Institute of Pharmaceutical Education and Research (NIPER), Kolkata, West Bengal, India

Kiran Bhopate
IES Institute of Pharmacy, IES University, Bhopal, Madhya Pradesh, India

Shabana Bibi
Department of Biosciences, Shifa Tameer-e-Millat University, Islamabad, Pakistan

Amrish Chandra
School of Pharmacy, Sharda University, Greater Noida, Uttar Pradesh, India

Samrat Chauhan
Chitkara College of Pharmacy, Chitkara University, Rajpura, Punjab, India

Hitesh Chopra
Department of Biosciences, Saveetha School of Engineering, Saveetha Institute of Medical and Technical Sciences, Chennai, Tamil Nadu, India

Soumarshi Das
Chitkara College of Pharmacy, Chitkara University, Rajpura, Punjab, India

Gabriele De Rubis
Discipline of Pharmacy, Graduate School of Health, University of Technology Sydney, Sydney, Australia; Faculty of Health, Australian Research Centre in Complementary and Integrative Medicine, University of Technology Sydney, Ultimo, NSW, Australia

Kondaveeti Devaki
KL College of Pharmacy, Koneru Lakshmaiah Education Foundation, Vaddeswaram, Guntur, Andhra Pradesh, India

Murali Dhanasekaran
Harrison College of Pharmacy, Auburn University, Auburn, AL, USA

Sanchit Dhankhar
Chitkara College of Pharmacy, Chitkara University, Rajpura, Punjab, India

Bhavesh Dharmani
Chitkara College of Pharmacy, Chitkara University, Rajpura, Punjab, India

Sonia Dhiman
Chitkara College of Pharmacy, Chitkara University, Rajpura, Punjab, India

Kamal Dua
Discipline of Pharmacy, Graduate School of Health, University of Technology Sydney, Sydney, NSW, Australia; Faculty of Health, Australian Research Centre in Complementary and Integrative Medicine, University of Technology Sydney, Ultimo, NSW, Australia

Madhukar Garg
Chitkara College of Pharmacy, Chitkara University, Chandigarh, Punjab, India

Nitika Garg
Chitkara College of Pharmacy, Chitkara University, Rajpura, Punjab, India

Vinod Kumar Gauttam
Department of Pharmacognosy, Shiva Institute of Pharmacy, Bilaspur, Himachal Pradesh, India

Bey Hing Goh
College of Pharmaceutical Sciences, Zhejiang University, Hangzhou, China; School of Medical and Life Sciences,'Sunway University, Sunway City, Malaysia

Navjyoti Goyal
M.M. College of Pharmacy, Maharishi Markandeshwar (Deemed to be University), Mullana, Ambala, Haryana, India

Sumeet Gupta
M.M. College of Pharmacy, Maharishi Markandeshwar (Deemed to be University), Mullana, Ambala, Haryana, India

Vaibhav Jaiswal
IES Institute of Pharmacy, IES University, Bhopal, Madhya Pradesh, India

Deepika Joshi
Siddhartha Institute of Pharmacy, Dehradun, Uttarakhand, India

Mohammad Amjad Kamal
Institutes for Systems Genetics, Frontiers Science Center for Disease-related Molecular Network/West China Nursing School, West China Hospital, Sichuan University, China; King Fahd Medical Research Center, King Abdulaziz University, Jeddah, Saudi Arabia; Department of Pharmacy, Faculty of Allied Health Sciences, Daffodil International University, Birulia, Bangladesh; Enzymoics, Hebersham, NSW, Australia Novel Global Community Educational Foundation, Hebersham, NSW, Australia

Divya Kanwar
Chitkara College of Pharmacy, Chitkara University, Rajpura, Punjab, India

Jasleen Kaur
Chitkara College of Pharmacy, Chitkara University, Chandigarh, Punjab, India

Jaspreet Kaur
School of Pharmaceutical Sciences, RIMT University, Mandi-Gobindgarh, Punjab, India

Loveleen Kaur
Chitkara College of Pharmacy, Chitkara University, Chandigarh, Punjab, India

Sofia Kokkinis
Discipline of Pharmacy, Graduate School of Health, University of Technology Sydney, Sydney, Australia; Faculty of Health, Australian Research Centre in Complementary and Integrative Medicine, University of Technology Sydney, Ultimo, Australia

Gauree Kukreti
School of Pharmaceutical Sciences and Technology, Sardar Bhagwan Singh University, Dehradun, Uttarakhand, India

B. Jeevan Kumar
KL College of Pharmacy, Koneru Lakshmaiah Education Foundation, Vaddeswaram, Guntur, Andhra Pradesh, India

Gautam Kumar
School of Pharmacy, Sharda University, Greater Noida, Uttar Pradesh, India

Shushank Mahajan
Chitkara College of Pharmacy, Chitkara University, Rajpura, Punjab, India

Raniya Malik
Discipline of Pharmacy, Graduate School of Health, University of Technology Sydney, Sydney, Australia; Faculty of Health, Australian Research Centre in Complementary and Integrative Medicine, University of Technology Sydney, Ultimo, Australia

Sakshi Malik
Acute and General Medicine, Hull University Teaching Hospitals NHS Trust, Hull, United Kingdom

Prachi Mall
School of Pharmacy, Graphic Era Hill University, Dehradun, Uttarakhand, India

Ashi Mannan
Chitkara College of Pharmacy, Chitkara University, Chandigarh, Punjab, India

Sanjana Mehta
Chitkara College of Pharmacy, Chitkara University, Rajpura, Punjab

Pooja Mittal
Chitkara College of Pharmacy, Chitkara University, Rajpura, Punjab, India

Vishnu Mittal
Guru Gobind Singh College of Pharmacy, Yamuna Nagar, Haryana, India

Dania Mughal
Complications of Excess Weight, Cambridge University Hospitals, Cambridge, United Kingdom

Kavita Munjal
Department of Pharmacy, Amity Institute of Pharmacy, Amity University, Noida, Uttar Pradesh, India

Parminder Nain
School of Pharmaceutical Sciences, RIMT University, Mandi-Gobindgarh, Punjab, India

Keshav Raj Paudel
Centre for Inflammation, Centenary Institute and University of Technology Sydney, Faculty of Science, School of Life Sciences, Sydney, Australia

Arvind Raghav
TMCOP, Teerthanker Mahaveer University, Moradabad, Uttar Pradesh, India

Himanshi Raheja
Drug Safety Department, Mumbai, Maharashtra, India

Deepika Raina
School of Pharmacy, Graphic Era Hill University, Dehradun, Uttarakhand, India

Vaibhav Rastogi
TMCOP, Teerthanker Mahaveer University, Moradabad, Uttar Pradesh, India

Monika Saini
MM College of Pharmacy, Maharishi Markandeshwar (Deemed to be University), Mullana, Ambala, India

Urvashi Saxena
TMCOP, Teerthanker Mahaveer University, Moradabad, Uttar Pradesh, India

Nidhi Semwal
School of Pharmaceutical Science, Shri Guru Ram Rai University, Dehradun, Uttarakhand, India

Himanshu Sharma
Chitkara College of Pharmacy, Chitkara University, Rajpura, Punjab, India

Mridul Sharma
Chitkara College of Pharmacy, Chitkara University, Chandigarh, Punjab, India

Sarita Sharma
M.M. College of Pharmacy, Maharishi Markandeshwar (Deemed to be University), Mullana, Ambala, Haryana, India

Sheenam Sharma
M.M. College of Pharmacy, Maharishi Markandeshwar (Deemed to be University), Mullana, Ambala, Haryana, India

Veerta Sharma
Chitkara College of Pharmacy, Chitkara University, Rajpura, Punjab, India

Nasir A Siddiqui
Department of Pharmacognosy, King Saud University, Riyadh, Saudi Arabia

Baljinder Singh
Chitkara College of Pharmacy, Chitkara University, Chandigarh, Punjab, India

Bhavana Singh
School of Pharmacy, Sharda University, Greater Noida, Uttar Pradesh, India

Thakur Gurjeet Singh
Chitkara College of Pharmacy, Chitkara University, Chandigarh, Punjab, India

Remya Sreedhar
School of Pharmacy, Sister Nivedita University, Newtown, Kolkata, West Bengal, India

Raghav Tandon
Chitkara College of Pharmacy, Chitkara University, Chandigarh, Punjab, India

Lavish Vaid
Chitkara College of Pharmacy, Chitkara University, Chandigarh, Punjab, India

Vandana
School of Pharmacy, Sharda University, Greater Noida, Uttar Pradesh, India

Chetan Vashist
IITM College of Pharmacy, IITM Group of Institutions, Sonipat, Haryana, India

Anurag Verma
TMCOP, Teerthanker Mahaveer University, Moradabad, Uttar Pradesh, India

Abbreviations

4Ms	monitoring, measurement, management, and motivation
4-PBA	4-phenylbutyrate
AACE	American Association of Clinical Endocrinologists
AASA	amino-adipic semi-aldehyde
ABC	ATP-binding cassette
ABCD-1	ABC transporter subfamily D member-1
ACC	American College of Cardiology
ACE	American College of Endocrinology
ACTH	adrenocorticotropic hormone
AEDs	antiepileptic drugs
AF-1	activation of function domain-1
AgRP	agouti-related protein
AHA	American Heart Association
ALD	adrenoleukodystrophy
ALDP	adrenoleukodystrophy protein
AMN	adrenomyeloneuropathy
AMPK	AMP-activated protein kinase
AOM	antiobesity medication
ASCVD	atherosclerotic cardiovascular disease
ASDs	antiseizure drugs
ATD	antithyroid drug
ATOX1	antioxidant 1
ATP	adenosine triphosphate
ATP7A	ATPase copper transporting alpha
ATRX	alpha thalassemia/mental retardation syndrome
BAT	brown adipose tissue
BBB	blood–brain barrier
BMI	body mass index
CAD	coronary artery disease
cALD	cerebral childhood ALD
cAMP	cyclic adenosine monophosphate
CaSRs	calcium-sensing receptors
CCCP	carboxy-carbonylcyanide m-chloro-phenyl-hydrazone
CD	Cushing's disease
CHI	congenital hyperinsulinism
CKD	chronic kidney disease

CNS	central nervous system
COPD	chronic obstructive pulmonary disease
COX17	cytochrome C oxidase copper chaperone
COX-2	cyclooxygenase-2
CPS	complex partial seizures
CRP	C-reactive protein
CT	computerized tomography
CTR1	copper transport protein 1
DA	dopamine agonist
DAG	diacylglycerol
DAXX	death domain-associated protein
DBH	dopamine-beta-hydroxylase
DDR	DNA damage response
EC	endothelial cells
ECM	extracellular matrix protein
EEG	electroencephalogram
ER	endoplasmic reticulum
ER	estrogen receptor
ERE	estrogen response element
ES-CU2+	elesclomol–copper
ETC	electron transport chain
FasL	fas ligand
FGF23	fibroblast growth factor-23
FOXO	forkhead box protein
FRIDs	fall-risk-inducing
FSH	follicle-stimulating hormone
GABA	gamma-aminobutyric acid
GC	glucocorticoids
GD	Graves' disease
GH	growth hormone
GHPA	growth hormone-secreting pituitary adenoma
GIP	glucose-dependent insulinotropic polypeptide
GLP-1	glucagon-like peptide 1
GLUT	glucose transporter
GM	gut microbiome
GPCR	G-protein-coupled receptors
GPER1	G-protein coupled
GR	glucocorticoid receptor
GRF	GH-releasing factor
GSA	glutamic semi-aldehyde
GSK3β	glycogen synthase kinase 3β
HD	hemodialysis

HDL	high-density lipoproteins
HHRH	hereditary hypophosphatemic rickets with hypercalciuria
HMG-CoA	3-hydroxy-3-methylglutaryl-coenzyme A
HPT	hypothalamic-pituitary-thyroid
IGF	insulin-like growth factor
IL	interleukin-6
IL-1RALPHA	interleukin-1 alpha
ILAE	International League Against Epilepsy
IP3	inositol trisphosphate
LBP	low back pain
LDL	low-density lipoprotein
LDL-R	LDL receptor
LEVO	levothyroxine
LH	luteinizing hormone
LRP1	low-density lipoprotein receptor-related protein
mAbs	monoclonal antibodies
MAPK	mitogen-activated protein kinase
MBDs	metabolic bone disorders
mbER	membrane-bound ER
MCP-1	monocyte chemoattractant protein-1
MD	Menkes disease
MEN	multiple endocrine neoplasia
mGPDH	mitochondrial glycerol-3-phosphate dehydrogenase
MLL1	mixed-lineage leukemia 1
MRI	magnetic resonance imaging
MTC	medullary thyroid carcinoma
mtDNA	mitochondrial DNA
mTOR	mammalian target of rapamycin
MUFAs	monounsaturated fatty acids
NAD+	nicotinamide adenine dinucleotide
NAFLD	nonalcoholic fatty liver disease
NDD	neurodegenerative disease
NENs	neuroendocrine neoplasms
nER	nuclear ER
NETs	neuroendocrine tumors
NF-κB	nuclear factor-kappa B
NMDA	*N*-methyl-D-aspartate
NSTEMI	nonsegment elevation myocardial infarction
OHS	occipital horn syndrome
OSX	osteoblast-specific transcription factor
OXPHOS	oxidative phosphorylation
PAI	plasminogen activator inhibitor

PAR	protease activation receptor
PCSK9	proprotein convertase subtilisin/kexin type 9
PD	peritoneal dialysis
PDB	Paget bone disease
PHPT	primary hyperparathyroidism
PI3K	phosphatidylinositol-3 kinase
PIP2	phosphatidylinositol 4,5-bisphosphate
PKB	protein kinase B
PKC	protein kinase C
PKM2	pyruvate kinase M2
PLS3	plastin 3
PP	pancreatic polypeptides
PPTD	pancreas-preserving total duodenectomy
PRL	prolactin
PTH	parathyroid hormone
PTU	propylthiouracil
PUFAs	polyunsaturated fatty acids
RAI	radioactive iodine
RANKL	receptor activator of NF-kB ligand
RBP	RNA binding protein
RCL	reactive centre loop
ROS	reactive oxygen species
RUNX2	runt-related transcription factor 2
SAP	serum alkaline phosphatase
SASP	senescence-associated secretory phenotype
SCFA	short-chain fatty acids
SCN1A	sodium voltage-gated channel alpha subunit 1
SCO	synthesis of cytochrome C oxidase
SGLT	sodium-glucose co-transporter
SOD	superoxide dis-mutases
SPS	simple partial seizures
SST2	somatostatin receptor subtype 2
STEMI	segment elevation myocardial infarction
T2DM	type 2 diabetes milletus
TC	total cholesterol
TFs	transcription factor
TGF	transforming growth factor
TGF	tumor growth factor
TGF-BETA	transforming growth factor-beta
TGN	trans-Golgi network
TNF	tumor necrosis factor
TNF-ALPHA	tumor necrosis factor alpha

TOS	The Obesity Society
tPA	tissue-type plasminogen activator
TRH	thyrotropin-releasing hormone
TRPV6	transient receptor potential vanilloid type 6
TSH	thyroid-stimulating hormone
TSI	thyroid-stimulating immunoglobulin
TTFA	they-trifluoro-acetone
UNL	upper normal limit
uPA	urokinase-type plasminogen activator
UTI	urinary tract infection
UVB	ultraviolet B
VEGFR	vascular endothelial growth factor receptor
VLCFA	very-long-chain fatty acids
VPA	valproic acid
WAT	white adipose tissues
WC	waist circumference
WHO	World Health Organization
Wnt	wingless-related integration
ZA	zoledronic acid

Foreword 1

It is with great pleasure that I introduce *Pharmacotherapeutic Approaches Toward Endocrine and Metabolic Diseases,* edited by Dr. Thakur Gurjeet Singh and Dr. Sanjana Mehta. This book represents a major milestone in the field of pharmacotherapy, offering an in-depth exploration of the latest advances in the management of endocrine and metabolic disorders.

The global rise in endocrine and metabolic diseases, such as diabetes, obesity, and thyroid dysfunctions, highlights the urgent need for innovative therapeutic solutions. Dr. Singh and Dr. Mehta have addressed this need by providing a comprehensive examination of pharmacological strategies to combat these conditions. Their book covers a wide range of topics, from the basic principles of pharmacotherapy to the most recent advancements, making it a valuable resource for healthcare providers.

Each chapter of this book is rich with evidence-based recommendations and practical insights, ensuring that readers gain a thorough understanding of both the theoretical and practical aspects of managing endocrine and metabolic diseases. The authors' meticulous approach to compiling the latest research and clinical guidelines makes this book an indispensable tool for clinicians, researchers, and students aiming to enhance their practice and improve patient outcomes.

I commend Dr. Singh and Dr. Mehta for their dedication and expertise in creating such a comprehensive and insightful resource. Their work will undoubtedly contribute to significant advancements in the field of endocrinology and metabolism, guiding healthcare professionals toward more effective treatments and better patient care.

Pharmacotherapeutic Approaches Toward Endocrine and Metabolic Diseases is a testament to the authors' commitment to advancing medical knowledge and improving healthcare delivery. It is a must-read for anyone involved in the care of patients with endocrine and metabolic disorders.

Sincerely,

Dr. Randhir Singh Dahiya
Associate Professor
Department of Pharmacology
School of Health Sciences, Central University of Punjab

Foreword 2

It is with great honor that I present the book, *Pharmacotherapeutic Approaches Toward Endocrine and Metabolic Diseases*, edited by Dr. Thakur Gurjeet Singh and Dr. Sanjana Mehta. This comprehensive work stands as a vital addition to the field of pharmacotherapy, addressing the pressing need for advanced treatment strategies in managing endocrine and metabolic disorders.

Endocrine and metabolic diseases, such as diabetes, obesity, and thyroid disorders, are among the most significant health challenges faced globally. The increasing prevalence of these conditions demands innovative therapeutic approaches and a profound understanding of their underlying mechanisms. In this book, Dr. Singh and Dr. Mehta have meticulously compiled the latest research and clinical practices, providing a thorough examination of pharmacological interventions. Each chapter delves deeply into the intricacies of these disorders, offering evidence-based recommendations and practical insights that are essential for optimizing patient care.

The strength of this book lies in its ability to bridge the gap between foundational knowledge and cutting-edge therapeutic strategies. It serves as an indispensable resource for clinicians, researchers, and students who are committed to enhancing their understanding and treatment of endocrine and metabolic diseases. The authors' dedication to compiling such a comprehensive and insightful text is commendable, and their work will undoubtedly inspire further advancements in the field.

I am confident that "Pharmacotherapeutic Approaches Toward Endocrine and Metabolic Diseases" will become an essential reference for healthcare professionals striving to improve the lives of patients affected by these challenging conditions. The expertise and dedication of Dr. Singh and Dr. Mehta shine through in every chapter, making this book a significant contribution to the field of pharmacotherapy.

Sincerely,

Dr. Puneet Kumar Bansal
Professor & Former HOD
Department of Pharmacology
School of Health Sciences, Central University of Punjab

Preface

Endocrine and metabolic diseases pose significant challenges to public health worldwide. From diabetes and obesity to thyroid disorders and adrenal diseases, these conditions affect millions of individuals, impacting their quality of life and increasing the burden on healthcare systems globally. This book, *Pharmacotherapeutic Approaches Toward Endocrine and Metabolic Diseases,* offers an exploration of therapeutic strategies and advancements in the management of endocrine and metabolic disorders. This comprehensive volume represents a collective effort of experts in the field to provide an in-depth exploration of pharmacological interventions for various endocrine and metabolic disorders.

This book aims to address these challenges by offering insights into the latest pharmacotherapy approaches for managing endocrine and metabolic diseases. Each chapter delves into specific disorders, discussing their pathophysiology, clinical manifestations, and cutting-edge therapeutic strategies. The diverse range of topics covered in this book reflects the complexity and multifaceted nature of endocrine and metabolic disorders. From hormonal regulation and epigenetics to nutritional interventions and emerging therapies, readers will gain a comprehensive understanding of the current landscape of pharmacotherapy in this field. The book is written in simple and clear text, and we also used many figures and tables to make the book easier to understand.

We hope that *Pharmacotherapeutic Approaches Toward Endocrine and Metabolic Diseases* serves as a valuable reference for advancing knowledge, improving patient care, and ultimately contributing to better health outcomes for individuals affected by these conditions.

We extend our heartfelt gratitude to all the authors who have contributed their expertise and insights to this book. Their dedication and commitment have been instrumental in creating a valuable resource for healthcare professionals, researchers, and students interested in endocrine and metabolic diseases. The editors are also thankful to Apple Academic Press and their team members for the opportunity to publish this volume.

Lastly, we thank our family members for their love, support, encouragement, and patience during the entire period of this work.

—Editors

Dr. Thakur Gurjeet Singh

Dr. Sanjana Mehta

CHAPTER 1

General Aspects and Therapeutic Relevance to the Thyroid Disorders

HITESH CHOPRA[1], VINOD KUMAR GAUTTAM[2], KAVITA MUNJAL[3*], KONDAVEETI DEVAKI[4], VAIBHAV JAISWAL[5], CHETAN VASHIST[6], and SHABANA BIBI[7]

[1]*Department of Biosciences, Saveetha School of Engineering, Saveetha Institute of Medical and Technical Sciences, Chennai, Tamil Nadu, India*

[2]*Department of Pharmacognosy, Shiva Institute of Pharmacy, Bilaspur, Himachal Pradesh, India*

[3]*Department of Pharmacy, Amity Institute of Pharmacy, Amity University, Noida, Uttar Pradesh, India*

[4]*KL College of Pharmacy, Koneru Lakshmaiah Education Foundation, Vaddeswaram, Guntur, Andhra Pradesh, India*

[5]*IES Institute of Pharmacy, IES University, Bhopal, Madhya Pradesh, India*

[6]*IITM College of Pharmacy, IITM Group of Institutions, Sonipat, Haryana, India*

[7]*Department of Biosciences, Shifa Tameer-e-Millat University, Islamabad, Pakistan*

*Corresponding author

ABSTRACT

Health and well-being are greatly affected by thyroid problems, which include hyperthyroidism and hypothyroidism. This chapter discusses thyroid problems' prevalence, diagnostic hurdles, and effective

Pharmacotherapy Approaches Toward Endocrine and Metabolic Diseases.
Thakur Gurjeet Singh and Sanjana Mehta (Eds.)

DOI: 10.1201/9781779640154-1

treatment techniques. These illnesses are significant in therapeutic practice because of their vast spectrum of symptoms, which include mental disorders and tiredness. Examining thyroid disorders alongside diabetes, cardiovascular issues, and autoimmune diseases emphasizes how interrelated health conditions are. Moving to therapy, the chapter discusses treatment options for thyroid issues. Thyroid hormone replacement and antithyroid medications are essential to thyroid function restoration. Surgery and radioactive iodine treatments are considered for thyroid cancer and severe hyperthyroidism. Lifestyle and dietary changes are also regarded as complementary to medical therapies. Regular blood testing of thyroid function is stressed to guarantee proper drug dosing and management. Additionally, thyroid diseases during pregnancy present particular complications, emphasizing the importance of effective therapy for maternal and fetal health. In conclusion, this chapter covers thyroid diseases' general and therapeutic relevance, emphasizing their health effects and the need for a multidisciplinary approach to therapy. It helps healthcare professionals, researchers, and thyroid-problem patients manage and improve their quality of life.

1.1 INTRODUCTION

Thyroid diseases indeed represent a significant health concern globally. The thyroid is a crucial endocrine gland controlling the body's metabolic processes. Thyroid illnesses affect an estimated 42 million individuals in India, which highlights the severity of the problem. Hypothyroidism (underactive thyroid) and hyperthyroidism (overactive thyroid) are the two most prevalent thyroid conditions. These conditions can result from various factors, including autoimmune disorders, iodine deficiency, genetics, and environmental influences. The accessibility of medical treatment for thyroid diseases is crucial for effective management. Thyroid disorders often require lifelong medication, particularly in cases of hypothyroidism, where thyroid hormone replacement therapy is necessary. Regular monitoring and adjustment of medication doses are essential to ensure optimal thyroid function. The relative visibility of thyroid conditions, such as a noticeable swelling (goiter), can aid in early diagnosis (Mansourian, 2011). Regular health check-ups, including thyroid function tests, are essential for detecting thyroid disorders in their early stages. Early intervention can prevent complications and improve the overall prognosis for individuals with thyroid diseases. Public awareness campaigns and healthcare initiatives can significantly educate people about the importance of thyroid health, the symptoms of thyroid disorders, and the need for timely medical attention (Rehni and Singh, 2011). Additionally, addressing iodine deficiency through public health measures can help prevent some thyroid disorders, as iodine is a significant mineral responsible for thyroid hormone biosynthesis. The management of thyroid-related diseases in India, as elsewhere, calls for a multifaceted strategy incorporating public awareness, accessible healthcare services, and early diagnosis and treatment. The collaborative efforts of healthcare professionals, policymakers, and the public are crucial for addressing the challenges posed by thyroid disorders nationally and globally (Tyagi et al., 2010; Unnikrishnan and Menon, 2011).

1.2 THYROID GLAND ANATOMY AND ITS ESSENTIAL ROLE IN HORMONE PRODUCTION AND REGULATION

1.2.1 ANATOMICAL PROFILE OF THYROID GLANDS

The thyroid gland forms during embryonic development from the germ layer known as endoderm. It is a butterfly-shaped structure with two lobes joined by a small isthmus at the front of the neck, close to the thyroid cartilage.

1.2.2 SIZE AND WEIGHT

The thyroid gland is one of the most prominent glands in the endocrine system. It is approximately 5 cm long and weighs approximately 25 g (Ostrowski et al., 2023).

1.2.3 PHYSIOLOGICAL SIGNIFICANCETHE THYROID GLAND IS ESSENTIAL IN THE ENDOCRINE SYSTEM BY PRODUCING SEVERAL HORMONES.

- **Important hormones of thyroid glands (T3 and T4):** These hormones, triiodothyronine (T3) and thyroxine (T4), are essential for regulating metabolism. They influence the body's energy production, heat generation, and overall metabolic rate.
- **Calcitonin:** This hormone controls blood calcium and phosphorus levels. It encourages calcium to be deposited in bone tissue, lowering blood calcium levels.

1.2.4 FUNCTIONS OF THYROID HORMONES

- **Metabolism regulations:** The hormones T3 and T4 are essential for controlling the body's metabolism. They affect the way that cells use the energy that comes from food.
- **Growth and development:** Hormones related to the thyroid are essential for healthy growth and development, particularly in the early years of life. They support both general physical growth and the development of the neurological system.
- **Electrolyte balance:** Thyroid hormones also impact electrolyte concentrations in the blood, helping to balance ions such as sodium and potassium (Fröhlich and Wahl, 2021).

1.2.5 THYROID GLAND ROLE IN HORMONE PRODUCTION AND REGULATIONS

- **Negative feedback control system:** The hypothalamic–pituitary–thyroid (HPT) axis operates as a negative feedback control system. Hypothalamic release of thyrotropin-releasing hormone (TRH) and the anterior pituitary glands thyrotropin thyroid-stimulating hormone (TSH) increase the thyroid gland's production and secretion of T3 and T4. Conversely, hormones from the thyroid inhibit the production and secretion of TRH and TSH. This intricate feedback system maintains serum thyroid hormone concentrations within narrow limits.

- **Regulation of thyroid hormones:** TSH secretion rises when thyroid hormone production declines, resulting in elevated thyroid hormone secretion. On the other hand, large doses of thyroid hormone or increased thyroid hormone production suppress TSH secretion, causing blood thyroid hormone concentrations to drop and return to normal (Ren and Zhu, 2022).
- **Triiodothyronine (T3) production:** In extrathyroidal tissues, de-iodination of T4 produces a significant portion of the daily generation of T3. Adverse situations include malnourishment, injuries, illness, infections, and the use of some medicines like amiodarone, which reduces the conversion of T4–T3.
- **Adaptation to starvation and illness:** The decrease in T3 production during adverse conditions like starvation and illness is considered a beneficial adaptation. By reducing the rate at which proteins break down and nutrients are used for heat generation, this reduction helps maintain tissue integrity and conserve energy resources (Thapa et al., 2021).
- **Fetal thyroid development:** The fetal thyroid gland starts functioning around 12 weeks of gestation, with its activity increasing progressively. TSH secretion spikes shortly after birth, raising the levels of T4 and T3 in the serum. These concentrations steadily decrease over time, reaching adult values during puberty.
- **Thyroid hormones in pregnancy:** Because pregnant women secrete more thyroid hormone than nonpregnant women, women with thyroid deficiencies typically need greater dosages of thyroid hormone during pregnancy.
- **Thyroid secretion in older adults:** Regarding thyroid secretion, older persons do not differ much from younger adults. The delicate balance maintained by the HPT axis is essential for adequately functioning various physiological processes in the body (Brown et al., 2023; Hoermann et al., 2017).

1.3 THYROID DISORDERS AND THEIR ASSOCIATION WITH OTHER MEDICAL CONDITIONS

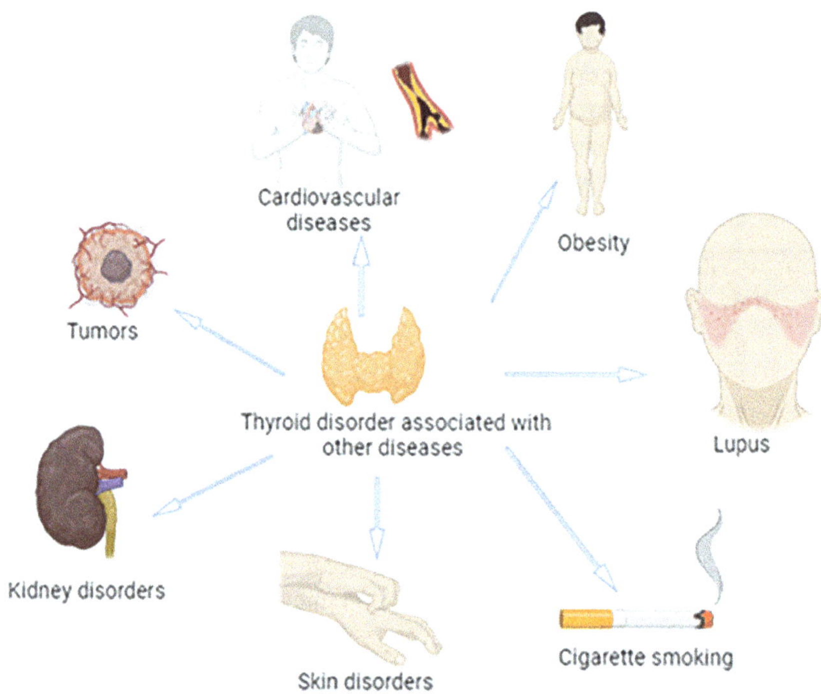

FIGURE 1.1 Thyroid disorders with other diseases association.

1.3.1 THYROID HORMONE ALTERATION IN CKD

Peripheral thyroid hormone metabolism and the hypothalamus-pituitary-thyroid axis are impacted by chronic kidney disease (CKD). Low T3 is the most frequent laboratory finding, and subclinical hypothyroidism is common. Although there is a disruption in the circadian rhythm, TSH levels are often normal. Uremia in CKD can blunt the pituitary response to TRH, leading to decreased TSH release. Abnormal serum constituents in uremia can displace T3 and T4 from normal protein binding sites. Low T4 levels may result from altered mono-deiodinase action and the formation of reverse T3. Transient increases in T4 levels after hemodialysis (HD) are attributed to heparin's effect on T4 binding (Basu and Mohapatra, 2012).

- **Factors contributing to low T3 in CKD:** Factors such as fasting, chronic metabolic acidosis, and protein malnutrition in CKD affect iodothyronine deiodinase, impacting T3 synthesis from T4. Inflammatory cytokines like TNF-alpha and IL-1 decrease peripheral conversion of T4 to T3 by inhibiting 1,5′-deiodinase expression. Low free T3 levels are independently associated with mortality in HD patients. Low T3 levels before renal transplant are linked to posttransplant risks of graft loss (Lim et al., 1977).
- **Goiter in CKD:** There is an increased prevalence of goiter (0–9%) in CKD patients. This may be due to decreased clearance of inorganic iodides, which causes thyroid hypertrophy and goiter. Decreased clearance of goitrogenic substances like aryl acid in CKD may also contribute. Increased serum iodine levels can prolong the Wolff-Chaikoff effect.
- **Physiological compensation in CKD:** Physiological compensation for low T3/T4 with normal TSH levels in CKD reduces protein catabolism, increasing nitrogen waste overload (Iglesias and Díez, 2009).

1.3.2 THYROID HORMONES AND GLOMERULONEPHRITIS

Renal pathophysiology in these situations is influenced by the participation of thyroglobulin and the deposition of immunological complexes. It is crucial to monitor and manage both thyroid disorders and renal illnesses because of their relationship. These pathophysiological conditions are described as:

- **Association with glomerulonephritis:** Numerous forms of glomerulonephritis are associated with thyroid disorders, including hypo- and hyperthyroidism. The glomerulonephritis types, membranous, IgA, mesangial-capillary, membranoproliferative, and minimal change glomerulonephritis, are linked to thyroid disorders.
- **Prevalence of membranous glomerulonephritis:** Among the mentioned types, membranous glomerulonephritis is the most frequent one associated with thyroid disease.

- **Histological changes:** One of the histological alterations seen is the thickening of the glomerular basement membrane due to immune complex deposition. Moreover, elevated mesangial and endocapillary cellularity is noted (Iglesias et al., 2017).
- **Role of thyroglobulin:** According to specific research, thyroglobulin is deposited in the glomeruli's basement membrane.
- **Similar effects in other autoimmune disorders:** Other autoimmune diseases, including systemic lupus erythematosus and diabetes, have similar effects, including immune complex deposition and changes in renal function (Iglesias et al., 2017).

1.3.3 THYROID DISEASE AND NEPHROTIC SYNDROME

Reduced blood T4 and total T3 levels result from proteinuria in nephrotic syndrome, which causes the loss of binding of thyroxine-binding globulin, transthyretin, and albumin proteins. Most people continue to be euthyroid despite protein losses because the thyroid keeps average amounts of free T3 and T4 to compensate for proteinuria. The role of levothyroxine in replacing thyroid hormone in nephrotic syndrome is controversial (Mohamedali et al., 2014).

1.3.4 KIDNEY ILLNESS AND THYROID CANCER

Thyroid cancer is becoming increasingly commonplace worldwide, with women three times more likely to receive a diagnosis. Individuals with thyroid cancer are more likely to develop other cancers, such as renal cell carcinoma, particularly if they have papillary, follicular, or anaplastic thyroid cancer (Grimm, 2022).

1.3.5 DIALYSIS'S IMPACT ON THYROID HORMONES

- **Hemodialysis:** Most people with HD are euthyroid and have low T3 levels, which are associated with systemic acidity, duration of dialysis, indicators of endothelial damage, and inflammation. In 20% of HD patients, elevated TSH may be a compensatory strategy (Wiederkehr et al., 2004).

- **Peritoneal dialysis (PD):** Subclinical hypothyroidism and low T3 levels are linked to Parkinson's disease. Inflammation, malnutrition, and decreased iodide clearance in advanced CKD contribute to low T3 levels. T4 and T3 losses in PD are minor and easily compensated; thyroid hormone supplementation is unnecessary (Fan et al., 2016).

1.4 TYPES OF THYROID DISORDERS

1.4.1 CONGENITAL HYPOTHYROIDISM

Congenital hypothyroidism is the term for a condition in which a baby has an insufficient amount of thyroid hormones; this disease can arise prior to or during delivery. This deficiency can be attributed to various factors, as outlined in Table 1.1. The main reasons include abnormalities in the enzymes synthesizing T4 and maldevelopment of the thyroid gland or the HPT system. One noteworthy feature is that thyroid hormones (T4 and T3) and TSH are mainly incapable of passing through the placenta. As such, problems with thyroid gland development or the HPT system are usually the cause of hypothyroidism in babies. In some cases, maternal factors can contribute to congenital hypothyroidism. For instance, if a pregnant woman experiences an iodine deficiency or uses antithyroid drugs for treating thyrotoxicosis during the first trimester, these substances can be transferred across the placenta, potentially affecting the average growth of the fetal thyroid gland. Given the critical role, thyroid hormones play in the average growth and development of the newborn's central nervous system and other organs, it is imperative to diagnose and treat congenital hypothyroidism as soon as possible. Early detection and treatment are crucial to avoid difficulties and guarantee the best possible growth. Regular screening programs are often in place to identify infants with congenital hypothyroidism shortly after birth, enabling timely intervention (Miculan et al., 1993; Rastogi and LaFranchi, 2010).

TABLE 1.1 Hypothyroidism-Associated Disease (Das et al., 2022)

Serial No.	Types of Disease Caused by Hypothyroidism	Risks	Clinical Symptoms	Management
2	Hashimoto's thyroiditis	An excess of iodine and elevated levels of thyroid antibody (Ab)	Low iron absorption, low heart rate, cutaneous myxedema, hashitoxicosis	Monitoring thyroid function, receiving appropriate medical treatment, and regular follow-ups with a healthcare professional are crucial for managing Hashimoto's thyroiditis and its potential complications
2	Cretinism	Iodine deficiency	Rheumatic aches, myopathy, macroglossia, and mental impairment	Early identification and management are essential for MPS sufferers to manage their symptoms and enhance their quality of life. Treatment approaches may include enzyme replacement therapy and supportive care to address specific symptoms
3	Myxedema	Gender, thyroid gland removal	Impaired mental stress, cardiovascular depression	Rewarming the person, providing warm fluids, and monitoring vital signs are essential to emergency care
4	Thyroiditis	Autoimmune disease	Frequent urination, sexual dysfunction, and water retention	Early diagnosis and management are crucial to addressing the symptoms and preventing potential complications

Congenital hypothyroidism frequently results in full-term gestations, with deliveries occurring after 40 weeks. These infants may also weigh more than 4 kg at birth, which is more significant than average for their gestational age. This larger size might be due to the lack of thyroid hormones affecting growth regulation during fetal development. The skeletal maturation defects and growth impairments that these neonates experienced during their stay in the womb are indicative of hypothyroidism. Affected neonates have clinical signs and symptoms of thyroid dysfunction. It is important to note that some infants may not exhibit noticeable symptoms, or their symptoms may be subtle and nonspecific. Care should be taken while diagnosing hypothyroidism in babies, particularly those born prematurely. Congenital hypothyroidism affects newborns in different ways; the degree of thyroid function, the way thyroid hormones interact, and other physiological processes all play a role in how severe the clinical manifestations are. Regular screening programs are often in place to identify affected infants shortly after birth, allowing for prompt treatment (Kirsten, 2000).

A complete approach, comprising a detailed history, physical examination, and specific diagnostic tests, is required to diagnose hypothyroidism in babies. Newborn screening programs are the primary means by which hypothyroidism is diagnosed in the United States and Canada. Most North American programs follow either an initial screening approach to measure thyroid hormone values or a two-tiered approach. The two-tiered technique measures T4 first, then evaluates TSH levels in newborns whose T4 levels are deficient. Blood is usually drawn between the second and fifth days of life when postnatal physiologic TSH rises. It is noteworthy that samples obtained between 24 and 48 h after birth, during this TSH rise, might occasionally result in falsely positive results for hypothyroidism, necessitating re-evaluation. It is recommended to do additional laboratory tests, as previously mentioned, on infants displaying physical signs of hypothyroidism before receiving the results of the neonatal screen. X-rays of the long bones can be helpful in addition to laboratory tests to determine bone age. These X-rays can determine the length and degree of thyroid dysfunction. The presence, size, and form of ossification centers in the foot and knee, along with the degree of skull maturation, are used to assess the extent of bone maturation. The information provided by these imaging techniques is beneficial in evaluating the infant's thyroid function and how it affects bone growth overall (Büyükgebiz, 2013).

1.4.2 HYPERTHYROIDISM

A rare disorder known as pediatric hyperthyroidism is typified by the thyroid gland secreting too much thyroid hormone. Like hypothyroidism, hyperthyroidism can occur spontaneously or develop over time. Congenital hyperthyroidism, also known as newborn thyrotoxicosis, is most commonly found in babies born to moms who have either Hashimoto's disease or Graves' disease (GD). This illness could be short-lived, lasting a few weeks, or long lived, lasting more than six months. The fundamental reason is linked to the autoantibody of class G immunoglobulin, thyroid-stimulating immunoglobulin (TSI), passing through the placenta. TSH that has been radiolabeled can be removed from TSH receptors on the thyroid membrane by TSI. Treatment must be started very early in order to reduce excess thyroid hormone production and relieve symptoms. Neonatal thyrotoxicosis is usually treated with medications, such as propylthiouracil (PTU), propranolol, and Lugol's solution (5% iodine and 10% potassium iodide). PTU is taken orally in divided dosages, whereas Lugol's solution is delivered in specified doses. In early PTU therapy, adverse reactions are possible, including rash, hives, joint discomfort, and arthritis, which are frequent side effects. Leukopenia that is transient is a common and often benign medication effect. More severe side effects include agranulocytosis, toxic hepatitis, collagen-vascular-like syndrome, thrombocytopenia, and diffuse interstitial pneumonitis. Fever, bacterial infection, and a granulocyte count $<250\ mm^{-3}$ indicate agranulocytosis. PTU should be stopped if there is a fever, upper respiratory illness, or oral infection. Healthcare providers must work together to manage congenital hyperthyroidism in newborns with close supervision to achieve the best potential results and reduce the chance of treatment-related side effects (Table 1.2) (De Leo et al., 2016).

1.4.3 T3 SYNDROME IN PREMATURE NEONATES

Premature babies have a physiological issue known as low T3 syndrome. T3 levels are lower in this phenomenon than in full-term newborns. With increasing gestational age, there is a tendency for the peak responses of T4 and T3 and the rise of TSH in neonates. Because of their early birth, premature babies frequently exhibit reduced T3 readings as a temporary developmental feature (LaFranchi, 2021).

This syndrome is characterized by a transient "decrease" in T3 levels. The relative undernutrition and feeding issues that are prevalent in preterm newborns throughout the neonatal period are probably connected to this decline. Several illnesses, such as infections, acidosis, hypoxia, hypoglycemia, and hypocalcemia, cause these difficulties (Singh et al., 2020; Bhatt et al., 2024). These elements may prevent T4 from being converted to

TABLE 1.2 Hyperthyroidism-Associated Disease (Das et al., 2022)

Serial Number	Disease Caused by Hyperthyroidism	Risk Associated	Clinical Symptoms	Management
1	Grave's disease	Iodine consumption increased, smoking, and vitamin D deficiency	Lymphocyte infiltration, aberrant cytokine release, and tissue injury	Diagnostic procedures, such as biopsies, imaging studies, or blood tests can reveal the presence of immune cells in tissues and altered cytokine profiles
2	Thyroid storm	Infection, acute illness, trauma, cardiovascular disease, thyroid surgery	Arrhythmia, seizure	Pharmacotherapeutic therapy
3	Thyroid nodules	Iodine deficiency	Neck lump, thyroid enlargement	Increase iodine intake
4	Goiter	Alcohol use, oral contraceptives, iodine deficiency, and tobacco use	Dysphagia, dyspnea, superior vena cava	Iodine intake increases; avoid tobacco and alcohol use
5	Thyroid cancer	Gender, age, breast cancer, poor iodine consumption, and radiation	Hoarseness, enlarged cervical lymph nodes, asymptomatic thyroid nodule	Increase iodine consumption. CT scans or MRIs may be ordered to assess the extent of lymph node enlargement and any impact on surrounding structures

T3, which would exacerbate the low T3 levels that are currently present. Premature babies may experience low serum T3 levels for one to two months. Not only do serum T3 levels tend to be low, but total T4 concentrations are usually low or average. However, free T4 readings typically fall within the range of healthy preterm newborns of the same weight and gestational age. Additionally, these newborns' serum TSH values stay within the normal range. Low T3 syndrome in premature infants typically does not require special medical care. This disorder is considered a natural component of the infant's development and usually goes away as the child ages. Healthcare professionals carefully monitor premature infants for various physiological parameters, and understanding the normal variations in thyroid hormone levels helps ensure appropriate care for these vulnerable neonates (Weiss et al., 2020).

1.4.4 DYSLIPIDEMIA

Thyroid hormones significantly influence the production, mobilization, and metabolism of lipids. Increased total cholesterol (TC) levels are a sign of hypercholesterolemia, which is linked to both overt and subclinical hypothyroidism. High levels of low-density lipoprotein (LDL) cholesterol are the leading cause of the rise in cholesterol. On the other hand, high-density lipoprotein cholesterol levels are often average or higher. The leading cause of dyslipidemia in hyperthyroidism is excess lipid production over breakdown (Duntas, 2002). Oxidative stress is caused by elevated TC levels, particularly LDL, a substrate for lipid peroxidation by reactive oxygen species (Garg et al., 2022). TSH levels have been identified as the primary cause of dyslipidemia in thyroid dysfunction cases. The atherosclerotic disease may emerge due to the detrimental effects of overt and subclinical hypothyroidism on the serum lipid profile (Swiger et al., 2014). Studies indicate that variations in lipid profiles may occur at various times for men and women. Before midlife, men may have higher amounts of LDL cholesterol, but women may show higher LDL cholesterol levels after midlife (Garg et al., 2021). Dyslipidemia is associated with menopause; this may be because of the metabolic alterations brought on by the sudden decrease in estrogen levels (Kant et al., 2020). The paragraph highlights the necessity of long-term studies to properly comprehend the relationship between thyroid illness and dyslipidemia. This implies that additional investigation is necessary to examine lipid profile alterations' long-term effects and trends in people with thyroid dysfunction (Fonseca et al., 2017).

1.5 THERAPEUTIC APPROACHES

1.5.1 PHARMACOTHERAPY FOR THYROID DISORDERS

1.5.1.1 THE STANDARD APPROACH TO TREATING HYPOTHYROIDISM

The standard approach to treating hypothyroidism mainly involves taking different formulations of levothyroxine sodium (LEVO sodium).

- **Levothyroxine:** The synthetic sodium salt of the levo-isomer of T4, known as LEVO sodium, is used to replace natural thyroid hormone. It has different strengths, and the patient's body weight determines the starting dosage. Patients are monitored regularly, and dosage adjustments are made based on laboratory results and clinical response. Frequently administered as a tablet, this absorbs best when taken on an empty stomach first thing in the morning (Liu et al., 2023).
- **Levothyroxine with liothyronine:** Some studies have explored combining liothyronine and LEVO for patients with persistent symptoms of LEVO alone. The combination therapy was effective in restoring euthyroidism in animal models but did not show superiority in humans over LEVO alone (Clyde et al., 2003).
- **Levothyroxine soft gel:** Soft gel and liquid formulations of LEVO have been investigated for improved bioavailability compared to conventional tablets. These formulations may benefit patients requiring frequent dose adjustments or those having difficulty taking tablets with food (Benvenga, 2019).
- **Levothyroxine injection:** In severe cases of noncompliance, weekly intramuscular injections of LEVO sodium have proven effective. Injections subcutaneous have also been investigated as a potential substitute for people unable to achieve the appropriate thyroid levels with oral LEVO (Liu et al., 2023).

- **Suppository formulations:** Suppositories have been investigated as a rectal administration method instead of oral delivery, particularly for individuals who are unable to swallow pills. A study in thyroidectomized rats showed lower bioavailability with a LEVO suppository than oral LEVO. Due to the nature of delivery, patient compliance with rectal administration may be challenging (Azarbayjani et al., 2010).

1.5.1.2 *ALTERNATIVE THERAPY FOR HYPOTHYROIDISM*

- **Implants:** In a variety of applications, implanted drug delivery systems have proven successful in providing prolonged and sustained drug release. Implants, such as pellet systems or osmotic pumps, have been used to deliver thyroid hormones (T3) in rodents. These systems provide stable amounts of T3 over a predefined period. Biodegradable subcutaneous poly (caprolactone) implants have been created for persistent LEVO release. T3 and ethylene-vinyl acetate are combined to form the solid rod ProNeura®, intended for subcutaneous administration. Preclinical studies have demonstrated six months of continuous T3 release (Donnelly et al., 2011; Magill et al., 2023; Rani et al., 2023).

1.5.1.3 *CONVENTIONAL TREATMENT OF HYPERTHYROIDISM*

- **Thyroidectomy:** Thyroidectomy, the surgical removal of the thyroid gland, is one of the oldest and preferred treatments for GD, a common cause of hyperthyroidism. LEVO therapy is necessary for patients following a complete thyroidectomy to replenish lost thyroid hormones (Smithson et al., 2019).
- **Oral administration of antithyroid drug regimens (ATDs):** Thiamazole (methimazole), PTU, and carbimazole are commonly used antithyroid drugs (ATDs). Thiamazole is preferred for treating GD due to its better efficacy, prolonged duration/half-life, and once-daily administration. There are two approaches for ATD treatment: titration (adjusting dose over time) and "block and replace" (higher doses with levothyroxine). Titration is preferred

due to a lower incidence of side effects than "block and replace." Initial dosage varies based on thyroid gland size and severity of the condition. The maintenance dose of thiamazole (5–10 mg) is continued for up to 18 months or longer to prevent relapse. Limitations include high relapse rates after discontinuation of treatment (Abraham et al., 2010).

- **Radioactive iodine therapy:** Since the 1940s, radioactive iodine (RAI) therapy has been extensively utilized to treat thyroid conditions. Iodine-131 is a radionuclide that emits beta particles and has specific energy properties that make it useful for therapeutic purposes. Its half-life is just over eight days. The way that RAI works is physiological. Iodide transporters in the thyroid process RAI similarly to natural iodine. The released beta-particles destroy the follicular cells and control thyrotoxicosis by gradually decreasing volume. RAI is generally safe, although adverse side effects might happen to patients. There is a significant chance of developing hypothyroidism, especially after GD therapy (Nixon et al., 2020). The symptoms of hyperthyroidism may momentarily intensify due to radiation thyroiditis. It has been demonstrated that lithium carbonate works well as an adjuvant therapy. It reduces the release of preformed thyroid hormone and enhances the therapeutic benefits of RAI. Adjunctive antithyroid drugs are frequently utilized right after radioiodine therapy to lessen the hyperthyroidism's biochemical exacerbation. Because RAI crosses the placenta readily, it should not be used when pregnant. According to the passage, minor prenatal exposure does not justify termination, and a maximum dosage of 15 mCi given up to 10 weeks of gestation has no adverse effects on fetal thyroid function. If pregnant women get RAI before the 10th week of their pregnancy, there is no increased risk of malignancies or congenital disabilities in their offspring (Mayson et al., 2021).

1.5.2 LIFESTYLE MODIFICATIONS

Stressful settings, increased chemical exposure, and less healthful lifestyles could all be contributing factors to the rising prevalence of thyroid cancer, particularly in the United States.

- **Impact of stress:** Stress is considered a significant factor that can lead to the development of autoimmune diseases, including thyroid disorders. Stressful conditions such as family sickness, financial problems, loss of job, and political instability contribute to anxiety, potentially linking to autoimmune diseases.
- **Toxic exposure:** Environmental toxins, including those present in polluted air and water, are highlighted as contributors to thyroid disease. Synthetic compounds with estrogenic activity, particularly xenoestrogens found in cosmetics and personal care products, are mentioned as potential culprits.
- **Caffeine and diet choice:** Consuming caffeine-filled foods like coffee may increase heart rate and worsen thyroid conditions (Danailova et al., 2022).
- **Coping strategies:** There is promising evidence for healthy lifestyles, gluten-free diets, and probiotics in treating thyroid diseases, but further research is needed. Understanding the root causes of thyroid diseases is crucial for developing effective preventive measures. Regardless of the conditions, annual health check-ups and blood tests for early detection are also important (Feng et al., 2022).

1.6 CONCLUSION

Given the prevalence of CKD and thyroid diseases in the United States, it is essential to take into account their physiological relationship. Thyroid-related alterations in CKD frequently include subclinical hypothyroidism and low T3 levels. It is essential to take into account both clinical characteristics and thyroid symptoms in individuals with CKD since hyperthyroidism speeds up the disease. While treating thyroid disease appropriately reduces the risk of developing or aggravating renal impairment, treating minor TSH increases requires careful consideration by clinicians in order to prevent negative nitrogen balance. They are essential to monitoring low T3 levels before renal transplant, as they are associated with graft loss.

The broad impact of both hypothyroidism and hyperthyroidism on multiple organ systems, emphasizing the potential for severe perioperative complications such as predisposition to anemia, electrophysiologic disturbances, hypotension, potential for cardiovascular collapse during surgery, renal and pulmonary changes, decreased gastrointestinal motility, promoting the development of ileus, thyrotoxicosis can trigger arrhythmias and fever, potential for gastrointestinal complications. So, it is essential to minimize the severe complications and risks before surgery, and it includes careful management and a multidisciplinary approach in the perioperative care of patients with thyroid dysfunctions.

KEYWORDS

- **thyroid disorders**
- **hormones**
- **surgery**
- **radioactive iodine**
- **hyperthyroidism**

REFERENCES

Abraham, P., Avenell, A., McGeoch, S.C., Clark, L.F., Bevan, J.S. (2010). Antithyroid drug regimen for treating Graves' hyperthyroidism. Cochrane Database of Systematic Reviews, 2010(1), CD003420. https://doi.org/10.1002/14651858.CD003420.pub4.

Azarbayjani, A.F., Venugopal, J.R., Ramakrishna, S., Lim, P.F., Chan, Y.W., Chan, S.Y. (2010). Smart polymeric nanofibers for topical delivery of levothyroxine. Journal of Pharmacy & Pharmaceutical Sciences, 13(3), 400–410. https://doi.org/10.18433/j3ts3g

Basu, G., Mohapatra, A. (2012). Interactions between thyroid disorders and kidney disease. Indian Journal of Endocrinology and Metabolism, 16(2), 204–213. https://doi.org/10.4103/2230-8210.93737

Benvenga, S. (2019). Liquid and softgel capsules of l-thyroxine results lower serum thyrotropin levels more than tablet formulations in hypothyroid patients. Journal of Clinical & Translational Endocrinology, 18, 100204. https://doi.org/10.1016/j.jcte.2019.100204

Bhatt, S., Anitha, K., Chellappan, D.K., Mukherjee, D., Shilpi, S., Suttee, A., Gupta, G., Singh, T.G., Dua, K. (2024). Targeting inflammatory signaling in obsessive compulsive disorder: A promising approach. Metabolic Brain Disease, 39(2), 335–346. https://doi.org/10.1007/s11011-023-01314-3

Brown, E.D.L., Obeng-Gyasi, B., Hall, J.E., Shekhar, S. (2023). The thyroid hormone axis and female reproduction. International Journal of Molecular Sciences, 24(12), 9815. https://doi.org/10.3390/ijms24129815

Büyükgebiz, A. (2013). Newborn screening for congenital hypothyroidism. Journal of Clinical Research in Pediatric Endocrinology, 5(Suppl 1), 8–12. https://doi.org/10.4274/jcrpe.845

Clyde, P.W., Harari, A.E., Getka, E.J., Shakir, K.M. (2003). Combined levothyroxine plus liothyronine compared with levothyroxine alone in primary hypothyroidism: A randomized controlled trial. JAMA, 290(22), 2952–2958. https://doi.org/10.1001/jama.290.22.2952

Danailova, Y., Velikova, T., Nikolaev, G., Mitova, Z., Shinkov, A., Gagov, H., Konakchieva, R. (2022). Nutritional management of thyroiditis of Hashimoto. International Journal of Molecular Sciences, 23(9), 5144. https://doi.org/10.3390/ijms23095144

Das, D., Banerjee, A., Jena, A.B., Duttaroy, A.K., Pathak, S. (2022). Essentiality, relevance, and efficacy of adjuvant/combinational therapy in the management of thyroid dysfunctions. Biomedicine & Pharmacotherapy = Biomedecine & Pharmacotherapie, 146, 112613. https://doi.org/10.1016/j.biopha.2022.112613

De Leo, S., Lee, S.Y., Braverman, L.E. (2016). Hyperthyroidism. Lancet (London, England), 388(10047), 906–918. https://doi.org/10.1016/S0140-6736(16)00278-6

Donnelly, R.F., Majithiya, R., Singh, T.R., Morrow, D.I., Garland, M.J., Demir, Y.K., Migalska, K., Ryan, E., Gillen, D., Scott, C.J., Woolfson, A.D. (2011). Design, optimization and characterisation of polymeric microneedle arrays prepared by a novel laser-based micromoulding technique. Pharmaceutical Research, 28(1), 41–57. https://doi.org/10.1007/s11095-010-0169-8

Duntas, L.H. (2002). Thyroid disease and lipids. Thyroid, 12(4), 287–293. https://doi.org/10.1089/10507250252949405

Fan, J., Yan, P., Wang, Y., Shen, B., Ding, F., Liu, Y. (2016). Prevalence and clinical significance of low T3 syndrome in non-dialysis patients with chronic kidney disease. Medical Science Monitor, 22, 1171–1179. https://doi.org/10.12659/msm.895953

Feng, X., Wang, F., Yang, W., Zheng, Y., Liu, C., Huang, L., Li, L., Cheng, H., Cai, H., Li, X., Chen, X., Yang, X. (2022). Association between genetic risk, adherence to healthy lifestyle behavior, and thyroid cancer risk. JAMA Network Open, 5(12), e2246311. https://doi.org/10.1001/jamanetworkopen.2022.46311

Fonseca, M.I.H., da Silva, I.T., Ferreira, S.R.G. (2017). Impact of menopause and diabetes on atherogenic lipid profile: Is it worth to analyse lipoprotein subfractions to assess cardiovascular risk in women. Diabetology & Metabolic Syndrome, 9, 22. https://doi.org/10.1186/s13098-017-0221-5

Fröhlich, E., Wahl, R. (2021). Physiological role and use of thyroid hormone metabolites—potential utility in COVID-19 patients. Frontiers in Endocrinology, 12, 587518. https://doi.org/10.3389/fendo.2021.587518

Garg, C., Khan, H., Kaur, A., Singh, T.G., Sharma, V.K., Singh, S.K. (2022). Therapeutic implications of sonic hedgehog pathway in metabolic disorders: Novel target for effective treatment. Pharmacological Research, 179, 106194. https://doi.org/10.1016/j.phrs.2022.106194

Garg, N., Singh, T.G., Khan, H., Arora, S., Kaur, A., Mannan, A. (2021). Mechanistic interventions of selected Ocimum species in management of diabetes, obesity and liver disorders: Transformative developments from preclinical to clinical approaches. Biointerface Research in Applied Chemistry, 12(1), 1304–1323.

Grimm, D. (2022). Recent advances in thyroid cancer research. International Journal of Molecular Sciences, 23(9), 4631. https://doi.org/10.3390/ijms23094631

Hoermann, R., Midgley, J.E.M., Larisch, R., Dietrich, J.W. (2017). Recent advances in thyroid hormone regulation: toward a new paradigm for optimal diagnosis and treatment. Frontiers in Endocrinology, 8, 364. https://doi.org/10.3389/fendo.2017.00364

Iglesias, P., Díez, J.J. (2009). Thyroid dysfunction and kidney disease. European Journal of Endocrinology, 160(4), 503–515. https://doi.org/10.1530/EJE-08-0837

Iglesias, P., Bajo, M.A., Selgas, R., Díez, J.J. (2017). Thyroid dysfunction and kidney disease: An update. Reviews in Endocrine & Metabolic Disorders, 18(1), 131–144. https://doi.org/10.1007/s11154-016-9395-7

Kant, R., Singh, T.G., Singh, S. (2020). Mechanistic approach to herbal formulations used for urolithiasis treatment. Obesity Medicine. 2020, 100266.

Kirsten, D. (2000). The thyroid gland: Physiology and pathophysiology. Neonatal Network: NN, 19(8), 11–26. https://doi.org/10.1891/0730-0832.19.8.11

LaFranchi, S.H. (2021). Thyroid function in preterm/low birth weight infants: Impact on diagnosis and management of thyroid dysfunction. Frontiers in Endocrinology, 12, 666207. https://doi.org/10.3389/fendo.2021.666207

Lim, V.S., Fang, V.S., Katz, A.I., Refetoff, S. (1977). Thyroid dysfunction in chronic renal failure. A study of the pituitary-thyroid axis and peripheral turnover kinetics of thyroxine and triiodothyronine. The Journal of Clinical Investigation, 60(3), 522–534. https://doi.org/10.1172/JCI108804

Liu, H., Li, W., Zhang, W., Sun, S., Chen, C. (2023). Levothyroxine: Conventional and novel drug delivery formulations. Endocrine Reviews, 44(3), 393–416. https://doi.org/10.1210/endrev/bnac030

Magill, E., Demartis, S., Gavini, E., Permana, A.D., Thakur, R.R.S., Adrianto, M.F., Waite, D., Glover, K., Picco, C.J., Korelidou, A., Detamornrat, U., Vora, L.K., Li, L., Anjani, Q.K., Donnelly, R.F., Domínguez-Robles, J., Larrañeta, E. (2023). Solid implantable devices for sustained drug delivery. Advanced Drug Delivery Reviews, 199, 114950. https://doi.org/10.1016/j.addr.2023.114950

Mansourian, A.R. (2011). Metabolic pathways of tetraidothyronine and triidothyronine production by thyroid gland: A review of articles. Pakistan Journal of Biological Sciences, 14(1), 1–12. https://doi.org/10.3923/pjbs.2011.1.12

Mayson, S.E., Chan, C.M., Haugen, B.R. (2021). Tailoring the approach to radioactive iodine treatment in thyroid cancer. Endocrine-related Cancer, 28(10), T125–T140. https://doi.org/10.1530/ERC-21-0161

Miculan, J., Turner, S., Paes, B.A. (1993). Congenital hypothyroidism: Diagnosis and management. Neonatal Network : NN, 12(6), 25–38.

Mohamedali, M., Reddy Maddika, S., Vyas, A., Iyer, V., Cheriyath, P. (2014). Thyroid disorders and chronic kidney disease. International Journal of Nephrology, 2014, 520281. https://doi.org/10.1155/2014/520281

Nixon, I.J., Shah, J.P., Zafereo, M., Simo, R.S., Hay, I.D., Suárez, C., Zbären, P., Rinaldo, A., Sanabria, A., Silver, C., Mäkitie, A., Vander Poorten, V., Kowalski, L.P., Shaha, A.R., Randolph, G.W., Ferlito, A. (2020). The role of radioactive iodine in the management of patients with differentiated thyroid cancer—An oncologic surgical perspective. European Journal of Surgical Oncology, 46(5), 754–762. https://doi.org/10.1016/j.ejso.2020.01.010

Ostrowski, P., Bonczar, M., Iwanaga, J., Michalczak, M., Dziedzic, M., Del Carmen Yika, A., Gil, A., Sporek, M., Szczepanek, E., Niemczyk, K., Walocha, J., Koziej, M. (2023). The prevalence and anatomy of the pyramidal lobe of the thyroid gland: A meta-analysis with implications for thyroid surgery. Clinical Anatomy (New York, NY), 36(6), 937–945. https://doi.org/10.1002/ca.24062

Rani, I., Munjal, K., Singla, R.K., Gautam, R.K.J.B.T.f.P.D.P.D. (2023). Artificial intelligence and machine learning-based new drug discovery process with molecular modelling. In: *Bioinformatics Tools for Pharmaceutical Drug Product Development*. pp. 19–35.

Rastogi, M.V., LaFranchi, S.H. (2010). Congenital hypothyroidism. Orphanet Journal of Rare Diseases, 5, 17. https://doi.org/10.1186/1750-1172-5-17

Rehni, A.K., Singh, T.G. (2011). Modulation of leukotriene D4 attenuates the development of seizures in mice. Prostaglandins, Leukotrienes, and Essential Fatty Acids, 85(2), 97–106. https://doi.org/10.1016/j.plefa.2011.04.003

Ren, B., Zhu, Y. (2022). A new perspective on thyroid hormones: Crosstalk with reproductive hormones in females. International Journal of Molecular Sciences, 23(5), 2708. https://doi.org/10.3390/ijms23052708

Singh, R., Rao, H.K., Singh, T.G. (2020). Advanced glycated end products (ages) in diabetes and its complications: An insight. Plant Arch, 20(1), 3838–3841.

Smithson, M., Asban, A., Miller, J., Chen, H. (2019). Considerations for thyroidectomy as treatment for graves disease. Clinical Medicine Insights. Endocrinology and Diabetes, 12, 1179551419844523. https://doi.org/10.1177/1179551419844523

Swiger, K.J., Martin, S.S., Blaha, M.J., Toth, P.P., Nasir, K., Michos, E.D., Gerstenblith, G., Blumenthal, R.S., Jones, S.R. (2014). Narrowing sex differences in lipoprotein cholesterol subclasses following mid-life: The very large database of lipids (VLDL-10B). Journal of the American Heart Association, 3(2), e000851. https://doi.org/10.1161/JAHA.114.000851

Thapa, K., Singh, T.G., Kaur, A. (2021). Cyclic nucleotide phosphodiesterase inhibition as a potential therapeutic target in renal ischemia reperfusion injury. Life Sciences, 282, 119843. https://doi.org/10.1016/j.lfs.2021.119843

Tyagi, S., Singh, U., Kalra, T., Munjal, K. (2010). Applications of metabolomics—A systematic study of the unique chemical fingerprints: An overview. International Journal of Pharmaceutical Sciences Review and Research, 3(1).

Unnikrishnan, A.G., Menon, U.V. (2011). Thyroid disorders in India: An epidemiological perspective. Indian Journal of Endocrinology and Metabolism, 15(Suppl 2), S78–S81. https://doi.org/10.4103/2230-8210.83329

Weiss, S.L., Peters, M.J., Alhazzani, W., Agus, M.S.D., Flori, H.R., Inwald, D.P., Nadel, S., Schlapbach, L.J., Tasker, R.C., Argent, A.C., Brierley, J., Carcillo, J., Carrol, E.D., Carroll, C.L., Cheifetz, I.M., Choong, K., Cies, J.J., Cruz, A.T., De Luca, D., Deep, A., … Tissieres, P. (2020). Surviving sepsis campaign international guidelines for the management of septic shock and sepsis-associated organ dysfunction in children. Intensive Care Medicine, 46(Suppl 1), 10–67. https://doi.org/10.1007/s00134-019-05878-6

Wiederkehr, M.R., Kalogiros, J., Krapf, R. (2004). Correction of metabolic acidosis improves thyroid and growth hormone axes in haemodialysis patients. Nephrology, Dialysis, Transplantation, 19(5), 1190–1197. https://doi.org/10.1093/ndt/gfh096

CHAPTER 2

Hormonal Regulation of Plasma Calcium, Parathyroid Gland, and Bone Metabolism

BALJINDER SINGH[1], RAGHAV TANDON[1], GEETANSH ALLAWADHI[1], LOVELEEN KAUR[1*], DEEPIKA RAINA[2*], KAMAL DUA[3,4], SANJANA MEHTA[1], and THAKUR GURJEET SINGH[1]

[1]*Chitkara College of Pharmacy, Chitkara University, Chandigarh, Punjab, India*

[2]*School of Pharmacy, Graphic Era Hill University, Dehradun, Uttarakhand, India*

[3]*Discipline of Pharmacy, Graduate School of Health, University of Technology Sydney, Sydney, NSW, Australia*

[4]*Faculty of Health, Australian Research Centre in Complementary and Integrative Medicine, University of Technology Sydney, Ultimo, NSW, Australia*

*Corresponding author

ABSTRACT

Maintaining plasma calcium within a narrow physiological range is vital for numerous bodily functions, including nerve conduction, muscle contraction, and bone integrity. This regulation relies on a dynamic interplay among hormones, the parathyroid gland, and bone metabolism. The parathyroid hormone (PTH), secreted by the parathyroid glands in response to low calcium levels, plays a central role in restoring balance

Pharmacotherapy Approaches Toward Endocrine and Metabolic Diseases.
Thakur Gurjeet Singh and Sanjana Mehta (Eds.)

DOI: 10.1201/9781779640154-2

by stimulating osteoclast-mediated bone resorption, enhancing renal calcium reabsorption, and promoting the activation of vitamin D. Active vitamin D (calcitriol) further facilitates calcium absorption from the intestines. Conversely, the thyroid hormone calcitonin counteracts these effects by inhibiting osteoclasts and promoting calcium storage in bones, although its role is secondary to that of PTH. Disruptions in this finely tuned system—such as in hyperparathyroidism, hypoparathyroidism, or vitamin D deficiency—can result in serious conditions like osteoporosis, nephrolithiasis, and neuromuscular disturbances. Understanding the mechanisms governing calcium homeostasis is crucial not only for diagnosing and managing such disorders but also for developing targeted therapies to correct hormonal imbalances and maintain bone health. Thus, the study of these regulatory pathways holds significant clinical relevance in addressing calcium-related diseases.

2.1 INTRODUCTION

Calcium is essential to many physiological functions, such as muscular contraction and nerve transmission. Its exact monitoring in the bloodstream is critical to preserving the integrity of these biological functions (Soetan et al., 2010). As a signaling molecule, calcium causes muscles to contract, allowing movement. Muscles could not function correctly without sufficient calcium, resulting in weakness and tiredness (Berchtold et al., 2000). Effective interaction within the nervous system becomes possible through calcium, which assists with electrical signals transmitting information between neurons (Burgoyne et al., 2019). Medical identities describing deficient and high serum calcium concentrations are hypocalcemia and hypercalcemia. Although neither hypercalcemia nor hypocalcemia independently represents calcium balance, both signal a significant impairment of calcium homeostasis (Aggarwal et al., 2023). Low calcium levels may cause problems with this function, potentially leading to weakness, tingling, seizure, and central nervous system disorders. In addition, calcium is necessary for various other processes, like developing and maintaining strong bones and teeth (Zhu and Prince, 2012). They ensure the blood clots appropriately to stop excessive bleeding and support several enzymes involved in various metabolic processes as cofactors (D, n.d.). The delicate equilibrium of calcium in the blood must be managed for optimal wellness (Sood et al., 2023). Too low (hypocalcaemia) could result in tetany, seizures, and muscle cramps, while too high (hypercalcemia) may cause kidney stones, muscle weakness, and possibly a state of coma (Tinawi, 2021).

Calcium metabolism is governed by the following main mechanisms: intestinal absorption, renal reabsorption, and bone turnover. The rate of calcium metabolism dictates the necessary quantity of calcium. It is then controlled by a group of interconnected hormones, such as ionized calcium, 1,25-dihydroxy vitamin D, parathyroid hormone (PTH), and the receptors of these hormones throughout the renal system, bone, and gastrointestinal tract (Khan, 2014). The parathyroid glands increase PTH synthesis in response to an alarm signal whenever blood calcium level falls below the specified range (Vanhouten et al., 2004). Conversely, elevated calcium levels mute the warning signal, decreasing PTH release. This constant interaction of PTH, calcium-sensing receptors (CaSRs), and parathyroid glands sustains a dynamic calcium equilibrium in the blood. Several functions, such as bone health, neuron transmission, and muscle contraction, depend on this balance (Hill et al., 2019). Since bones continuously rebuild themselves through a cyclic combination of resorption and creation, they are not stable structures. Specialized bone-resorbing cells called osteoclasts break down aging bone tissue while reintroducing calcium and other minerals into the blood circulation. As new bone tissue begins to be put down, osteoblasts—the cells that make new bone—integrate the released calcium and minerals (Safadi et al., 2009).

In this chapter, we will learn how the kidney regulates the body's calcium levels, how gastrointestinal absorption influences calcium metabolism, and how calcium is transported through the blood. We will also discuss how bone metabolism and PTH regulate calcium levels. Additionally, we will investigate the condition associated with an imbalance in hormones that impacts the calcium level in the body.

2.2 CALCIUM METABOLISM

Calcium is an essential mineral for many physiological processes in the human body. The intestine is one of the central locations where calcium is absorbed, and a sophisticated and tightly controlled mechanism guarantees the best possible absorption of this vital vitamin (Hoenderop et al., 2005).

2.2.1 ABSORPTION OF CALCIUM IN THE INTESTINE

Mammals absorb calcium via two pathways: a paracellular, concentration-dependent diffusion process that occurs throughout the intestine and a transcellular mechanism that is mainly found in the duodenum and is controlled by vitamin D. The amount of calcium transported paracellularly is inversely related to the rate of intestinal propulsion and is directly related to the chyme's duration in a particular intestinal segment. Calcium absorption takes place via a combination of both active and passive diffusion or mechanisms (Strom et al., 2017).

2.2.1.1 ACTIVE DIFFUSION MECHANISM

2.2.1.1.1 TRPV6 Protein

A specific protein known as transient receptor potential vanilloid type 6 (TRPV6) aids in the active absorption of calcium. TRPV6 primarily occurs in the duodenum, which is essential for calcium absorption from food. TRPV6 belongs to the family of TRP, which is highly selective for calcium ions (Fecher-Trost et al., 2014). When calcium ions enter the enterocytes from the intestinal lumen, the active transport of calcium starts. TRPV6 functions as a calcium channel, allowing calcium ions to pass through the enterocytes' apical membrane and into their cytoplasm via the intestinal lumen (Hong and Jeung, 2013). They act as a buffer, moving calcium ions to the basolateral membrane across the cell. Calcium ions are rapidly transferred from the cells into the bloodstream at the basolateral membrane of the enterocytes. Other transport proteins are involved in this basolateral transport and work jointly to pump calcium out of the enterocytes (Cashman and Flynn, 1999).

2.2.1.1.2 Calcium-Binding Proteins

Certain proteins, such as calbindin-D9k and calbindin-D28k, are bound by calcium ions within intestinal epithelial cells. These calcium-binding proteins depend on intracellular calcium transport across the epithelial cells (Hong and Jeung, 2013).

2.2.1.2 PASSIVE DIFFUSION

Although active transport is prominent in calcium absorption, passive diffusion also plays a role, especially in the jejunum (Cashman and Flynn, 1999). The calcium concentration gradient between the intestinal lumen and the epithelial cells affects this process. The solubility of calcium salts in the intestinal fluid is one of the elements that affect calcium absorption through passive diffusion.

2.2.1.3 ROLE OF VITAMIN D

Vitamin D is an essential modulator of calcium absorption. The active element of vitamin D is calcitriol, which the skin and liver manufacture in response to exposure to sunshine or food intake. When exposed to calcitriol, intestinal epithelial cells produce more calcium-binding proteins. A sufficient amount of vitamin D is necessary for adequate calcium absorption; a lack of it can result in reduced calcium uptake and possible problems with bone health (Tangpricha, 2014).

2.2.1.4 IMPACT OF HORMONES

The parathyroid glands release PTH in response to low blood calcium levels. PTH improves calcium reabsorption in the kidneys and triggers calcium release from bone. It also encourages the transformation of vitamin D into its active form, which aids in the intestinal absorption of calcium. Thyroid-produced calcitonin works against PTH. It prevents bone resorption, lowers intestinal calcium absorption, and regulates calcium levels (Bhattarai et al., 2020).

2.2.2 ROLE OF KIDNEY IN CALCIUM REGULATION

To maintain calcium homeostasis, the kidneys are essential for controlling calcium levels in the body. Calcium is necessary for many physiological functions, such as bone health, muscular contraction, nerve transmission, and blood clotting. The kidneys play a vital role in maintaining the proper mineral balance by controlling calcium's reabsorption, excretion, and synthesis of active vitamin D (Jeon, 2008). The following are essential components of the kidneys' function in regulating calcium.

2.2.2.1 GLOMERULUS FILTRATION

The glomerulus, where blood is filtered to create the glomerular filtrate, is the first stage of renal calcium regulation. The glomerular capillaries allow calcium to filter and enter the renal tubules readily (Jeon, 2008).

2.2.2.2 PASSIVE REABSORPTION IN THE PROXIMAL TUBULE

The proximal tubule of the nephron passively reabsorbs most of the filtered calcium. The electrochemical gradient created by the reabsorption of water and salt powers this process. In the proximal tubule, between 60% and 70% of the filtered calcium is reabsorbed and added back to the bloodstream.

2.2.2.2.1 Active Reabsorption in the Distal Tubule and Collecting Ducts

The filtered residual calcium reaches the distal tubule and collecting ducts, where active calcium reabsorption occurs in sections. Hormones, specifically PTH and calcitriol, monitor the active reabsorption of calcium.

2.2.2.2.1.1 Parathyroid hormone

PTH increases calcium reabsorption in the collecting ducts and distal tubule (Ayers et al., 2018). Additionally, PTH increases phosphate excretion in the urine, which lowers the production of insoluble calcium phosphate and indirectly affects calcium levels.

2.2.2.2.1.2 Calcitriol production

Calcitriol, the active form of vitamin D, primarily depends on the kidneys. The kidneys change inactive vitamin D (calcidiol) into its active form, calcitriol, in response to low blood calcium levels (Tangpricha, 2014). Calcitriol affects the intestines, improving the absorption of calcium from food. Additionally, it facilitates calcium reabsorption in the kidney's collecting ducts and distal tubules.

2.2.2.2.1.3 Excess calcium excretion

When blood calcium levels are raised, the kidneys expel extra calcium into the urine. This procedure helps avoid hypercalcemia and maintains proper calcium levels in the blood.

2.2.3 CALCIUM TRANSPORT IN BLOOD

Ionized and bound calcium are the two main calcium types in circulation. In contrast to bound calcium, mainly linked to proteins like albumin, ionized calcium is the physiologically active component necessary for cellular processes (Najar et al., 2022). It acts as a reservoir to preserve stability. The ionized calcium, also known as free calcium, is the active ingredient in cellular functions. It is essential for blood coagulation, neuronal transmission, muscle contraction, and the activation of several enzymes. Ionized calcium concentration is carefully controlled to maintain these essential processes. About half of the calcium in the blood is incorporated into proteins, mainly albumin. As a reserve, this bound calcium ensures that ionized calcium is always available (Rutala et al., 2019). The interaction with transport proteins facilitates the solubility and circulation of calcium. Hormones play a graceful ballet in controlling blood calcium levels, especially PTH and calcitonin. PTH increases bone resorption, renal reabsorption, and calcitriol production. It is secreted in response to low calcium levels. In contrast, calcitonin promotes renal excretion while preventing bone resorption. The active form of vitamin D, calcitriol, is essential for improving the small intestine's ability to absorb calcium (Hill et al., 2019). Calcitriol, produced in reaction to sunlight or acquired through nutrition, ensures that the body always has enough calcium to meet its needs. Calcium interacts with several blood proteins, including globulins and albumin. These proteins support calcium transport by preserving its solubility and easing its passage through the circulation. Variations in these proteins' concentrations can affect the blood's overall calcium content. Calcium transport in the blood is a dynamic process that is carefully regulated. It is not a static process. Blood calcium levels are kept within the ideal range for cellular functions via the interaction of binding and ionized calcium and the coordinated actions of hormones and vitamin D (Tangpricha, 2014).

2.3 PARATHYROID HORMONE

2.3.1 PHYSIOLOGY OF THE PARATHYROID GLAND

The parathyroid glands, four tiny glands in the neck below the thyroid gland, are the leading producers of PTH. Eighty-four amino acids constitute the peptide hormone PTH. The active PTH molecule is generated by breaking down the pre-pro-PTH precursor produced in the parathyroid central cells (Riccardi and Brown, 2010).

Serum calcium levels are monitored by feedback mechanisms that precisely regulate PTH secretion. PTH is released when serum calcium levels are low and suppressed when levels are high. The surface calcium-sensing receptor on parathyroid cells is crucial for detecting fluctuations in extracellular calcium and regulating PTH secretion (Potts, 2005).

PTH has a significant impact on the metabolic function of bone. Elevated osteoclast activity promotes bone resorption and calcium release into the bloodstream. PTH directly stimulates their proliferation, durability, and function, which all rise due to the elevated calcium release. Infrequent or irregular PTH secretion stimulates the production of new bone, whereas continuous increases in PTH may lead to decreased bone density. Hyperparathyroidism, characterized by persistently high PTH levels, can harm bone health. Net bone loss and lower bone density are due to increased bone resorption surpassing bone production.

Whereas PTH does not directly affect intestinal calcium absorption, the stimulating action of vitamin D via PTH indirectly improves calcium absorption in the small intestine.

The particular receptors found on the surface of parathyroid chief cells continuously sense variations in blood calcium levels, functioning as the orchestra conductor. It causes a spike in PTH release when blood calcium levels drop below normal. On the other hand, increased calcium levels cause a reduction in PTH release, resulting in a negative feedback loop that maintains an exact calcium balance. Furthermore, the activity of the parathyroid gland is directly impacted by the vitamin D endocrine system, which emphasizes the intricate interaction between hormones and signaling pathways in the control of calcium metabolism.

2.3.2 SECRETION AND REGULATION OF PARATHYROID HORMONE

The parathyroid gland's central cells carry CaSR at the outermost layer. As shown in Figure 2.1, alteration in extracellular calcium concentration may influence these receptors. CaSRs detect a drop in blood calcium levels and initiate the release of PTH. Conversely, CaSRs reduce PTH production as a reaction to rising calcium levels (Chen and Goodman, 2004). It comprises a negative feedback loop that controls PTH secretion (Review, n.d.).

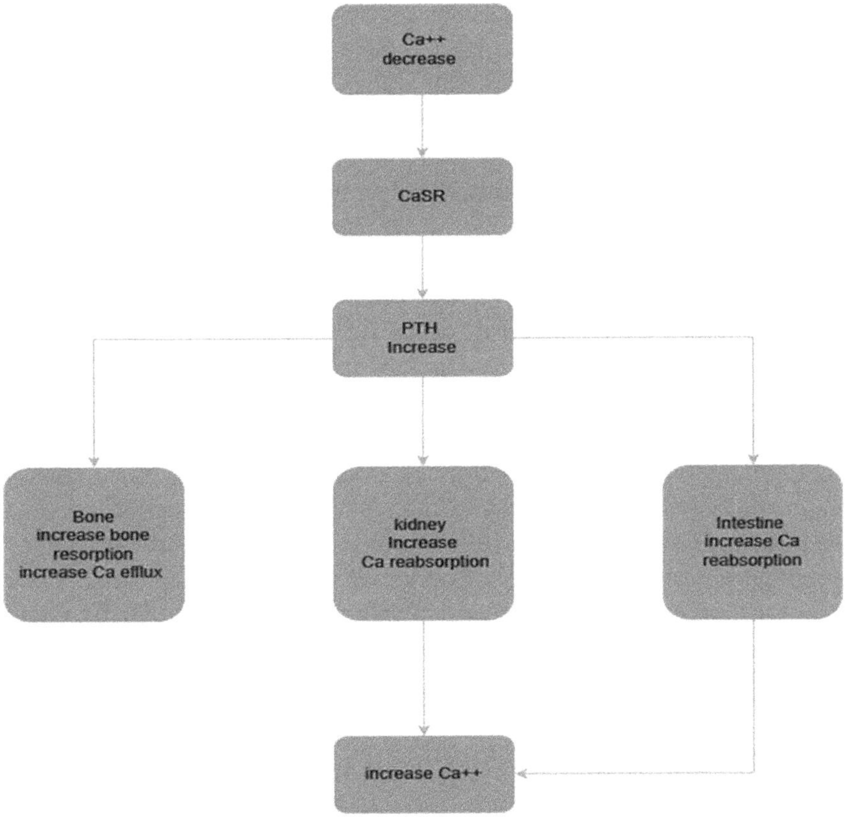

FIGURE 2.1 Flowchart depicts the effect of alteration in the extracellular calcium concentration.

Magnesium levels impact PTH secretion alongside calcium, and low magnesium levels may promote PTH release. By stimulating phosphate excretion by the kidneys, PTH helps maintain phosphate homeostasis (Devi et al., 2024). PTH increases phosphate excretion by directly inhibiting the renal tubules' potential to reabsorb the mineral. Magnesium may directly interact with parathyroid cell CaSRs to simulate the effects of low calcium and trigger PTH production (Rodríguez-ortiz et al., 2014).

PTH is necessary to activate vitamin D, which indirectly affects its secretion. PTH enables the kidneys to transform inactive vitamin D (calcidiol) into its active form (calcitriol) as a reaction to low blood calcium levels (Sharma and Singh, 2020). PTH stimulates the kidney's proximal tubules to express more of the enzyme 1-alpha hydroxylase, which transforms calcidiol into calcitriol. The metabolic processes of PTH to increase blood calcium levels are additionally aided by active vitamin D, which boosts calcium absorption in the intestines (Healy et al., 2005).

Alongside blood calcium levels, other factors may influence PTH secretion. These hormonal parameters, such as low estrogen levels in postmenopausal women, can boost PTH secretion. It is believed that this is due to estrogen's encouraging effects on calcium metabolism and bone health (Singh et al., 2020). This equilibrium might get altered by estrogen loss following menopause, which might end up in secondary hyperparathyroidism (Paoletti et al., 1996). Certain medications and diseases impacting the parathyroid glands can also impact PTH secretion. Several medications, including lithium, magnesium deficits, and diuretics, may activate the parathyroid glands directly or change the calcium or magnesium levels, indirectly affecting PTH release (Bhargava et al., 2022).

Production of PTH follows a circadian cycle, suggesting that it rises at night and lowers during the day. Although the specific procedures behind PTH's circadian rhythm are still being investigated, several factors may be at play: Gene clocks: The parathyroid glands include certain clock genes that control PTH synthesis cyclically (Egstrand et al., 2020). Other hormones, such as growth hormone, melatonin, and cortisol, all have circadian rhythms and interact with PTH to affect how it is released.

2.4 HORMONAL REGULATION OF PLASMA CALCIUM

Calcitonin, 1,25-dihydroxy vitamin D-3, and PTH are the primary hormones.

2.4.1 CALCITONIN AND ITS ROLE IN CALCIUM HOMEOSTASIS

A hormone called calcitonin is involved in maintaining calcium homeostasis or a steady concentration of calcium in the extracellular fluid. The essential elements of calcitonin's function in calcium homeostasis are as follows:

2.4.1.1 BLOCKING THE RESORPTION OF BONE

By preventing bone resorption—the process by which osteoclasts break down bone tissue and release calcium into the bloodstream—calcitonin works to lower blood calcium levels. It accomplishes this by directly preventing osteoclasts from breaking down bone through reduced activity.

2.4.1.2 ACTIVATION OF BONE'S CALCIUM INCORPORATION

Calcitonin prevents bone resorption and encourages calcium to be incorporated into the bone matrix, which helps the bone mineralize. This function helps maintain the overall calcium balance, making it particularly significant when blood calcium levels are elevated. However, calcitonin plays a limited role in the intestinal absorption of calcium. In contrast to PTH, calcitonin plays a very minor role in controlling the intestinal absorption of calcium. The primary hormone increasing the amount of calcium absorbed from the intestines is PTH (Kim et al., 2021).

2.4.1.3 ACTIONS INVERSED BY PARATHYROID HORMONE

PTH and calcitonin have different effects on how the body regulates calcium levels in the blood. PTH raises blood calcium levels, whereas calcitonin reduces them. These two hormones interact dynamically, aiding in regulating calcium homeostasis (Zhang and Li, 2020).

2.4.1.4 CONTROL OF SECRETION OF CALCITONIN

The amount of calcium in the blood essentially controls the release of calcitonin. Increased calcium levels in the blood cause the thyroid gland to secrete calcitonin. Other elements, including hormonal signals and specific drugs, can also influence calcitonin secretion.

2.4.2 VITAMIN D AND CALCIUM ABSORPTION

Calcium and vitamin D absorption have a complex and multi-step connection (Fleet, 2022). An outline of how vitamin D aids in the absorption of calcium is provided below.

2.4.2.1 ABSORPTION IN THE INTESTINE

Calcium is mainly absorbed in the duodenum and jejunum of the small intestine. Only 10–15% of the ingested calcium is absorbed without vitamin D. However, vitamin D amplifies this absorption considerably (Fleet, 2022).

2.4.2.2 CALCITRIOL PRODUCTION

Sunlight's UVB rays change the skin's 7-dehydrocholesterol to previtamin D3, which is then transformed into vitamin D3. After additional hydroxylation in the liver, vitamin D3 becomes calcidiol (25-hydroxyvitamin D), which is then converted into calcitriol (1,25-dihydroxy vitamin D) in the kidney (Khazan et al., 2022).

2.4.2.3 CALCIUM ABSORPTION AND CALCITRIOL

Calcitriol improves calcium absorption by upregulating the production of calcium-binding proteins in the gut epithelium. These proteins bind to calcium and aid in the passage of calcium from the intestinal epithelial cells into circulation (Khazan et al., 2022).

2.4.2.4 INTERACTION WITH PARATHYROID HORMONE

Vitamin D interacts with PTH to control calcium levels. PTH improves intestinal absorption of calcium by inducing the kidneys to produce more calcitriol (Clinical et al., 2011).

2.4.2.5 BONE HEALTH

Sufficient quantities of vitamin D are necessary to sustain healthy bone structure. By ensuring enough calcium is available for bone mineralization, vitamin D helps shield against diseases like osteomalacia in adults and rickets in youngsters.

2.4.2.6 EQUILIBRIUM OF CALCIUM

Vitamin D is essential for preserving calcium homeostasis by controlling the ratio of calcium release from bones, calcium reabsorption in the kidneys, and calcium absorption from the intestines (Fenn and Rahn, 1979).

2.4.3 INTERPLAY OF HORMONES IN CALCIUM REGULATION

PTH promotes bone resorption while calcitonin inhibits it; these are the opposing actions of PTH and calcitonin on bone resorption (Zhang and Li, 2020). Together, PTH and vitamin D enhance the kidneys' calcitriol synthesis. The balance between these hormones depends on maintaining the right amounts of calcium in the blood and good bone health. Blood calcium levels affect the secretion of PTH, calcitonin, and calcitriol by providing feedback to the kidneys, thyroid, and parathyroid glands.

The complex and strictly regulated system of hormone interactions is involved in calcium regulation. PTH, calcitonin, and vitamin D collaborate and compete to keep blood calcium levels within the limited physiological range required for different cellular processes and general skeletal health.

2.5 BONE METABOLISM

The endochondral and intramembranous ossification processes form bone. At each stage, mesenchymal progenitors gather and initiate developmental programs, including osteoblastogenesis and chondrogenesis (Galea et al., 2021).

During endochondral ossification, mesenchymal cells undergo chondrocyte differentiation, forming the cartilage growth plate. Then, the bone gradually replaces the cartilage growth plate. In the human skeleton, endochondral ossification produces the majority of the bones. These comprise the irregular, short, and long bones (Long and Ornitz, 2013). Intramembranous ossification is the process that creates flat bones, such as those found in the pelvis, skull, and face bones. Mesenchymal stem cells directly develop into osteoblasts during this phase, resulting in structured bone (Lin et al., 2020).

Osteoblastic bone development is the same in both methods. Osteoblasts need type 1 collagen to begin the process of synthesizing bone matrix. Type 1 collagen makes up most of the extracellular matrix protein in bone, giving it strength and suppleness. It also acts as a scaffold to deposit other matrix elements like hydroxyapatite (Lin et al., 2020).

Many signaling pathways regulate the homeostasis of the bones. Accordingly, osteoblasts express two essential transcription factors—osteoblast-specific transcription factor, or OSX—and runt-related transcription factor 2 (RUNX2), both required and sufficient for osteoblast development. Although it is clear that RUNX2 controls osteogenesis, several studies have demonstrated that OSX and RUNX2 alone are not enough to cause osteoblast maturation (Shahi et al., 2017).

2.5.1 BONE COMPOSITION

Bone generally consists of 40% organic matrix, 50–70% minerals, 5–10% water, and not more than 3% lipids. Minor quantities of magnesium, carbonate, and acid phosphate make up the majority of the minerals in bone. These minerals lack the usually common hydroxyl groups. The most significant dimension of bone hydroxyapatite crystals is around 200 Å, significantly less than that of geologic hydroxyapatite crystals.

The organic matrix gives bone flexibility and elasticity, whereas the bone mineral gives bone mechanical rigidity and load-bearing strength. The first "hole" zones where bone mineral is deposited are those found between the ends of collagen fibrils. Extracellular matrix vesicles in bone may aid in this process, much as they do in the calcification of cartilage and mineralization of the turkey tendon. Since hydroxyapatite is not often supersaturated in the extracellular fluid, it does not precipitate on its own. Proteins, an acidic phospholipid, calcium, and an inorganic phosphate complex comprise the nucleation core of matrix extracellular vesicles (Ferreira, 2022).

2.5.2 BONE STRUCTURE

As a mineralized connective tissue, bone contains four distinct cell types: osteoblasts, osteocytes, osteoclasts, and bone lining cells. In addition to allowing movement, storing calcium and phosphate, and housing bone marrow, bones also play essential roles in the body. Although bone may appear inactive, osteoclasts and osteoblasts constantly resorb and neo-form it, making bone an extremely dynamic organ. It has been demonstrated that osteoclasts coordinate and serve as mechanical sensors. Although the exact function of bone-lining cells is unclear, they play a critical role in bridging the gap between bone resorption and growth.

1. Osteoblasts are cells with cuboidal shape present on the surface of bones and comprise 4–6% of all resident bone cells. Their capacity to generate new bone is what makes them most well-known. These cells have the external characteristics of cells that make proteins, including a robust Golgi apparatus, a growing rough endoplasmic reticulum, and a plethora of secretory vesicles.
2. Additionally, gap junctions between osteocytes and adjacent cells that line the bone are observed. Cells with processes extending into canaliculi exist (Florencio-Silva et al., 2015).
3. Osteocytes, the most common and longest-living bone cells, may survive up to 25 years. They comprise 90–95% of all bone cells. Osteocytes were formerly distinguished from osteoblasts and osteoclasts by their specific roles during bone formation and resorption, respectively, based on their shape and location.
4. Numerous mechanisms lead to the development of multinucleated, terminally differentiated cells called osteoclasts. These include macrophage colony-stimulating factor, secreted by osteoprogenitor mesenchymal cells and osteoblasts, and receptor activator of nuclear factor κ B (RANK) ligand, released by osteoblasts, osteocytes, and stromal cells. These components work together to promote transcription factor activation and gene expression in osteoclasts (Dorozhkin, 2009).

2.5.2.1 ROLE OF CALCIUM IN BONE HEALTH

The human body accommodates 99% calcium, essential for bone health, strength, and muscle tone. However, its quantity should be ideal. Calcitropic hormones make this possible.

It is a necessary component. Over 99% of bone comprises calcium-phosphate complexes, including most mineral calcium (Dorozhkin, 2009).

For all life phases, optimal calcium intake is necessary for bone health.

2.5.3 INFLUENCE OF HORMONE ON BONE METABOLISM

Both progestins and estrogens significantly impact bone metabolism and, consequently, bone health. This is usually observed in early postmenopausal women or premenopausal women on GnRH treatment. Estrogens influence osteoclasts' ability to resorb bone, osteoclastogenesis, and osteoclast apoptosis, which mediates some of these effects.

Studies in the laboratory and clinic have provided proof that estrogens have a direct impact on osteoblast activity. Nonetheless, research on how estrogens affect osteoblasts' proliferative and synthetic activities has shown inconsistent findings, possibly due to the variety of *in-vitro* systems employed. When postmenopausal women receive estrogen therapy *in vivo*, their bone resorption and formation indicators rapidly decline, and their apparent bone mineral density increases concurrently (Herrmann and Seibel, 2010).

At physiological levels, insulin has anabolic effects on bone. It prevents bone resorption and lessens PTH's capacity to activate protein kinase C in osteoblasts. Furthermore, insulin encourages osteoblasts to produce collagen.

Regularly measuring blood calcium concentration is the first step in identifying calcium imbalance since hyper- or hypocalcemic individuals may not exhibit any symptoms. It is strongly advised that the albumin, phosphate, and calcium concentrations be tested concurrently with serum. Furthermore, PTH should be tested as the initial hormone.

When hypoalbuminemia is present, serum calcium concentration cannot accurately represent serum ionized calcium concentration. Therefore, albumin correction should always be applied to serum calcium concentration.

2.6 CLINICAL IMPLICATIONS

2.6.1 DISORDER RELATED TO CALCIUM IMBALANCE

2.6.1.1 DISORDERS RELATED TO HYPERCALCEMIA

Calcium concentrations greater than 10.5 mg/dL are considered hypercalcemia. Finding the cause of hypercalcemia is the next step after a diagnosis; a correct diagnosis enables efficient and frequently life-saving treatment. Primary hyperparathyroidism and hypercalcemia due to malignancy are the most frequent causes. We should first investigate these two differential diagnoses to lower healthcare expenses and standardize diagnostic evaluation.

A slightly or moderately raised blood calcium concentration implies hyperparathyroidism, while a high calcium concentration frequently indicates hypercalcemia connected to cancer. PTH production is high in primary hyperparathyroidism. Hyperparathyroidism is caused in roughly 80% of instances by benign enlargement of one parathyroid gland. Overproduction occurs in two or three glands in 20% of instances, and hyperplasia occurs in all four glands in a tiny percentage of individuals. Parathyroid cancer accounts for less than 1% of instances, with an equal frequency in males and females; patients are often younger, between the ages of 40 and 50.

About 20% of instances of malignancy-associated hypercalcemia are caused by bone metastases, which rank as the second most frequent cause. Moreover, some metastases, such as those from breast cancer, may increase the synthesis of PTHrp locally.

Non-Hodgkin and Hodgkin lymphoma breast cancer are the tumors most commonly associated with this sort of mechanism.

2.6.1.2 DISORDERS RELATED TO HYPOCALCEMIA

Regular chemical panels include Ca^{2+}, which makes hypocalcemia easy to detect. Similar to hypercalcemia, Ca^{2+} needs to be adjusted in cases of hypoalbuminemia or hyperalbuminemia. To confirm the diagnosis, it is preferable to obtain ionized Ca^{2+}, particularly in critically ill patients when Ca^{2+} binding to albumin is affected by pH changes. As mentioned earlier, metabolic alkalosis reduces ionized Ca^{2+} while increasing Ca^{2+} binding to albumin. PTH release from hypocalcemia promotes renal calcitriol production; both hormones boost serum Ca^{2+} through the abovementioned mechanism.

While other factors result in excessive PTH, PTH deficiency causes hypocalcemia, associated with low or average PTH and hyperphosphatemia. Acute pancreatitis, Mg^{2+} deficiency, hungry bone syndrome, and vitamin D deficiency are the causes of hypocalcemia with normal or low serum phosphate. The majority of people with persistent hypocalcemia have no symptoms. The clinical signs of hypocalcemia are determined by the severity and speed with which it develops. Muscle weakness, weariness, disorientation, sadness, and memory loss are all symptoms of hypoglycemia. Anxiety, tetany, paresthesias, laryngospasm, seizures, and QT interval prolongation are among the severe signs of acute hypocalcemia (Tinawi, 2021).

2.6.2 OSTEOPOROSIS AND HORMONAL IMBALANCE

An imbalance between bone resorption and bone creation causes rapid bone loss, brought on by increased bone turnover. Overuse of glucocorticoids may result in osteoporosis by demineralizing the bone and significantly altering its microscale spatial heterogeneities, which may increase the risk of fracture.

Osteocytes, osteoblasts, and osteoclasts are rich in estrogen receptors, which protect the bone. Estrogen binds to endogenous receptors, which control the expression of target genes for estrogen that encode proteins like transforming growth factor (TGF), insulin-like growth factor (IGF-1), and interleukin-1 (IL-1). Moreover, estrogen receptors (ERs) can inhibit nuclear factor-ligand (RANKL) activity, which lowers osteoclast proliferation and bone resorption. In the absence of estrogen, the expression of genes targeted by estrogen is altered, leading to an increased production of pro-inflammatory cytokines such as IL-1, IL-6, and tumor necrosis factor (TNF). Additionally, it has been shown that the absence of estrogen directly affects cell differentiation and death. Osteoporosis is the net outcome of decreased estrogen levels due to accelerated bone turnover and increased bone resorption.

Estrogens boost the synthesis of IGF1 and TGF by osteoblasts, promoting bone growth. Estrogens also inhibit osteoclast differentiation and promote osteoclast death by increasing TGF production. RANKL expression is increased in the presence of estrogen deprivation, which leads to osteoclastogenesis (Cheng et al., 2022).

While glucocorticoids (GCs) do not appear to alter the metabolism of osteoclasts, they do appear to influence bone metabolism primarily through osteoblasts. Thus, the primary explanation for GC-induced osteoporosis has been suggested to be inhibiting bone formation. Dexamethasone at 10-8 M was found to suppress the phosphorylation of the PI3K/AKT pathway, which in turn reduced osteogenesis and the production of osteogenic proteins (such as osteocalcin and alkaline phosphatase) in an *in-vitro* study. GCs may hamper osteoblast development, lifespan, and function. Males produce far more testosterone than females do, yet testosterone still has strong androgenic and anabolic effects that affect both sexes equally. In other words, androgens help young men form their skeletons and help older men avoid losing bone mass. Several case studies revealed severe osteoporosis in guys with mutations in the aromatase or estrogen receptor genes, indicating that testosterone's aromatization to estradiol contributes to at least some of its effects on the male skeleton. The three primary types of bone cells control the intricate remodeling process. Hormones, cytokines, minerals, and nutritional constituents can all send messages to these bone cells. These cells are responsive to both sex hormones because some of them express both ERs and androgen receptors. Deregulation of the remodeling process results from malfunctions in these cells. Net bone loss occurs in osteoporosis when the rate of bone resorption outpaces the rate of bone formation.

2.6.3 DIAGNOSIS AND TREATMENT OF HYPERCALCEMIA

Hypercalcemia and hypercalciuria, which are similar to hypercalcemia from any other cause, are the clinical symptoms of vitamin D intoxication, in addition to gastrointestinal symptoms like anorexia, nausea, vomiting, and constipation; cardiovascular symptoms like ectopy; and renal symptoms like polyuria and renal colic brought on by renal stone passage; and neuropsychiatric symptoms. For the treatment of hypercalcemia brought on by hypervitaminosis D, the vitamin D preparation is withheld. When taking 1-hydroxylated vitamin D analogs, those with chronic renal failure may be able to get by without the medication. It will be helpful to take a loop of diuretic and isotonic fluids.

2.6.3.1 TREATMENT OF HYPOCALCEMIA

Vitamin D supplementation of 1000–2000 IU/day is advised for people with vitamin D insufficiency. To avoid hypercalciuria and nephrocalcinosis. There will be no response to hypocalcemia therapy unless hypomagnesemia is first treated. Rapid intravenous magnesium infusion must be avoided due to the danger of arrhythmias (Vuralli, 2019).

2.6.3.2 DIAGNOSIS OF OSTEOPOROSIS

Osteoporosis screening should be performed on all women over 65. Risk factors for osteoporosis include anorexia, smoking, alcohol abuse, prolonged use of certain medications, early menopause (45 years of age), and other conditions. Men and women over 65 should be evaluated for these risk factors.

2.6.3.3 TREATMENT OF OSTEOPOROSIS

Numerous interventions, including vitamin D and calcium supplements, physical activity, and interdisciplinary treatments to lower the risk of falls, are available to prevent osteoporosis and its aftereffects. Both *in vivo* and *in vitro*, bisphosphonates directly impact crystal formation. They prevent the formation of new crystals, the conversion of hydroxyapatite from amorphous calcium phosphate, and the apatite crystals' aggregation into larger clusters. They also postpone the dissolution of crystals. While changes in hydroxyapatite crystals brought on by bisphosphonates may increase bone's resistance to resorption, these changes do not seem to have any bearing on the effects of bisphosphonates on bone (Bernabei et al., 2014).

2.7 CURRENT RESEARCH AND FUTURE PERSPECTIVES

Scientific advances and discoveries constantly influence our understanding of the complex hormonal interconnections that control bone metabolism, parathyroid function, and calcium homeostasis.

To provide insight into future possibilities for therapeutic intervention and preventing illness, epigenetic studies attempt to comprehend how environmental factors and lifestyle choices influence the regulation of PTH. Epigenetic alterations affect gene expression without altering the underlying DNA sequence. A few of these modifications include histone modifications, DNA methylation, and noncoding RNAs. Environmental elements and lifestyle options can be impacted by dietary elements such as calcium and vitamin D; smoking and exposure to environmental contaminants can alter PTH gene expression through epigenetic alterations, resulting in novel approaches to treating conditions, including osteoporosis and primary hyperparathyroidism.

Short-chain fatty acids produced by specific strains of bacteria can reduce gut pH, enhancing calcium solubility and improving absorption. Furthermore, the management of calcium homeostasis can be affected through the interaction between gut bacteria and vitamin D metabolism (Sharma et al., 2022). The delicate equilibrium of calcium in the body is preserved significantly by the gut bacteria, which governs hormone regulation, metabolism, and absorption. This broad knowledge makes it possible to develop therapies to address various health problems connected to calcium and gut bacteria (Cheng et al., 2022).

Implementing nanoparticles with ligands that attach to bone cells or other target tissue receptors in a particular manner guarantees that therapeutic drugs are adequately delivered while minimizing off-target effects. Nanoparticles may reduce the necessary dosage and eliminate potential adverse outcomes while boosting local medication concentration and optimizing therapy efficacy. Numerous conditions connected to the metabolism of calcium and bone, such as osteoporosis, hypercalcemia, and bone infections, may be managed using this treatment method (Baranwal et al., 2023).

The development of chronotherapeutic methodologies that adjust medication circulation or treatment schedules to correspond with the body's natural rhythms, potentially increasing efficacy while reducing adverse effects, could be impacted by understanding the timing of PTH oscillations with circadian rhythm. The complicated interactions between internal clocks, hormone control, and other physiological systems have been explained by studies regarding circadian rhythms, which enriches the current understanding of overall wellness and health (el-Hajj Fuleihan et al., 1997).

Massive databases incorporating hormone measurements, genetic data, and clinical data can be examined by machine learning and artificial intelligence algorithms, which can discover fragile connections and trends that are difficult to recognize. The capacity to break down complicated connections enables investigators to recognize novel regulatory mechanisms controlling the interactions between hormones, providing knowledge about previously unidentified pathways impacting human health (Yadav et al., 2023).

Evaluating every individual's unique hormonal profile—which offers variations in PTH, calcium, and vitamin D levels—allows physicians to more effectively personalize therapy regimens and adjust dosage schedules to accomplish better symptom control and greater efficacy (Singh et al., 2020). Discovering gene changes related to parathyroid diseases, like primary hyperparathyroidism (resulting from gene mutations in parathyroid cells), can help diagnose, anticipate the condition's seriousness, and guide therapy options (Bilezikian et al., 2021).

2.8 CONCLUSION

Conclusively, the comprehensive review of the chapter related to the hormonal regulation of plasma calcium, the parathyroid gland, and bone metabolism highlights the complex systems that supervise the delicate equilibrium of calcium homeostasis within the human body.

With PTH secretion, the parathyroid gland becomes essential in this regulatory symphony. For the body to maintain ideal plasma calcium concentrations, PTH acts as a critical mediator, coordinating a dynamic interaction between the skeletal and renal systems. The primary objective in bone metabolism is to boost osteoclast activity, which raises bone resorption and distributes more calcium into the blood. In addition to helping maintain plasma calcium levels, PTH improves calcium reabsorption through the renal tubules.

Another vital hormone discussed in this chapter, calcitonin works opposite PTH by improving bone calcium deposition and suppressing osteoclast activity. Their complex antagonistic relationship emphasizes the complexity of the regulatory systems implicated and provides accurate oversight over plasma calcium concentrations.

Commonly termed the "sunshine vitamin," vitamin D is essential for maintaining calcium homeostasis. Its active form, calcitriol, strengthens the systemic control of this vital mineral by facilitating intestinal absorption of calcium. The mutually beneficial effects of vitamin D and PTH highlight the intricate interplay of endocrine signals influencing calcium metabolism.

This regulation mechanism is much more significant than simply maintaining the balance of minerals; it influences essential physiological functions like cell signaling, blood clotting, and neuromuscular excitability. Defects in these delicately functioning systems may lead to various illnesses, such as hyper- and hypocalcemia, which can severely impact general health.

The chapter describes the pathophysiology of disorders associated with calcium imbalance and bone health, highlighting the complexity of hormone control in this context. Furthermore, it creates opportunities for further research and medical therapies to optimize such complex regulatory systems.

To put it briefly, analyzing hormone regulation of bone metabolism, the parathyroid gland, and plasma calcium provides a comprehensive perspective on the physiological complexities behind maintaining calcium homeostasis.

KEYWORDS

- **calcitonin**
- **parathyroid hormone**
- **bone metabolism**
- **calcium regulation**
- **vitamin D**
- **thyroid gland**

REFERENCES

Aggarwal, G., Gupta, S., Sardana, O., Kumari, P., Kaur, R., Singh, T.G., Singh, R. (2023). Comparison of efficacy of metformin and D-chiro-inositol on clinical biomarkers in patients with polycystic ovarian syndrome: An open label study. Global Health Journal, 7(3), 147–152.

Ayers, K.L., Glicksberg, B.S., Garfield, A.S., Longerich, S., White, J.A., Yang, P., Du, L., Chittenden, T.W., Gulcher, J.R., Roy, S., Fiedorek, F., Gottesdiener, K., Cohen, S.,

North, K.E., Schadt, E.E., Li, S.D., Chen, R., Van der Ploeg, L.H.T. (2018). Melanocortin 4 receptor pathway dysfunction in obesity: Patient stratification aimed at MC4R agonist treatment. The Journal of Clinical Endocrinology and Metabolism, 103(7), 2601–2612. https://doi.org/10.1210/jc.2018-00258

Baranwal, J., Barse, B., Di Petrillo, A., Gatto, G., Pilia, L., Kumar, A. (2023). Nanoparticles in cancer diagnosis and treatment. Materials (Basel, Switzerland), 16(15), 5354. https://doi.org/10.3390/ma16155354

Berchtold, M.W., Brinkmeier, H., Müntener, M. (2000). Calcium ion in skeletal muscle: Its crucial role for muscle function, plasticity, and disease. Physiological Reviews, 80(3), 1215–1265. https://doi.org/10.1152/physrev.2000.80.3.1215

Bernabei, R., Martone, A.M., Ortolani, E., Landi, F., Marzetti, E. (2014). Screening, diagnosis and treatment of osteoporosis: A brief review. Clinical Cases in Mineral and Bone Metabolism, 11(3), 201–207.

Bhargava, S.K., Singh, T.G., Mannan, A., Singh, S., Gupta, S. (2022). Pharmacological evaluation of Thuja occidentalis for the attenuation of nephropathy in streptozotocin-induced diabetes rats. Obesity Medicine, 31, 100391.

Bhattarai, H.K., Shrestha, S., Rokka, K., Shakya, R. (2020). Vitamin D, calcium, parathyroid hormone, and sex steroids in bone health and effects of aging. Journal of Osteoporosis, 2020, 9324505. https://doi.org/10.1155/2020/9324505

Bilezikian, J.P., Formenti, A.M., Adler, R.A., Binkley, N., Bouillon, R., Lazaretti-Castro, M., Marcocci, C., Napoli, N., Rizzoli, R., Giustina, A. (2021). Vitamin D: Dosing, levels, form, and route of administration: Does one approach fit all. Reviews in Endocrine & Metabolic Disorders, 22(4), 1201–1218. https://doi.org/10.1007/s11154-021-09693-7

Bilezikian, J.P., Khan, A.A., Potts, Jr J.T. (2014). Guidelines for managing asymptomatic primary hyperparathyroidism: Summary statement from the third international workshop. Journal of Clinical Endocrionology & Metabolism 94(2), 335–339. https://doi.org/10.1210/jc.2008-1763

Bronner, F. (1973). Calcium homeostasis. IFAC Proceedings Volumes, 6(4), 44–48. https://doi.org/10.1016/S1474-6670(17)67967-9

Burgoyne, R.D., Helassa, N., McCue, H.V., Haynes, L.P. (2019). Calcium sensors in neuronal function and dysfunction. Cold Spring Harbor Perspectives in Biology, 11(5), a035154. https://doi.org/10.1101/cshperspect.a035154

Cashman, K.D., Flynn, A. (1999). Optimal nutrition: Calcium, magnesium and phosphorus. The Proceedings of the Nutrition Society, 58(2), 477–487. https://doi.org/10.1017/s0029665199000622

Chen, R.A., Goodman, W.G. (2004). Role of the calcium-sensing receptor in parathyroid gland physiology. American Journal of Physiology. Renal Physiology, 286(6), F1005–F1011. https://doi.org/10.1152/ajprenal.00013.2004

Cheng, C.H., Chen, L.R., Chen, K.H. (2022). Osteoporosis due to hormone imbalance: An overview of the effects of estrogen deficiency and glucocorticoid overuse on bone turnover. International Journal of Molecular Sciences, 23(3), 1376. https://doi.org/10.3390/ijms23031376

Devi, S., Chauhan, S., Mannan, A., Singh, T.G. (2024). Targeting cardiovascular risk factors with eugenol: An anti-inflammatory perspective. Inflammopharmacology, 32(1), 307–317. https://doi.org/10.1007/s10787-023-01392-w

Dorozhkin, S.V. (2009). Calcium orthophosphates in nature, Biology and Medicine, 399–498. https://doi.org/10.3390/ma2020399

Egstrand, S., Nordholm, A., Morevati, M., Mace, M.L., Hassan, A., Naveh-Many, T., Rukov, J.L., Gravesen, E., Olgaard, K., Lewin, E. (2020). A molecular circadian clock operates in the parathyroid gland and is disturbed in chronic kidney disease associated bone and mineral disorder. Kidney International, 98(6), 1461–1475. https://doi.org/10.1016/j.kint.2020.06.034

el-Hajj Fuleihan, G., Klerman, E.B., Brown, E.N., Choe, Y., Brown, E.M., Czeisler, C.A. (1997). The parathyroid hormone circadian rhythm is truly endogenous—a general clinical research center study. The Journal of Clinical Endocrinology and Metabolism, 82(1), 281–286. https://doi.org/10.1210/jcem.82.1.3683.

Fecher-trost, C., Weissgerber, P., Wissenbach, U. (2014). TRPV6 Channels. https://doi.org/10.1007/978-3-642-54215-2

Fenn, W., Rahn, H. (1979). 1893—1971.

Ferreira, C.J. (2022). ScholarWorks @ UMass Amherst Controlled Codelivery of miR-26a and antagomiR-133a with Osteoconductive Scaffolds to Promote Healing of Large Bone Defects. March.

Fleet, J.C. (2022). Vitamin D-mediated regulation of intestinal calcium absorption. Nutrients, 14(16), 3351. https://doi.org/10.3390/nu14163351

Florencio-Silva, R., Sasso, G.R., Sasso-Cerri, E., Simões, M.J., Cerri, P.S. (2015). Biology of bone tissue: Structure, function, and factors that influence bone cells. BioMed Research International, 2015, 421746. https://doi.org/10.1155/2015/421746

Galea, G.L., Zein, M.R., Allen, S., Francis-West, P. (2021). Making and shaping endochondral and intramembranous bones. Developmental Dynamics, 250(3), 414–449. https://doi.org/10.1002/dvdy.278

Healy, K.D., Vanhooke, J.L., Prahl, J.M., DeLuca, H.F. (2005). Parathyroid hormone decreases renal vitamin D receptor expression in vivo. Proceedings of the National Academy of Sciences of the United States of America, 102(13), 4724–4728. https://doi.org/10.1073/pnas.0501312102

Herrmann, M., Seibel, M.J. (2010). The effects of hormonal contraceptives on bone turnover markers and bone health. Clinical Endocrinology, 72(5), 571–583. https://doi.org/10.1111/j.1365-2265.2009.03688.x

Hill, T.R., Verlaan, S., Biesheuvel, E., Eastell, R., Bauer, J.M., Bautmans, I., Brandt, K., Donini, L.M., Maggio, M., Mets, T., Seal, C.J., Wijers, S.L., Sieber, C., Cederholm, T., Aspray, T.J., PROVIDE Consortium (2019). A vitamin D, calcium and leucine-enriched whey protein nutritional supplement improves measures of bone health in sarcopenic non-malnourished older adults: The provide study. Calcified Tissue International, 105(4), 383–391. https://doi.org/10.1007/s00223-019-00581-6

Hoenderop, J.G., Nilius, B., Bindels, R.J. (2005). Calcium absorption across epithelia. Physiological Reviews, 85(1), 373–422. https://doi.org/10.1152/physrev.00003.2004

Hollis, B.W., Johnson, D., Hulsey, T.C., Ebeling, M., Wagner, C.L. (2011). Vitamin D supplementation during pregnancy: double-blind, randomized clinical trial of safety and effectiveness, Randomized Controlled Trial, 26(10), 2341–2357. https://doi.org/10.1002/jbmr.498

Hong, E.J., Jeung, E.B. (2013). Biological significance of calbindin-D9k within duodenal epithelium. International Journal of Molecular Sciences, 14(12), 23330–23340. https://doi.org/10.3390/ijms141223330

Jeon, U.S. (2008). Kidney and calcium homeostasis. Electrolyte & Blood Pressure: E & BP, 6(2), 68–76. https://doi.org/10.5049/EBP.2008.6.2.68

Khazan, N., Kim, K.K., Hansen, J.N., Singh, N.A., Moore, T., Snyder, C.W.A., Pandita, R., Strawderman, M., Fujihara, M., Takamura, Y., Jian, Y., Battaglia, N., Yano, N., Teramoto, Y., Arnold, L.A., Hopson, R., Kishor, K., Nayak, S., Ojha, D., Sharon, A., … Moore, R.G. (2022). Identification of a vitamin-D receptor antagonist, MeTC7, which inhibits the growth of xenograft and transgenic tumors *In Vivo*. Journal of Medicinal Chemistry, 65(8), 6039–6055. https://doi.org/10.1021/acs.jmedchem.1c01878

Kim, B., Cho, Y.J., Lim, W. (2021). Osteoporosis therapies and their mechanisms of action (Review). Experimental and Therapeutic Medicine, 22(6), 1379. https://doi.org/10.3892/etm.2021.10815

Lin, X., Patil, S., Gao, Y.G., Qian, A. (2020). The bone extracellular matrix in bone formation and regeneration. Frontiers in Pharmacology, 11, 757. https://doi.org/10.3389/fphar.2020.00757

Long, F., Ornitz, D.M. (2013). Development of the endochondral skeleton. Cold Spring Harbor Perspectives in Biology, 5(1), a008334. https://doi.org/10.1101/cshperspect.a008334

Najar, I.A., Bhat, M.H., Qadrie, Z.L., Amaldoss, M.J.N., Kushwah, A.S., Singh, T.G., Kabra, A., Khan, N., Kumar, M. (2022). Cardioprotection by citrus grandis (L.) peel ethanolic extract in alloxan-induced cardiotoxicity in diabetic rats. BioMed Research International, 2022, 2807337. https://doi.org/10.1155/2022/2807337

Paoletti, A.M., Serra, G.G., Cagnacci, A., Vacca, A.M., Guerriero, S., Solla, E., Melis, G.B. (1996). Spontaneous reversibility of bone loss induced by gonadotropin-releasing hormone analog treatment. Fertility and Sterility, 65(4), 707–710.

Potts, J.T. (2005). Starling review parathyroid hormone: Past and present. Journal of Endocrinology, 187, 311–325. https://doi.org/10.1677/joe.1.06057

Review, M. (n.d.). Calcium-sensing receptor: Role in health and disease, Indian Journal of Endocrinology and Metabolism, 16, 213–216. https://doi.org/10.4103/2230-8210.104041

Riccardi, D., Brown, E.M. (2010). Physiology and pathophysiology of the calcium-sensing receptor in the kidney. American Journal of Physiology. Renal Physiology, 298(3), F485–F499. https://doi.org/10.1152/ajprenal.00608.2009

Rodríguez-Ortiz, M.E., Canalejo, A., Herencia, C., Martínez-Moreno, J.M., Peralta-Ramírez, A., Perez-Martinez, P., Navarro-González, J.F., Rodríguez, M., Peter, M., Gundlach, K., Steppan, S., Passlick-Deetjen, J., Muñoz-Castañeda, J.R., Almaden, Y. (2014). Magnesium modulates parathyroid hormone secretion and upregulates parathyroid receptor expression at moderately low calcium concentration. Nephrology, Dialysis, Transplantation, 29(2), 282–289. https://doi.org/10.1093/ndt/gft400

Rutala, W.A., Weber, D.J., Hill, C. (2019). Guideline for Disinfection and Sterilization in Healthcare Facilities, 2008. May.

Safadi, F.F., Barbe, M.F., Abdelmagid, S.M., Rico, M.C., Aswad, R.A. (2009). Bone structure, development and bone biology: Bone pathology bone structure, Development and Bone Biology (Issue December). https://doi.org/10.1007/978-1-59745-347-9

Shahi, M., Peymani, A., Sahmani, M. (2017). Regulation of bone metabolism. Reports of Biochemistry & Molecular Biology, 5(2), 73–82.

Sharma, V.K., Singh, T.G. (2020). Chronic stress and diabetes mellitus: Interwoven pathologies. Current Diabetes Reviews, 16(6), 546–556. https://doi.org/10.2174/15733 99815666191111152248

Sharma, V.K., Singh, T.G., Dhiman, S., Garg, N. (2022). Mechanisms of beneficial effects of probiotics in diabetes mellitus. In: *Probiotic Research in Therapeutics: Volume 5: Metabolic Diseases and Gut Bacteria.* Singapore: Springer Nature Singapore, pp. 97–124.

Singh, R., Rao, H.K., Singh, T.G. (2020). Advanced glycated end products (ages) in diabetes and its complications: An insight. Plant Arch, 20(1), 3838–3841.

Singh, R., Rao, H.K., Singh, T.G. (2020). Neuropathic pain in diabetes mellitus: Challenges and future trends. Obesity Medicine, 18, 100215.

Soetan, K.O., Olaiya, C.O., Oyewole, O.E. (2010). The importance of mineral elements for humans, domestic animals and plants: A review. African Journal of Food Science, 4(May), 200–222.

Sood, A., Baishnab, S., Gautam, I., Choudhary, P., Lang, D.K., Jaura, R.S., Singh, T.G. (2023). Exploring various novel diagnostic and therapeutic approaches in treating diabetic retinopathy. Inflammopharmacology, 31(2), 773–786. https://doi.org/10.1007/s10787-023-01143-x

Strom, S.C., Garcia-olmo, D., Martino, V. Di, Farkas, D.T., Firpi, R.J., Gazouli, M., Kramvis, A., Kruis, W., Lee, H.C., Mcdonald, C., Mendez-sanchez, N., Renteln, D. Von, Sangiovanni, A., Seo, D., Stanley, A.J., Feinle-bisset, C., Horowitz, M. (2017). World Journal of Gastroenterology, 9327(16), 2819–3010.

Tangpricha, V. (2014). NIH Public Access. June. https://doi.org/10.1007/s11926-008-0020-y

Tinawi, M. (2021). Disorders of calcium metabolism: Hypocalcemia and hypercalcemia. Cureus, 13(1), e12420. https://doi.org/10.7759/cureus.12420

VanHouten, J., Dann, P., McGeoch, G., Brown, E.M., Krapcho, K., Neville, M., Wysolmerski, J.J. (2004). The calcium-sensing receptor regulates mammary gland parathyroid hormone-related protein production and calcium transport. The Journal of Clinical Investigation, 113(4), 598–608. https://doi.org/10.1172/JCI18776

Vuralli, D. (2019). Clinical approach to hypocalcemia in newborn period and infancy: Who should be treated. International Journal of Pediatrics, 2019, 4318075. https://doi.org/10.1155/2019/4318075

Yadav, N., Mohan, B., Chettri, D., Pulwani, C., Velusamy, P., Iyer, M., Vellingiri, B. (2023). Artificial intelligence in heavy metals detection: Methodological and ethical challenges. Hygiene and Environmental Health Advances, 7(July), 100071. https://doi.org/10.1016/j.heha.2023.100071

Zhang, G., Li, F. (2020). Disorders of calcium and phosphorus metabolism and the proteomics/metabolomics-based research. Frontiers in Cell and Developmental Biology, 8(September). https://doi.org/10.3389/fcell.2020.576110

Zhu, K., Prince, R.L. (2012). Calcium and bone. Clinical Biochemistry, 45(12), 936–942. https://doi.org/10.1016/j.clinbiochem.2012.05.006

CHAPTER 3

Epigenetics in Adrenoleukodystrophy

VEERTA SHARMA[1], THAKUR GURJEET SINGH[1*], SANJANA MEHTA[1], and SOFIA KOKKINIS[2,3]

[1]*Chitkara College of Pharmacy, Chitkara University, Rajpura, Punjab, India*

[2]*Discipline of Pharmacy, Graduate School of Health, University of Technology Sydney, Sydney, NSW, Australia*

[3]*Faculty of Health, Australian Research Centre in Complementary and Integrative Medicine, University of Technology Sydney, Ultimo, NSW, Australia*

*Corresponding author

ABSTRACT

Adrenoleukodystrophy (ALD) is a rare and fatal X-linked hereditary condition characterized by an aberrant build-up of very long-chain fatty acids, resulting in demyelination in the brain and adrenal insufficiency. While the genetic basis of ALD has received much attention, emerging evidence reveals that epigenetic pathways play an essential role in disease development. Thus, it is crucial to create effective and safe treatment methods. This review gives a complete overview of the present epigenetic landscape in ALD, focusing on the pathological events present in the disease. The influence of epigenetic changes on critical genes involved in the metabolism of very long-chain fatty acids, peroxisomal function, and inflammatory responses is examined, illumining how epigenetic dysregulation may contribute to the variability of clinical symptoms seen in ALD patients. The study also emphasizes the potential diagnostic and

Pharmacotherapy Approaches Toward Endocrine and Metabolic Diseases.
Thakur Gurjeet Singh and Sanjana Mehta (Eds.)

DOI: 10.1201/9781779640154-3

prognostic significance of epigenetic markers in ALD, underlining the need for a better knowledge of the epigenetic fingerprints associated with disease development. Finally, this review synthesizes existing knowledge on the epigenetic aspects of ALD, laying the groundwork for future research directions and developing personalized therapeutic strategies to mitigate the impact of epigenetic dysregulation in individuals suffering from this devastating disorder.

3.1 INTRODUCTION

Adrenoleukodystrophy (ALD) is a neurodegenerative disease (NDD) characterized by progressive demyelination in the brain, adrenal insufficiency, and build-up of very-long-chain fatty acids (VLCFA) due to impaired transport and subsequent β-oxidation in peroxisomes. The most common peroxisomal disease affects one in every 17,000 homozygous males and heterozygous females (Moser et al., 2007). Mutations in the ABC transporter subfamily D member-1 (ABCD-1) gene lead to the adrenoleukodystrophy protein (ALDP) loss of function. ALDP is a peroxisomal ATP-binding cassette (ABC) half-transporter that imports VLCFA into the peroxisome for breakdown (Kemp and Wanders, 2010). The same nuclear family can have extensive clinical variance in ALD, suggesting genetic, environmental, and stochastic variables. It is classified into cerebral childhood ALD (cALD) and adreno-myeloneuropathy (AMN). cALD affects boys between the ages of five and 10 years, is associated with a robust inflammatory reaction in the CNS white matter, and may involve auto-immune mechanisms. AMN affects adult males 20–52 years of age and heterozygous women after 42. However, cerebral demyelination may develop in around 20% of people having AMN over 10 years (Mahmood et al., 2005). The common feature of the two main phenotypes is axon loss with destruction of myelin sheath occurring as a first event for cALD and as a subsequent phase in AMN patients (Kemp et al., 2016). Too far, the only therapy is allogeneic bone marrow transplantation, which is linked with substantial morbidity and mortality and is only given to children with cALD who are mainly asymptomatic. According to accumulating data, epigenetic pathways play a significant role in disease development (Singh and Singh, 2021). As a result, developing effective and safe treatment approaches is critical. Therefore, this review gives a complete overview of the present epigenetic landscape in ALD, focusing on the pathological events present in the disease (Singh et al., 2020). Furthermore, it provides insights into the biochemical and genetic aspects involved in ALD, the various epigenetic markers in ALD, and the clinical aspects of drugs, laying the groundwork for future research directions and the development of personalized therapeutic strategies aimed at mitigating the impact of epigenetic dysregulation in individuals suffering from this devastating disorder (Khan et al., 2022).

3.2 PATHOLOGICAL EVENTS UNDERLYING THE DISEASE

3.2.1 OXIDATIVE STRESS

It is described as a redox imbalance resulting in excess reactive oxygen species (ROS). ROS reacts and causes chemical changes in deoxyribose nucleic acid (DNA), lipids, and proteins due to their extreme instability. These modifications are harmful if the changed residues are required for the protein's function or the turnover (Sharma et al., 2020; Rotariu et al., 2022). Furthermore, oxidative damage can change lipids' characteristics and cause DNA mutations, causing mitochondrial dysfunction and disease (Thapa et al., 2023; Islam, 2017). Examining the postmortem brains of ALD patients and the rodent model, where it occurs very early in life, it was found that oxidative stress is a common feature in ALD patients (Singh et al., 2021; Deon et al., 2016). In both presymptomatic spinal cords and ALD human fibroblasts, quantitative indicators of protein carbonylation (glutamic semi-aldehyde [GSA] and amino-adipic semi-aldehyde [AASA]), glycoxidation and lipoxidation (carboxy-ethyl-lysine and carboxy-ethyl-lysine), and protein lipoxidation (malondialdehyde-lysine) accumulate. At three months of age, ALD animals' spinal cords have lower levels of superoxide dismutases (SOD)-1 and 2, and their fibroblasts are more susceptible to glutathione depletion (Sharma et al., 2023). In addition, Hexacosanoic acid exclusively damages proteins and lipids in ALD fibroblasts, showing a deficiency in antioxidant defense. Both lines of evidence reveal an impaired antioxidant response, which leads to oxidative damage in the illness (Baarine et al., 2012). VLCFA build-up in ALD was initially recorded 355 years ago, but its toxicity was just discovered (Vishwakarma et al., 2022; Aubourg, 2007). Excess VLCFA causes enhanced levels of ROS and mitochondrial membrane potential dissipation and reduced glutathione levels. Similar investigations in rodent primary brain cell cultures revealed that VLCFA might depolarize mitochondria and elevate intracellular Ca^{2+} levels in oligo-dendrocytes (Schlüter et al., 2012).

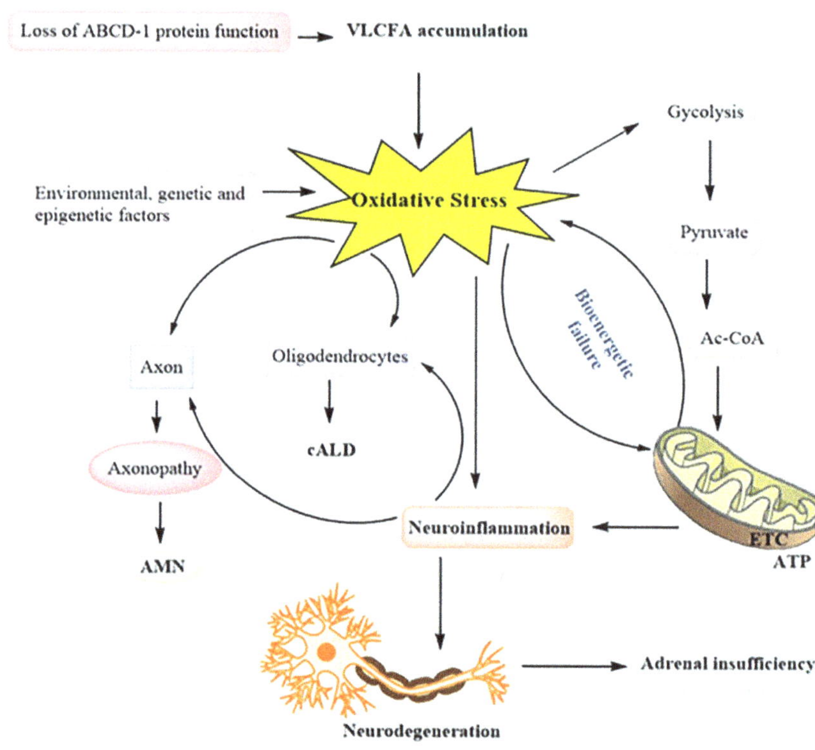

FIGURE 3.1 The X-ALD pathogenesis.3.2.2 mitochondrial dysfunction.

Axonal degeneration in various NDDs is caused by a lack of redox homeostasis linked to mitochondria dysfunction (Panchal and Tiwari, 2019). Mitochondria are the leading producers of ROS and are vulnerable to oxidative stress, especially when the (mitochondrial) electron transport chain (ETC) fails. As a result, the accumulation of damaged mitochondria is often associated with the progression of the disease. Mitochondria produce most ROS in ALD fibroblasts when exposed to excess hexacosanoic acid (Rehni et al., 2009; Vargas et al., 2004). The mitochondrial uncoupler carboxy-carbonylcyanide *m*-chloro-phenyl-hydrazone (CCCP) and various oxidative-phosphorylation (OXPHOS) system inhibitors like rotenone for complex-1 and they-trifluoro-acetone (TTFA) for complex-2 can inhibit C26:0-induced ROS production, suggesting that complex-1 and 2 of ETC are the primary ROS sources in fibroblasts with excess hexacosanoic acid. Incubated with VLCFA, 158N oligo-dendroidal cells showed mitochondrial ROS (López-Erauskin et al., 2013; Baarine et al., 2012). However, there is a chance that the observed ROS generation by mitochondria is caused by signals originating in peroxisomes. Indeed, the mitochondrial redox state is altered in catalase-deficient cells and when oxidative stress is induced in peroxisomes, demonstrating a direct cross-talk between these two organelles (Rehni and Singh, 2010; Fransen et al., 2012). In more relevant rodent models for the illness, xanthine oxidase, peroxisomes, and NADPH oxidases must be systematically assessed. VLCFA are typically present in complex lipids absorbed into membranes, increasing microviscosity and rupturing them (Whitcomb et al., 1988). By altering mitochondrial membrane lateral chains of phospholipids, hexacosanoic acid may physically interfere with the OXPHOS process, causing the production of ROS. Using high-resolution respirometry, it was found that the decreased OXPHOS function results in ALD (Ho et al., 1995).

3.3 BIOCHEMICAL AND GENETIC ASPECTS IN ALD

The peroxisomal matrix degrades the saturated, unbranched VLCFA by β-oxidation pathway enzyme activities. ALD patients' tissues and body fluids acquire saturated VLCFA, particularly C26:0, a diagnostic marker (Bezman et al., 2001). The ABCD-1 gene on chromosome Xq28 is mutated in all ALD patients (Kemp et al., 2001). ABCD-1's ATP-binding domain is exposed to the cytosol, and substrates are transferred from the cytosol into the peroxisome via ATP consumption. CoA-activated VLCFA, including C26:0, C24: and C22:0, are suitable substrates for the human ABCD-1 protein, and the breakdown of these fatty acids by peroxisomal β-oxidation is strongly inhibited in cultured ALD fibroblasts (van Roermund et al., 2008, 2011; Wiesinger et al., 2013).

In addition to ABCD-1, the peroxisomal membrane has two more ABC transporters, ABCD-2 and ABCD-3. In the peroxisomal membrane, the ABCD-1 transporter dimerizes to form a homodimer; *in vivo*, although it heterodimer with ABCD-2 and -3, the other two peroxisomal ABCD family members (Berger and Gärtner, 2006). In all tissues investigated, the β-oxidation of VLCFA was never wholly abolished by ABCD-1 mutations, not even those causing a complete loss of function. Researchers have found that X-ALD primary fibroblast's residual activity depends primarily on the homologous peroxisomal ABC transporter (ABCD-3). However, ABCD-3 was 45 times less effective than ABCD-1 at transporting C26:0-CoA over the peroxisomal membrane. ABCD-2, the relative homolog of ABCD-1, is expected to compensate more effectively than ABCD-3. However, it is not expressed significantly in fibroblasts, limiting its contribution to residual β-oxidation activity under normal circumstances. The metabolic deficiency in ALD may vary based on the cell type-specific expression profiles of ABCD-1, -2, and -3, as they all contribute to VLCFA transport and degradation through ω-oxidation.

The three significant findings show that X-ALD has no generalized genotype–phenotype correlation: first, the same ABCD-1 mutation can cause all clinical phenotypes within a kindred (Berger et al., 1994); second, a complete loss of ABCD-1 protein (e.g., early frameshift, non-sense mutations and large deletions); and third, a two-base pair deletion in exon-5 has been found in patients with the entire clinical spectrum of X-ALD. However, specific mutations that produce a stable, appropriately localized protein that may form dimers and facilitate residual transporter function may be unique to the AMN phenotype (Guimarães et al., 2001).

Interestingly, standard VLCFA diet limitation in X-ALD patients did not reduce plasma C26:0 (Bezman et al., 2001). Recent investigations have shown that X-ALD's VLCFA is partially absorbed from the food but mainly synthesized endogenously by VLCFA elongation (Kemp et al., 2005). In addition, X-ALD patients' fibroblasts stimulate this elongation mechanism. This would explain why C22:0 does not accumulate and is frequently somewhat decreased in X-ALD tissues and cells, even though C22:0–CoA is a strong ABCD-1 substrate (Wiesinger et al., 2013).

3.4 EPIGENETIC MARKERS IN ALD

Epigenetic factors can cause disease by altering gene expression without changing DNA sequence. DNA methylation, histone methylation, acetylation, phosphorylation, and noncoding RNA regulation are epigenetic changes.

DNA methylation regulates gene expression and cell differentiation, and several studies have demonstrated the association between changes in DNA methylation and disease pathogenesis. Schlüter and colleagues compared the genome-wide DNA methylation pattern of unaffected frontal brain white matter patients with AMN and cALD with cerebral involvement. They found hypermethylation of genes involved in oligodendrocyte differentiation, which can impair precursor cell differentiation to remyelinating oligodendrocytes, and hypomethylation of genes involved in immune function, such as interferon-induced genes (Schlüter et al., 2018). This supports cerebral X-ALD neuropathological findings of demyelination and immunological activation. This study also found that SPG-20, UNC45-A, and COL9-A3 methylation and ID4 and MYRF expression might distinguish CALD from AMN.

Aberrant expression of micro-RNAs (miRNAs), short noncoding RNAs that regulate posttranscriptional gene expression, may contribute to neurons' inflammation and degeneration (Shah and Singh, 2017). In cALD, miR-196a expression dropped while ELOVL, IKKα/β, mitogen-activated protein kinase (MAP-4K3 and MAP-3K2) expression increased compared to AMN and control fibroblasts, suggesting miR-196a regulates inflammatory signaling pathways in cALD brains.

3.5 CLINICAL ASPECTS OF DRUGS

3.5.1 IMMUNOSUPPRESSANTS

White matter alterations in the cerebral type of illness appear to be linked to cytokine or immune-mediated brain inflammation. All therapeutic studies have been conducted to modify the inflammatory response to β-interferon, cyclophosphamide, pentoxifylline, immunoglobulins, thalidomide, and cyclosporin (Berger and Gärtner, 2006).

3.5.2 CHOLESTEROL REDUCING DRUGS

VLCFA build-up in human X-ALD fibroblasts is normalized by either cholesterol depletion or therapy with the cholesterol-lowering medication lovastatin (Weinhofer et al., 2002). Thus, there is a link between VLCFA breakdown and cholesterol levels. Lovastatin, which lowers cholesterol levels by blocking hydroxymethyl-glutaryl-CoA reductase enzyme, appeared as a promising therapy for X-ALD since it reduced VLCFA in X-ALD patients (Pai et al., 2000). However, in comparable clinical research using simvastatin, the VLCFA levels in patients' plasma could not be normalized. Differences in research design or using a different statin might account for the different outcomes. The X-ALD rodent model has shown that ALDP deficiency and VLCFA are linked to cholesterol, although species variations make evaluating cholesterol-lowering medicines problematic (Weinhofer et al., 2005).

3.5.3 4 PHENYLBUTYRATE

Phenyl acetate's prodrug 4-phenylbutyrate (4-PBA) reduced VLCFA in X-ALD (fibroblast), attributed to higher peroxisomal β-oxidation rates in preliminary investigations with cultured cells. Kemp and colleagues observed enhanced ABCD-2 mRNA and peroxisome proliferation in cultured human and mouse primary fibroblasts following 4-PBA therapy. The amount of ALDR protein increased in ABCD-1-deficient mouse fibroblasts but not in wild-type mice fibroblasts (Berger et al., 2010). Most notably, following 4–6 weeks of dietary 4-PBA therapy, a significant decrease of VLCFA was obtained in the brain and adrenal glands of ABCD-1 deficient animals. The effect of 4-PBA in human X-ALD fibroblasts was reported first to increase the β-oxidation of LCFA, followed by enhanced peroxisomal VLCFA β-oxidation, which preceded the up-regulation of the levels of ABCD-2 mRNA (McGuinness et al., 2001).

3.5.4 ARGININE BUTYRATE

The half-life of 4-phenyl butyrate leads to rapid liver metabolism and tachyphylaxis *in vivo*. An interval treatment regimen may mitigate these effects. Research suggests testing pharmacological compounds similar to 4-PBA but with longer lasting pharmacokinetic qualities to address VLCFA build-up in X-ALD fibroblasts (McGuinness et al., 2001). To overcome the issue of oral 4-PBA medication quantities, an intermittent pulsed intravenous (IV) arginine butyrate regime was created for hemoglobinopathies (McGovern et al., 2003). A test was conducted in a four-month open trial of IV arginine butyrate infusion for one patient with juvenile cALD, with occasional days off therapy. Well-tolerated, the therapy immediately reduced plasma VLCFA levels in humans. However, in this individual, neurological impairment worsened during therapy, presumably due to CNS inflammation at the start of the experiment. Further clinical research is needed to evaluate dose and interval and determine if early therapy can prevent brain deterioration.

3.5.5 VALPROIC ACID

Valproic acid (VPA), a class 1-selective HDAC inhibitor, is widely used in epilepsy therapy due to its anticonvulsant properties. It crosses the blood–brain barrier and is well tolerated. ABCD-2 is one of numerous cholesterol and fatty acid metabolism genes. ABCD-2 was highly up-regulated by VPA in primary cultures of rat cortical neurons, which may be relevant to neurodegeneration (Fukuchi et al., 2009).

Recently, Pujol and coworkers evaluated the neuroprotective potential of VPA in X-ALD, focusing on AMN. They found that VPA inhibits HDAC and increases ABCD-2 expression in human X-ALD fibroblasts, decreasing oxidative damage to proteins (Fourcade et al., 2010). Thus, it was expected that VPA would lower VLCFA levels. While VPA increased ABCD-2 expression in rat and mouse hippocampus slices, as well as human cortical slices, it did not alleviate saturated VLCFA build-up in ABCD-1 or ABCD-1/ABCD-2 double-deficient slice cultures (Fourcade et al., 2010).

3.5.6 ANTIOXIDANT STRATEGIES

Postmortem brain tissues from cALD patients show oxidative damage in X-ALD. In astrocytes and microglia from the damaged white matter, iNOS and nitrotyrosine levels rise, indicating oxidative damage (Moser et al., 2005). X-ALD patients' plasma thiobarbituric acid test suggests oxidative damage may be a broader process and a potential disease biomarker. Current research shows that hexacosanoic acid build-up causes excessive free radical generation and impaired antioxidant defense response to oxidative assaults (Vargas et al., 2004; Fourcade et al., 2008).

Although epidemiological evidence is intriguing, antioxidant treatments have been applied to several NDDs with limited success. Pitfalls include the endogenous antioxidant levels in the treated patients, which were not controlled. This is significant because individuals may react differently to antioxidants, depending on their baseline levels. Both the antioxidant effects of the medicine in living organisms and the patient's compliance with the treatment were not monitored. The exact nature of the causal relationship between oxidative stress and illness has not been determined. Experiments were carried out on individuals with significant diseases, meaning preventative actions could have been too late to be effective. Antioxidants tend to reduce oxidative damage and slow disease development better in rodent models than in humans (Moser et al., 2007).

Studies on X-ALD physio-pathogenesis in mice support preclinical investigations exploring oxidative damage reduction (Fourcade et al., 2010). Moreover, susceptible and quantitative indicators of oxidative damage, initially found in the murine model and subsequently confirmed in the lymphoblasts of X-ALD patients, were used to faithfully monitor the positive effects of antioxidants. VPA has been found to have antioxidant effects in X-ALD patients, suggesting that it may assist them by combining HDAC inhibitory characteristics with antioxidant activities (Fourcade et al., 2010).

A new antioxidant combination reduces ROS generation *in vitro* and normalizes oxidative damage to proteins *in vivo* in X-ALD mice's spinal cords (López-Erauskin et al., 2011). It will be determined by the work being done whether or not this correction coincides with the prevention or arrest of neurodegeneration in this rodent model. Preclinical research with antioxidants would prove the function of oxidative stress in X-ALD development as a contributor rather than a cause. Before patients can be given a rational strategy with a good chance of success, much experimental data is needed on the intracellular sources of ROS, the organelles and enzymes involved, and the cell types that generate and maintain ROS in the X-ALD rodent model. It is pretty likely that this therapy approach will only be practical for individuals with AMN and, at best, for those who are in the very early stages of myelin sheath degeneration (Berger et al., 2010).

3.6 ONGOING CLINICAL TRIALS

More agents that help treat ALD need to be explored. Therefore, Table 3.1 contains all the information on ongoing clinical trials on ALD to explore their effects.

TABLE 3.1 Ongoing Clinical Trials

Sr. No.	The Official Title of the Study	Drug/Treatment/ Intervention	NCT Number
1	National registry study: ALD	Biospecimen sample collection	NCT03789721
2	Registry of X-linked ALD		NCT05939232
3	SMART-ALD: A new lifestyle intervention to improve quality of life in women with X-ALD	SMART-ALD (behavioral)	NCT04687007
4	Validation of a prognostic biomarker using brain diffusion MRI in X-ALD (CALDIFF)	Brain-quant module of brain-tale care platform (device)	NCT05911919
5	Gene therapy (Lentiviral) for ALD	Intracerebral LV gene therapy	NCT03727555
6	A phase-3 trial of Lorenzo's oil in ALD	Lorenzo oil	NCT00545597
7	A pilot study of vitamin D in boys with X-linked ALD	Vitamin D3	NCT02595489
8	MT2022-01: MSCs for ALD	Mesenchymal stem cells (IV-MSC)	NCT06030648
9	A study to assess the pharmacodynamics of VK0214 in male patients	VK0214	NCT04973657

3.7 CONCLUSION AND FUTURE PERSPECTIVES

Over 100 years of study on pathological, biochemical, clinical, and genetic aspects of X-ALD, theories to explain molecular pathways responsible for symptoms have changed several times. Despite this, the primary patient's need for effective and all-available treatment has not yet been satisfied. The epigenetic landscape in ALD involves alterations in DNA methylation patterns, histone modifications, and the dysregulation of noncoding RNAs. These epigenetic modifications contribute to the aberrant expression of genes associated with peroxisomal function and VLCFA metabolism, critical factors in the progression of ALD. Therefore, current research should concentrate on identifying the natural substrate for ALD and gaining a deeper understanding of the molecular pathways responsible for brain inflammation and axonal degeneration. This will allow for the development of these urgently needed innovative, effective therapies.

Furthermore, identifying specific epigenetic modifiers and exploring their roles in ALD have opened new avenues for understanding the molecular underpinnings of the disease. Targeting these epigenetic markers emerges as a promising therapeutic strategy, offering potential interventions to modulate gene expression and ameliorate the devastating effects of ALD.

KEYWORDS

- **adrenoleukodystrophy**
- **epigenetics**
- **demyelination**
- **ABC transporter**
- **oxidative stress**

REFERENCES

Aubourg, P. (2007). Adrénoleucodystrophie liée à l'X [X-linked adrenoleukodystrophy]. Annales D Endocrinologie, 68(6), 403–411. https://doi.org/10.1016/j.ando.2007.04.002.

Baarine, M., Andréoletti, P., Athias, A., Nury, T., Zarrouk, A., Ragot, K., Vejux, A., Riedinger, J.M., Kattan, Z., Bessede, G., Trompier, D., Savary, S., Cherkaoui-Malki, M., Lizard, G. (2012). Evidence of oxidative stress in very long chain fatty acid--treated oligodendrocytes and potentialization of ROS production using RNA interference-directed knockdown of ABCD1 and ACOX1 peroxisomal proteins. Neuroscience, 213, 1–18. https://doi.org/10.1016/j.neuroscience.2012.03.058.

Berger, J., Gärtner, J. (2006). X-linked adrenoleukodystrophy: Clinical, biochemical and pathogenetic aspects. Biochimica Et Biophysica Acta, 1763(12), 1721–1732. https://doi.org/10.1016/j.bbamcr.2006.07.010.

Berger, J., Molzer, B., Faé, I., Bernheimer, H. (1994). X-linked adrenoleukodystrophy (ALD): A novel mutation of the ALD gene in 6 members of a family presenting with 5 different phenotypes. Biochemical and Biophysical Research Communications, 205(3), 1638–1643. https://doi.org/10.1006/bbrc.1994.2855. PMID: 7811247.

Berger, J., Pujol, A., Aubourg, P., Forss-Petter, S. (2010). Current and future pharmacological treatment strategies in X-linked adrenoleukodystrophy. Brain Pathology, 20(4), 845–856. https://doi.org/10.1111/j.1750-3639.2010.00393.x.

Bezman, L., Moser, A.B., Raymond, G.V., Rinaldo, P., Watkins, P.A., Smith, K.D., Kass, N.E., Moser, H.W. (2001). Adrenoleukodystrophy: Incidence, new mutation rate, and results of extended family screening. Annals of Neurology, 49(4), 512–517. https://doi.org/10.1002/ana.101

Deon, M., Marchetti, D.P., Donida, B., Wajner, M., Vargas, C. (2016). Oxidative stress in patients with X-Linked adrenoleukodystrophy. Cellular and Molecular Neurobiology, 36(4), 497–512. https://doi.org/10.1007/s10571-015-0234-2.

Fourcade, S., López-Erauskin, J., Galino, J., Duval, C., Naudi, A., Jove, M., Kemp, S., Villarroya, F., Ferrer, I., Pamplona, R., Portero-Otin, M., Pujol, A. (2008). Early oxidative damage underlying neurodegeneration in X-adrenoleukodystrophy. Human Molecular Genetics, 17(12), 1762–1773. https://doi.org/10.1093/hmg/ddn085.

Fourcade, S., Ruiz, M., Guilera, C., Hahnen, E., Brichta, L., Naudi, A., Portero-Otín, M., Dacremont, G., Cartier, N., Wanders, R., Kemp, S., Mandel, J.L., Wirth, B., Pamplona, R., Aubourg, P., Pujol, A. (2010). Valproic acid induces antioxidant effects in X-linked adrenoleukodystrophy. Human Molecular Genetics, 19(10), 2005–2014. https://doi.org/10.1093/hmg/ddq082.

Fransen, M., Nordgren, M., Wang, B., Apanasets, O. (2012). Role of peroxisomes in ROS/RNS-metabolism: Implications for human disease. Biochimica Et Biophysica Acta, 1822(9), 1363–1373. https://doi.org/10.1016/j.bbadis.2011.12.001.

Fukuchi, M., Nii, T., Ishimaru, N., Minamino, A., Hara, D., Takasaki, I., Tabuchi, A., Tsuda, M. (2009). Valproic acid induces up- or down-regulation of gene expression responsible for the neuronal excitation and inhibition in rat cortical neurons through its epigenetic actions. Neuroscience Research, 65(1), 35–43. https://doi.org/10.1016/j.neures.2009.05.002.

Guimarães, C.P., Lemos, M., Menezes, I., Coelho, T., Sá-Miranda, C., Azevedo, J.E. (2001). Characterisation of two mutations in the ABCD1 gene leading to low levels of normal ALDP. Human Genetics, 109(6), 616–622. https://doi.org/10.1007/s00439-001-0632-z.

Ho, J.K., Moser, H., Kishimoto, Y., Hamilton, J.A. (1995). Interactions of a very long chain fatty acid with model membranes and serum albumin. Implications for the pathogenesis of adrenoleukodystrophy. Journal of Clinical Investigation, 96(3), 1455–1463. https://doi.org/10.1172/JCI118182.

Islam, M.T. (2017). Oxidative stress and mitochondrial dysfunction-linked neurodegenerative disorders. Neurological Research, 39(1), 73–82. https://doi.org/10.1080/01616412.2016.1251711.

Kemp, S., Huffnagel, I.C., Linthorst, G.E., Wanders, R.J., Engelen, M. (2016). Adrenoleukodystrophy - neuroendocrine pathogenesis and redefinition of natural history. Nature Reviews Endocrinology, 12(10), 606–615. https://doi.org/10.1038/nrendo.2016.90.

Kemp, S., Pujol, A., Waterham, H.R., van Geel, B.M., Boehm, C.D., Raymond, G.V., Cutting, G.R., Wanders, R.J., Moser, H.W. (2001). ABCD1 mutations and the X-linked adrenoleukodystrophy mutation database: Role in diagnosis and clinical correlations. Human Mutation, 18(6), 499–515. https://doi.org/10.1002/humu.1227. PMID: 11748843.

Kemp, S., Valianpour, F., Denis, S., Ofman, R., Sanders, R.J., Mooyer, P., Barth, P.G., Wanders, R.J. (2005). Elongation of very long-chain fatty acids is enhanced in X-linked adrenoleukodystrophy. Molecular Genetics and Metabolism, 84(2), 144–151. https://doi.org/10.1016/j.ymgme.2004.09.015. Erratum in: Mol Genet Metab. (2008). 93(3), 350. PMID: 15670720.

Kemp, S., Wanders, R. (2010). Biochemical aspects of X-linked adrenoleukodystrophy. Brain Pathology, 20(4), 831–837. https://doi.org/10.1111/j.1750-3639.2010.00391.x.

Khan, H., Garg, N., Singh, T.G., Kaur, A., Thapa, K. (2022). Calpain inhibitors as potential therapeutic modulators in neurodegenerative diseases. Neurochemical Research, 47(5), 1125–1149. https://doi.org/10.1007/s11064-021-03521-9.

López-Erauskin, J., Fourcade, S., Galino, J., Ruiz, M., Schlüter, A., Naudi, A., Jove, M., Portero-Otin, M., Pamplona, R., Ferrer, I., Pujol, A. (2011). Antioxidants halt axonal degeneration in a mouse model of X-adrenoleukodystrophy. Annals of Neurology, 70(1), 84–92. https://doi.org/10.1002/ana.22363.

López-Erauskin, J., Galino, J., Ruiz, M., Cuezva, J.M., Fabregat, I., Cacabelos, D., Boada, J., Martínez, J., Ferrer, I., Pamplona, R., Villarroya, F., Portero-Otín, M., Fourcade, S., Pujol, A. (2013). Impaired mitochondrial oxidative phosphorylation in the peroxisomal disease X-linked adrenoleukodystrophy. Human Molecular Genetics, 22(16), 3296–3305. https://doi.org/10.1093/hmg/ddt186.

Mahmood, A., Dubey, P., Moser, H.W., Moser, A. (2005). X-linked adrenoleukodystrophy: Therapeutic approaches to distinct phenotypes. Pediatric Transplantation, 9(Suppl 7), 55–62. https://doi.org/10.1111/j.1399-3046.2005.00447.x.

McGovern, M.M., Wasserstein, M.P., Aron, A., Perrine, S.P. (2003). Biochemical effect of intravenous arginine butyrate in X-linked adrenoleukodystrophy. Journal of Pediatrics, 142(6), 709–713. https://doi.org/10.1067/mpd.2003.201. PMID: 12838202.

McGuinness, M.C., Zhang, H.P., Smith, K.D. (2001). Evaluation of pharmacological induction of fatty acid beta-oxidation in X-linked adrenoleukodystrophy. Molecular Genetics and Metabolism, 74(1–2), 256–263. https://doi.org/10.1006/mgme.2001.3239. PMID: 11592822.

Moser, H.W., Mahmood, A., Raymond, G.V. (2007). X-linked adrenoleukodystrophy. Nature Reviews Neurology, 3(3), 140–151. https://doi.org/10.1038/ncpneuro0421.

Moser, H.W., Raymond, G.V., Dubey, P. (2005). Adrenoleukodystrophy: New approaches to a neurodegenerative disease. JAMA, 294(24), 3131–3134. https://doi.org/10.1001/jama.294.24.3131. PMID: 16380594.

Pai, G.S., Khan, M., Barbosa, E., Key, L.L., Craver, J.R., Curé, J.K., Betros, R., Singh, I. (2000). Lovastatin therapy for X-linked adrenoleukodystrophy: Clinical and biochemical observations on 12 patients. Molecular Genetics and Metabolism, 69(4), 312–322. https://doi.org/10.1006/mgme.2000.2977. PMID: 10870849.

Panchal, K., Tiwari, A.K. (2019). Mitochondrial dynamics, a key executioner in neurodegenerative diseases. Mitochondrion, 47, 151–173. https://doi.org/10.1016/j.mito.2018.11.002.

Rehni, A.K., Singh, T.G., Kalra, R., Singh, N. (2009). Pharmacological inhibition of inducible nitric oxide synthase attenuates the development of seizures in mice. Nitric Oxide, 21(2), 120–125. https://doi.org/10.1016/j.niox.2009.06.001.

Rehni, A.K., Singh, T.G. (2010). Levamisole-induced reduction in seizure threshold: A possible role of nicotinic acetylcholine receptor-mediated pathway. Naunyn-Schmiedebergs Archives of Pharmacology, 382(3), 279–285. https://doi.org/10.1007/s00210-010-0543-4.

Rotariu, D., Babes, E.E., Tit, D.M., Moisi, M., Bustea, C., Stoicescu, M., Radu, A.F., Vesa, C.M., Behl, T., Bungau, A.F., Bungau, S.G. (2022). Oxidative stress - Complex pathological issues concerning the hallmark of cardiovascular and metabolic disorders. Biomedicine & Pharmacotherapy, 152, 113238. https://doi.org/10.1016/j.biopha.2022.113238.

Schlüter, A., Espinosa, L., Fourcade, S., Galino, J., López, E., Ilieva, E., Morató, L., Asheuer, M., Cook, T., McLaren, A., Reid, J., Kelly, F., Bates, S., Aubourg, P., Galea, E., Pujol, A. (2012). Functional genomic analysis unravels a metabolic-inflammatory interplay in adrenoleukodystrophy. Human Molecular Genetics, 21(5), 1062–1077. https://doi.org/10.1093/hmg/ddr536.

Schlüter, A., Sandoval, J., Fourcade, S., Díaz-Lagares, A., Ruiz, M., Casaccia, P., Esteller, M., Pujol, A. (2018). Epigenomic signature of adrenoleukodystrophy predicts compromised oligodendrocyte differentiation. Brain Pathology, 28(6), 902–919. https://doi.org/10.1111/bpa.12595.

Shah, N., Singh, I. (2017). MicroRNA profiling identifies miR-196a as differentially expressed in childhood Adrenoleukodystrophy and adult adrenomyeloneuropathy. Molecular Neurobiology, 54(2), 1392–1403. https://doi.org/10.1007/s12035-016-9746-0.

Sharma, V., Kaur, A., Singh, T.G. (2020). Counteracting role of nuclear factor erythroid 2-related factor 2 pathway in Alzheimer's disease. Biomedicine & Pharmacotherapy, 129, 110373. https://doi.org/10.1016/j.biopha.2020.110373.

Sharma, V., Singh, T.G., Kaur, A., Mannan, A., Dhiman, S. (2023). Brain-derived neurotrophic factor: A novel dynamically regulated therapeutic modulator in neurological disorders. Neurochemical Research, 48(2), 317–339. https://doi.org/10.1007/s11064-022-03755-1.

Singh, S., Singh, T.G., Rehni, A.K. (2020). An insight into molecular mechanisms and novel therapeutic approaches in epileptogenesis. CNS Neurol Disord Drug Targets, 19(10), 750–779. https://doi.org/10.2174/1871527319666200910153827. PMID: 32914725.

Singh, S., Singh, T.G., Singh, M., Najda, A., Nurzyńska-Wierdak, R., Almeer, R., Kamel, M., Abdel-Daim, M.M. (2021). Anticonvulsive effects of chondroitin sulfate on pilocarpine and pentylenetetrazole induced epileptogenesis in mice. Molecules (Basel, Switzerland). 26(22), 6773. https://doi.org/10.3390/molecules26226773.

Singh, S., Singh, T.G. (2021). Emerging perspectives on mitochondrial dysfunctioning and inflammation in epileptogenesis. Inflammation Research, 70(10–12), 1027–1042. https://doi.org/10.1007/s00011-021-01511-9.

Thapa, K., Shivam, K., Khan, H., Kaur, A., Dua, K., Singh, S., Singh, T.G. (2023). Emerging targets for modulation of immune response and inflammation in stroke. Neurochemical Research, 48(6), 1663–1690. https://doi.org/10.1007/s11064-023-03875-2.

van Roermund, C.W., Visser, W.F., Ijlst, L., van Cruchten, A., Boek, M., Kulik, W., Waterham, H.R., Wanders, R.J. (2008). The human peroxisomal ABC half transporter ALDP functions as a homodimer and accepts acyl-CoA esters. FASEB Journal, 22(12), 4201–4208. https://doi.org/10.1096/fj.08-110866.

van Roermund, C.W., Visser, W.F., Ijlst, L., Waterham, H.R., Wanders, R.J. (2011). Differential substrate specificities of human ABCD1 and ABCD2 in peroxisomal fatty acid β-oxidation. Biochimica Et Biophysica Acta, 1811(3), 148–152. https://doi.org/10.1016/j.bbalip.2010.11.010.

Vargas, C.R., Wajner, M., Sirtori, L.R., Goulart, L., Chiochetta, M., Coelho, D., Latini, A., Llesuy, S., Bello-Klein, A., Giugliani, R., Deon, M., Mello, C.F. (2004). Evidence that oxidative stress is increased in patients with X-linked adrenoleukodystrophy. Biochimica Et Biophysica Acta, 1688(1), 26–32. https://doi.org/10.1016/j.bbadis.2003.10.004. PMID: 14732478.

Vishwakarma, S., Singh, S., Singh, T.G. (2022). Pharmacological modulation of cytokines correlating neuroinflammatory cascades in epileptogenesis. Molecular Biology Reports, 49(2), 1437–1452. https://doi.org/10.1007/s11033-021-06896-8.

Weinhofer, I., Forss-Petter, S., Kunze, M., Zigman, M., Berger, J. (2005). X-linked adrenoleukodystrophy mice demonstrate abnormalities in cholesterol metabolism. FEBS Letters, 579(25), 5512–5516. https://doi.org/10.1016/j.febslet.2005.09.014.

Weinhofer, I., Forss-Petter, S., Zigman, M., Berger, J. (2002). Cholesterol regulates ABCD2 expression: Implications for the therapy of X-linked adrenoleukodystrophy. Human Molecular Genetics, 11(22), 2701–2708. https://doi.org/10.1093/hmg/11.22.2701. PMID: 12374760.

Whitcomb, R.W., Linehan, W.M., Knazek, R. (1988). Effects of long-chain, saturated fatty acids on membrane microviscosity and adrenocorticotropin responsiveness of human adrenocortical cells in vitro. The Journal of Clinical Investigation, 81(1), 185–188. https://doi.org/10.1172%2FJCI113292

Wiesinger, C., Kunze, M., Regelsberger, G., Forss-Petter, S., Berger, J. (2013). Impaired very long-chain acyl-CoA β-oxidation in human X-linked adrenoleukodystrophy fibroblasts is a direct consequence of ABCD1 transporter dysfunction. Journal of Biological Chemistry, 288(26), 19269–19279. https://doi.org/10.1074/jbc.M112.445445.

CHAPTER 4

Drug Targeting: The Pituitary Gland

PRACHI MALL[1], DEEPIKA RAINA[1*], and GABRIELE DE RUBIS[2,3]

[1]*School of Pharmacy, Graphic Era Hill University, Dehradun, Uttarakhand, India*

[2]*Discipline of Pharmacy, Graduate School of Health, University of Technology Sydney, Sydney, NSW, Australia*

[3]*Faculty of Health, Australian Research Centre in Complementary and Integrative Medicine, University of Technology Sydney, Ultimo, NSW, Australia*

*Corresponding author

ABSTRACT

The pituitary gland plays a pivotal role in the endocrine system, regulating numerous hormones in essential physiological functions. These hormones are responsible for growth and development, reproduction, stress management, and so on. Dysfunction of the pituitary can lead to endocrine disorders and hormonal imbalances, requiring early diagnosis, management, and correct treatment. Drug targeting offers precise treatments for various pituitary disorders, commonly including adenomas, prolactinoma, and Cushing disease. Drug targeting provides the advantage of improved quality of life, fewer side effects, tailored medication, decreased toxicity, accuracy in hormone management, potential avoidance of surgery, and increased efficacy. Combination therapies are also becoming more popular. In the future, medicinal treatment alone for pituitary adenomas—especially macroadenomas—instead of surgery and radiation therapy may be possible due to an increasing understanding

Pharmacotherapy Approaches Toward Endocrine and Metabolic Diseases.
Thakur Gurjeet Singh and Sanjana Mehta (Eds.)

DOI: 10.1201/9781779640154-4

of all the processes governing pituitary secretion regulation and cellular growth. Furthermore, the treatment choice for pituitary tumors should be made individually, including the patient's quality of life, biochemical control, and tumor shrinking.

4.1 INTRODUCTION

The pituitary gland is also commonly called the master gland of the endocrine system. It plays a vital role in regulating and controlling different physiological functions through the secretion of hormones (Bangar et al., 2024). The primary functions of the pituitary gland in the endocrine system include the production of many hormones, regulation of other endocrine glands, growth and development, stress response, reproductive functions, and other critical functions . Dysfunction of the pituitary gland can lead to various endocrine disorders and hormonal imbalances. Therefore, early diagnosis, management, and correct treatment approach to these conditions are critical for overall health (Behera et al., 2023). The pituitary gland comprises three regions: anterior lobe (adenohypophysis), posterior lobe (neurohypophysis), and intermediate lobe. Most hormones are secreted from the anterior lobe. The hormones of the hypothalamus regulate the secretions of the pituitary gland. Disorders of the pituitary gland can significantly impact a person's health and lifestyle. Pituitary tumors can squeeze significant brain regions as they grow because of the pituitary gland's advantageous placement within the skull (Singh et al., 2022). The most frequent scenario is compression of the optic nerves, which results in a progressive loss of eyesight. Peripheral vision on both sides frequently deteriorates first in cases of this vision loss (Oki, 2014). Drug targeting in pituitary disorders has the potential to provide more precise and effective treatments for diseased conditions (Melmed, 2008).

4.1.1 DISEASES AND DISORDERS OF PITUITARY GLAND

Table 4.1 discusses the different diseases and disorders related to the pituitary gland and their conditions and effects.

TABLE 4.1 Diseases and Disorders of Pituitary Gland

Disease and Disorders	Condition	Effect
Pituitary adenoma	Tumors of the anterior pituitary	Impaired vision
Prolactinoma	Noncancerous tumor of the pituitary gland causes excess prolactin release	Decreased levels of sex hormones
Cushing disease	Excess growth or tumor of the pituitary gland	High blood pressure or bone loss, rarely type 2 diabetes
GH secreting adenoma	Tumors, secreting growth hormone	Acromegaly or gigantism in children
Stalk compression syndrome	Compression or distortion of the pituitary stalk	Chronic increase in cerebrospinal fluid vasopressin, oxytocin
Pituitary apoplexy	Hemorrhage, bleeding, or blockage in blood flow of the pituitary gland	Severe headache, vomiting, visual defect, and endocrine dysfunction
Sheehan syndrome	It damages the anterior pituitary gland due to significant blood loss, especially during childbirth	Insufficient hormone releases due to the death of some tissues of the pituitary gland
Lymphocytic hypophysitis	The autoimmune condition causes the pituitary gland to be infiltrated by lymphocytes	Hypopituitarism
Empty sella syndrome	The pituitary gland shrinks or flattens	Weight gain due to insufficient thyroid-stimulating hormone
Syndrome of inappropriate antidiuretic hormone (SIADH)	Condition in which the body retains water instead of excreting it generally in urine	Hyponatremia, low blood sodium levels
Craniopharyngiomas	A tumor that generally occurs above the pituitary gland grows by cell division and fluid accumulation	Compression of the average pituitary tissue results in pituitary deficiencies, especially anterior pituitary hormones
Rathke's cleft cyst	Tumors that develop due to fluid accumulation between the parts of the pituitary gland	Changes in vision

4.1.2 ROLE OF DRUG TARGETING

In one way or another, the pituitary gland tumors disturb the gland's secretions. Thus, there is a need to target the drugs to the gland and provide a sustainable treatment approach. Drug targeting offers several critical advantages in managing pituitary gland disorders:

- Enhanced efficacy
- Minimized side effects
- Improved patient compliance
- Personalized medicine
- Reduced toxicity
- Precision in hormone regulation
- Treatment for inoperable tumor
- Potentially avoiding surgery
- Improved quality of life
- Research and innovation (Tang et al., 2021)

Transsphenoidal surgery is the first-line therapy for pituitary adenomas with more advanced intraoperative visualization techniques such as neuronavigation, intraoperative magnetic resonance imagings, intraoperative computed tomography scans, and endoscopy. The new medical therapy approaches focus on targeting the tumors locally at the molecular level. Dopamine agonists (DAs) such as Cabergoline and Bromocriptine, somatostatin analogues, and adrenostatic drugs are the first-line chemotherapy treatment for prolactinomas and a potential alternative for growth hormone (GH)-secreting pituitary adenomas (Lu et al., 2019; Voellger et al., 2021).

4.2 THERAPEUTIC APPROACHES

4.2.1 PITUITARY ADENOMA

Pituitary adenomas are noncancerous tumors or growths of the pituitary gland that can interfere with the secretions and affect normal pituitary function. These tumors are categorized as macroadenomas ($\geq$10 mm) and microadenomas (<10 mm). Additionally, pituitary adenomas can also be classified as secreting or nonsecreting (nonfunctioning); hypersecretory adenomas cause a range of clinical manifestations. Hypersecretory pituitary adenomas cause acromegaly/gigantism in GH-secreting patients,

Cushing disease (CD) in adrenocorticotropic hormone (ACTH)-secreting patients, and Forbes–Albright syndrome in prolactin (PRL)-secreting patients. Further unusual diseases may occur when thyroid-stimulating hormone or follicle-stimulating hormone/luteinizing hormone-secreting adenomas are present. Nonfunctioning adenomas do not cause typical clinical signs and symptoms, but they can cause mass-effect symptoms like visual defects due to optic nerve compression and partial or total hypopituitarism (Solari et al., 2019). Macroadenomas can cause vision issues, hypopituitarism, headaches, and so on. The first-line therapy for pituitary adenomas is transsphenoidal pituitary surgery (Tritos and Miller, 2023). Somatostatin receptor ligands and DAs are well-established for treating pituitary adenomas. In the future, medicinal treatment alone for pituitary adenomas, especially macroadenomas instead of surgery and radiation therapy may be possible due to an increasing understanding of all the processes governing both pituitary secretion regulation and cellular growth (Gheorghiu et al., 2020; Ilie et al., 2023).

4.2.2 CUSHING DISEASE

CD is a rare endocrine disorder caused by a corticotroph tumor of the pituitary gland. It results in hypercortisolism and enhanced secretion of ACTH. The exact mechanisms at the molecular level of the disease are not known. The primary treatment of CD is adenoma resection, which has varying success rates (Molitch, 2017). However, some patients are not candidates for surgery due to clinical characteristics, such as severe comorbidities, tumor characteristics, such as large size or challenging environment, or decline or wish for a different surgery for personal purposes (Pivonello et al., 2015). The medical therapies include pituitary-directed, adrenal-directed, and glucocorticoid receptor (GR)-directed drugs (Störmann and Schopohl, 2018). Earlier, cabergoline was the only medication approved to treat CD that goes straight after the illness (Pivonello et al., 2020). With a better understanding of the disease, new and viable alternatives, that is, targeting the GR, somatostatin analogue, DAs, and pasireotide, are introduced (Bhargava et al., 2022). However, understanding the disease at its molecular level is necessary to target the drug. With the identification of the connection between GRs and transcriptional regulators like HSP90 and TR4, discoveries on the molecular mechanism causing partial glucocorticoid resistance in CD have been made. Inhibitors of HSP90 (Silibinin) and molecules connected to the TR4 signaling pathway are potentially promising and effective novel treatments for CD (Mannan et al., 2022). Based on the safety profile and potential chemotherapeutic action, silibinin is a viable medication for CD management (Ciato and Albani, 2020). The combined therapy of somatostatin analogue and DAs proved more efficacious. Table 4.2 discusses the different test compounds used to treat CD, their route of administration, target, molecular mechanism, therapeutic effect, and available formulations.

Phase III clinical trials have developed new drug moieties that inhibit adrenal steroidogenesis in treating CD (Theodoropoulou and Reincke, 2019).

Recent research has also drawn attention to vitamin A (retinoic acid) and thiazolidinediones, which reduce ACTH and corticosterone levels and tumor size. Osilodrostat and levoketoconazole, two novel steroidogenesis inhibitors, have demonstrated encouraging outcomes in recently concluded clinical trials. Similarly, levoketoconazole is hypothesized to show higher potency and lower hepatotoxicity (Theodoropoulou and Reincke, 2019).

Combination therapy may be a valuable substitute for patients who do not respond to a single medication. It is essential to understand that each patient's medical care should be customized based on their unique characteristics, such as hypercortisolism severity, acute hypercortisolism consequences, diabetes mellitus, and so on, and the characteristics of the medications used. Subsequent research endeavors should delve deeper into the ideal dosage and mix of accessible medications concerning their enduring effectiveness and safety (Simões Corrêa Galendiet al., 2021). Comorbidity should be evaluated and treated appropriately, focusing on cardiovascular risk factors. However, more extensive research is required to evaluate the safety and effectiveness of polypharmacotherapy for treating CD, particularly for novel combinations (Vilar et al., 2015). Cancer immunotherapy is an emerging therapeutic approach for refractory pituitary adenomas and pituitary carcinomas (Dai et al., 2020).

4.2.3 PROLACTINOMA

Prolactinomas are pituitary adenomas that release PRL and are usually benign but can be clinically significant. Prolactinoma is the most prevalent

TABLE 4.2 Drug Compounds Used in Cushing Disease

Test Compound	Route of Administration	Target	Molecular Mechanism	Therapeutic Effect	Formulation
Pasireotide	Subcutaneous, intramuscular	Corticotroph pituitary tumor	Somatostatin receptor	ACTH secretion inhibited	Subcutaneous injection (immediate-release ampoules, containing 300, 600, and 900 μg doses), pasireotide LAR (10, 20, 30, and 40 mg doses) intramuscularly
Cabergoline (DA)	Oral	Corticotroph pituitary tumor	Dopamine receptor agonist	Reduces ACTH secretion	Immediate-release tablet, 0.5 mg dose
Roscovitine	Oral (under investigation)	Inhibit cyclin-dependent kinases (CDKs) through direct competition at the ATP-binding site	CDKs inhibitor	ACTH secretion inhibited	Not available
Ketoconazole	Under clinical trial	Inhibit 17,20-lyase, 11β-hydroxylase, and 17β-hydroxylase	Steroidogenesis inhibitor	Decreased cortisol production	Immediate release tablet, 200 mg dose, max. 1200 mg/day
Levoketoconazole	Oral	Inhibit 11β-hydroxylase, 17α-hydroxylase, and aldosterone synthase	Steroidogenesis inhibitor	Decreased cortisol production	Immediate-release tablet 150 mg
Silibinin	Under investigation	HSP90 (molecular chaperone)	Enhanced release of mature GR when the protein's C-terminal domain is inhibited	ACTH secretion inhibited	Not available
MEK-162	Under investigation	TR4 (transcriptional factor)	MEK phosphorylating activity inhibition	ACTH secretion inhibited	Not available

TABLE 4.2 *(Continued)*

Test Compound	Route of Administration	Target	Molecular Mechanism	Therapeutic Effect	Formulation
Metyrapone	Oral (under investigation)	Block 11β-hydroxylase	Steroidogenesis inhibitor (inhibit 11-beta-hydroxylase)	Inhibit cortisol production	Immediate release capsule, 250 mg dose
Osilodrostat	Oral	Inhibit aldosterone synthase, 11β-hydroxylase	Steroidogenesis inhibitor	Decreased cortisol production	Immediate-release tablet (1, 5, 10 mg)
Mifepristone	Oral	Act on cortisol GR binding	Glucocorticoid receptor antagonist	Peripheral effects	Immediate-release capsule (300 mg) dose
ATR-101	Under investigation	Inhibit acyl-coenzyme A: cholesterol acyltransferase 1 (ACAT1)	Steroidogenesis inhibitor	Decreased cortisol levels	Immediate-release tablets (125, 250, and 500 mg) doses

secreting pituitary adenoma observed in clinical settings. Hyperprolactinemia is the clinical feature of prolactinoma (Cozzi et al., 2023). The general classification of prolactinomas by size is microadenomas (under 10 mm) or macroadenomas (over 10 mm). More than 90% of tiny intrasellar tumors called prolactinomas seldom grow. Sometimes, these adenomas can compress the critical structures, becoming aggressive or locally encroaching. Estrogen enhances PRL secretion, while dopamine inhibits it (Casanueva et al., 2006). Therefore, DAs are considered to be the primary treatment for most prolactinomas, with surgery as a backup (Inder and Jang, 2022). DA, such as bromocriptine and cabergoline, reduces the PRL levels, reducing the tumor volume. Rarely, temozolomide can be used as an alternative for rare cases of aggressive and malignant prolactinomas (Chanson and Maiter, 2019). Radiotherapy and surgery are the only available options for treating malignant prolactinomas or people who are DA-resistant or intolerant (Castinetti et al., 2021). Table 4.3 depicts the drug molecules used for prolactinoma, its source, and target receptors.

TABLE 4.3 Depicts the Drug Molecules used for Prolactinoma

Dopamine Agonists	Source	Target Receptors
Bromocriptine (Br)	Ergot derivative	D1R and D2R
Cabergoline (Cab)	Ergot derivative	D2R
Quinagolide	Non-ergot derivative	selective D2R

Cabergoline is the preferred DA for its effectiveness, tolerability, and persistent action. Cabergoline typically starts at 0.25–0.5 mg weekly, once or twice a week after dinner or bedtime. Bromocriptine is occasionally utilized due to its frequent daily doses. Specific mild side effects of DA include nausea, fatigue, vomiting, dizziness, and headache (Zamanipoor Najafabadi et al., 2020). Temozolomide is nowadays becoming popular to be used as a therapy against aggressive prolactinomas that are resistant to cabergoline and bromocriptine (Chen et al., 2017).

4.2.4 GROWTH HORMONE SECRETING ADENOMA

Acromegaly is an essential clinical feature in growth hormone-secreting pituitary adenomas (GHPAs) patients. The insidious clinical signs of acromegaly include menstruation difficulties, coarse facial features, thicker soft tissues and lips, erectile dysfunction, hyperhidrosis, and swollen limbs (Caulley et al., 2024). Some patients with large tumor masses may experience symptoms such as visual defects, headaches, and cranial neuropathies (Lopes, 2010). GH receptor antagonists, dopamine agonists, and somatostatin analogues are the medical therapies for GHPAs. However, transsphenoidal surgery is the primary treatment, and the medical therapies are used as adjuncts to the surgery (Torres et al., 2021). Transsphenoidal surgery removes cancer from the sella using an endonasal or microscopic technique to minimize harm to adjacent tissues and pituitary function. Stereotactic radiosurgery is an alternative for tumors that do not respond to surgery and medical interventions (Donoho et al., 2017). Table 4.4 shows the different drug categories for the treatment of GH-secreting adenoma.

TABLE 4.4 The Drug Molecules Used for Growth Hormone Secreting Adenoma, Their Targets, Associated Adverse Effects, and Examples

Drug Category	Examples	Target	Adverse Effects
Somatostatin analogs	Octreotide, lanreotide, and pasireotide	Bind to somatostatin receptors 1 and 5, suspending GH hypersecretion	Abdominal cramps, flatulence, diarrhea, gall bladder stones, and alopecia
Dopamine agonists	Bromocriptine and cabergoline	Bind to D2 (dopamine) receptors suppressing GH hypersecretions	Nausea, vomiting, constipation, dizziness, headache, and postural hypotension
GH-receptor antagonists	Pegvisomant	Inhibit GH action	Elevated hepatic transaminases, as well as local inflammation and lipodystrophy

4.2.5 STALK COMPRESSION SYNDROME

Stalk compression syndrome refers to a condition in which the pituitary stalk is compressed or distorted. It is characterized by moderately elevated PRL levels and a sellar or suprasellar mass. However, alteration of the pituitary stalk does not necessarily indicate hyperprolactinemia (Simander et al., 2023). No exact PRL concentration differentiates stalk compression from actual prolactinoma, but values of 2500–5000 mU/l are commonly cited despite exceptions in the literature (Samperi et al., 2019). The focus should be considered from the perspective of imaging. Dopamine agonists, especially bromocriptine, are the treatment approach for the syndrome. Surgical resection remains the mainstay of the syndrome (Samarasinghe et al., 2014).

4.2.6 PITUITARY APOPLEXY

It is a rare but fatal life condition in which the volume of the pituitary gland increases. It usually arises after pituitary lesion hemorrhage and infarction, having an incidence among pituitary adenomas. It is often accompanied by symptoms including nausea, vomiting, headache, vision degradation, cranial nerve palsies, and loss of consciousness, usually due to pituitary hormonal support loss (Almeida et al., 2019). Pituitary apoplexy can lead to loss of vision. Most patients had decreased pituitary function and ACTH insufficiency before apoplexy, requiring glucocorticoid supplementation. The primary intervention includes corticosteroid administration and electrolyte management (Glezer and Bronstein, 2015). However, transsphenoidal surgery is indicated if consciousness and vision are impaired (Sibal et al., 2004).

4.2.7 SHEEHAN SYNDROME

It is a scarce condition of ischemic pituitary necrosis. Hypopituitarism is one of the most common causes (Laway and Baba, 2021). Vasospasm of hypothalamic portal arteries after substantial postpartum hemorrhage causes anterior pituitary gland cell loss. Small sella turcica size, coagulation problems, and antipituitary antibodies also cause ischemia damage. The main symptoms of regular and complete Sheehan syndrome are lactation failure, failure to resume menstrual cycles following puerperium, loss of axillary and pubic hair, hypocortisolism, hypothyroidism, and neuropsychiatric and cardiac abnormalities less commonly. Hormone replacement therapies are given according to the deficient hormone of the pituitary to treat the syndrome (Laway and Baba, 2023).

4.2.8 LYMPHOCYTIC AND GRANULOMATOUS HYPOPHYSITIS

Lymphocytic hypophysitis is an inflammatory autoimmune condition of the pituitary gland. T and B lymphocyte infiltration into the pituitary tissue of T and B lymphocytes typically causes inflammation (Donegan et al., 2022). Granulomatous hypophysitis is a rare inflammatory condition mimicking pituitary adenoma (Elgamal et al., 2017). Central diabetes insipidus, anterior pituitary hormone deficits, and hyperprolactinemia are endocrine signs of pituitary failure (Naran and Can, 2023). The primary treatment is hormone replacement. High-dose corticosteroid transsphenoidal therapy and surgery are the first-line treatment for sella mass effect and surrounding structure compression. Immunosuppressants work for steroid-resistant patients or those with unacceptable side effects (Kluczyński et al., 2019).

4.2.9 RATHKE'S CLEFT CYST

Rathke cleft cysts are fluid-filled growths between pituitary gland components at the brain's base, arising from embryonic remnants of Rathke's pouch (Petersson et al., 2022). In symptomatic Rathke's cleft cyst patients, transsphenoidal surgery prevents future vision loss and usually restores some vision (Marcus et al., 2020). Other symptoms include hormonal disturbances and headaches. Hormonal replacement therapy is recommended for hormonal imbalances. Surgical removal may be recommended in cases where the cyst is causing clinical symptoms or compressing nearby structures (Ozoner et al., 2019). However, it has to be noted here that after pituitary surgery, persistent hypopituitarism has been observed, which is directly linked to higher mortality due to adrenal crisis.

4.3 ROUTE OF DRUG ADMINISTRATION

Different routes of drug administration can be used to target the medications to the pituitary gland. Figure 4.1 depicts the different routes of drug administration to the pituitary gland.

Intravenous administration is frequently employed to treat specific conditions associated with the pituitary gland, particularly in critical circumstances or when prompt therapeutic outcomes are required. Intramuscular or subcutaneous administration is frequently employed for hormonal therapies requiring a slow release into the circulation. However, implantable devices are also used when sustained release of the hormonal therapy is required. The oral route of drug administration is not suitable

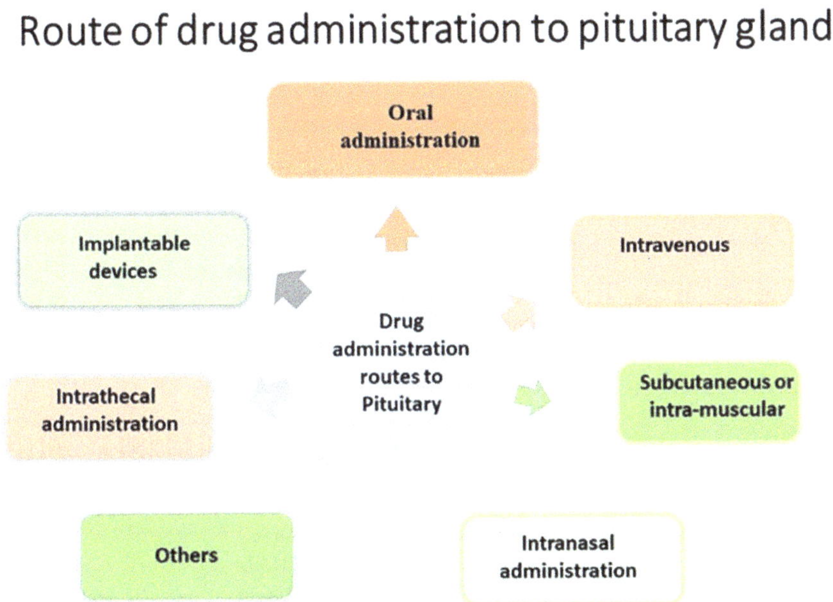

FIGURE 4.1 Routes of drug administration to the pituitary gland.

for all drug candidates due to the risk of degradation in the digestive system. The intranasal route can be very useful for drugs targeting the hypothalamus, which is closely connected to the pituitary gland (Gadhave et al., 2022). In some instances, drugs are injected directly into the cerebrospinal fluid around the brain and spinal cord, allowing targeted drug delivery to the central nervous system, including the hypothalamus and pituitary gland.

The choice of the route of administration depends on drug type, patient condition, desired therapeutic effect, and pharmacokinetics. Before choosing a route for pituitary-related medications, healthcare practitioners must carefully evaluate all the above aspects (Reglodi et al., 2018).

4.4 PATENTS

Table 4.5 enlists some patents related to pituitary diseases and disorders and their findings.

TABLE 4.5 List of Some Pituitary Diseases and Disorders of Patients and Their Findings

S. No.	Target Area	Findings	Reference No.
1.	Targeting pituitary tumors	Relacorilant can reduce the size of pituitary tumors, including hormone-secreting and nonsecreting ones. It can be administered before, during, or after surgery to improve surgical outcomes. Relacorilant can be administered orally to a fasted or fed patient and may be combined with other treatments like surgical, radiation, chemotherapy, and other pharmaceuticals	
2.	Targeting cancer and tumors	The disclosure focuses on methods and compositions for inhibiting or protecting against diseases arising from constitutively active G protein, specifically FR900359, YM-254890, which can be used in treating various cancers, including growth hormone-secreting pituitary tumors, uveal melanoma, and several other types of cancers	US20230130103A1. Pdf (n.d.)
3.	Targeted drug delivery	A method for targeted drug delivery has been developed, involving targeting molecules like hormones, a drug to be delivered, and a nanoparticle containing the drug and the targeting molecule. These compositions can be administered via injections, topically, orally, nasally, vaginally, rectally, or ocularly and can also be administered to the pulmonary system	
4.	Targeting pituitary adenylate cyclase-activating polypeptide (PACAP) for the treatment of migraine	The disclosure relates to peptide immunogen constructs targeting PACAP, compositions containing these constructs, antibodies elicited by them, and methods for creating and using them. These constructs stimulate the generation of particular antibodies for migraine prevention and treatment	US20230146694A1. Pdf (n.d.)

4.5 CONCLUSION

Early intervention is crucial for curing or controlling pituitary tumors and their side effects. Surgery is often the first line of treatment, but it is not always feasible in all cases. Postoperative hypopituitarism is associated with higher mortality due to adrenal crisis. Medical treatments have evolved to treat pituitary disorders, with new drug molecules allowing targeted targeting. Combination therapy of drugs is encouraged when monotherapy is not adequate. If medication or surgery cannot effectively treat the tumor, radiation therapy may be considered a viable option. High-dose X-ray radiation treats tumor cells, while medicine is used to shrink or eliminate the tumor.

KEYWORDS

- **pituitary gland**
- **drug targeting**
- **adenomas**
- **Cushing disease**
- **hormone regulation**
- **transsphenoidal surgery**

REFERENCES

Almeida, J.P., Sanchez, M.M., Karekezi, C., Warsi, N., Fernández-Gajardo, R., Panwar, J., Mansouri, A., Suppiah, S., Nassiri, F., Nejad, R., Kucharczyk, W., Ridout, R., Joaquim, A.F., Gentili, F., Zadeh, G. (2019). Pituitary apoplexy: Results of surgical and conservative management clinical series and review of the literature. World Neurosurgery, 130, e988–e999. https://doi.org/10.1016/j.wneu.2019.07.055.

Bangar, A., Khan, H., Kaur, A., Dua, K., Singh, T.G. (2024). Understanding mechanistic aspect of the therapeutic role of herbal agents on neuroplasticity in cerebral ischemic-reperfusion injury. Journal of Ethnopharmacology, 319(Pt 2), 117153. https://doi.org/10.1016/j.jep.2023.117153.

Behera, R., Sharma, V., Grewal, A.K., Kumar, A., Arora, B., Najda, A., Albadrani, G.M., Altyar, A.E., Abdel-Daim, M.M., Singh, T.G. (2023). Mechanistic correlation between mitochondrial permeability transition pores and mitochondrial ATP dependent potassium channels in ischemia reperfusion. Biomedicine & Pharmacotherapy, 162, 114599. https://doi.org/10.1016/j.biopha.2023.114599.

Bhargava, S.K., Singh, T.G., Mannan, A., Singh, S., Singh, M., Gupta, S. (2022). Pharmacological evaluation of Thuja occidentalis for the attenuation of neuropathy via AGEs and TNF-α inhibition in diabetic neuropathic rats. Environmental Science and Pollution Research International, 29(40), 60542–60557. https://doi.org/10.1007/s11356-022-20106-3.

Casanueva, F.F., Molitch, M.E., Schlechte, J.A., Abs, R., Bonert, V., Bronstein, M.D., Brue, T., Cappabianca, P., Colao, A., Fahlbusch, R., Fideleff, H., Hadani, M., Kelly, P., Kleinberg, D., Laws, E., Marek, J., Scanlon, M., Sobrinho, L.G., Wass, J.A., Giustina, A. (2006). Guidelines of the pituitary society for the diagnosis and management of prolactinomas. Clinical Endocrinology, 65(2), 265–273. https://doi.org/10.1111/j.1365-2265.2006.02562.x.

Castinetti, F., Albarel, F., Amodru, V., Cuny, T., Dufour, H., Graillon, T., Morange, I., Brue, T. (2021). The risks of medical treatment of prolactinoma. Annales D Endocrinologie, 82(1), 15–19. https://doi.org/10.1016/j.ando.2020.12.008.

Caulley, L., Quinn, J.G., Doyle, M.A., Alkherayf, F., Metzendorf, M.I., Kilty, S., Hunink, M.G.M. (2024). Surgical and non-surgical interventions for primary and salvage treatment of growth hormone-secreting pituitary adenomas in adults. Cochrane Database of Systematic Reviews (Online), 2(2), CD013561. https://doi.org/10.1002/14651858.CD013561.pub2.

Chanson, P., Maiter, D. (2019). The epidemiology, diagnosis and treatment of Prolactinomas: The old and the new. Best Practice & Research. Clinical Endocrinology & Metabolism, 33(2), 101290. https://doi.org/10.1016/j.beem.2019.101290.

Chen, C., Yin, S., Zhang, S., Wang, M., Hu, Y., Zhou, P., Jiang, S. (2017). Treatment of aggressive prolactinoma with temozolomide: A case report and review of literature up to date. Medicine, 96(47), e8733. https://doi.org/10.1097/MD.0000000000008733.

Ciato, D., Albani, A. (2020). Molecular mechanisms of glucocorticoid resistance in corticotropinomas: New developments and drug targets. Frontiers in Endocrinology, 11, 21. https://doi.org/10.3389/fendo.2020.00021.

Cozzi, R., Simona Auriemma, R., De Menis, E., Esposito, F., Ferrante, E., Iatì, G., Mazzatenta, D., Poggi, M., Rudà, R., Tortora, F., Cruciani, F., Mitrova, Z., Saulle, R., Vecchi, S., Basile, M., Cappabianca, P., Paoletta, A., Papini, E., Persichetti, A., Samperi, I., Scoppola, A., Bozzao, A., Caputo, M., Doglietto, F., Ferraù, F., Lania, A.G., Laureti, S., Lello, S., Locatelli, D., Maffei, P., Minniti, G., Peri, A., Ruini, C., Settanni, F., Silvani, A., Veronese, N., Grimaldi, F., Attanasio, R. (2023). Italian guidelines for the management of prolactinomas. Endocrine, Metabolic & Immune Disorders Drug Targets, 23(12), 1459–1479. https://doi.org/10.2174/1871530323666230511104045.

Dai, C., Liang, S., Sun, B., Kang, J. (2020). The progress of immunotherapy in refractory pituitary adenomas and pituitary carcinomas. Frontiers in Endocrinology, 11, 608422. https://doi.org/10.3389/fendo.2020.608422.

Donegan, D., Saeed, Z., Delivanis, D.A., Murad, M.H., Honegger, J., Amereller, F., Oguz, S.H., Erickson, D., Bancos, I. (2022). Outcomes of initial management strategies in patients with autoimmune lymphocytic hypophysitis: A systematic review and meta-analysis. Journal of Clinical Endocrinology and Metabolism, 107(4), 1170–1190. https://doi.org/10.1210/clinem/dgab839.

Donoho, D.A., Bose, N., Zada, G., Carmichael, J.D. (2017). Management of aggressive growth hormone secreting pituitary adenomas. Pituitary, 20(1), 169–178. https://doi.org/10.1007/s11102-016-0781-7.

Elgamal, M.E., Mohamed, R.M.H., Fiad, T., Elgamal, E.A. (2017). Granulomatous hypophysitis: Rare disease with challenging diagnosis. Clinical Case Reports, 5(7), 1147–1151. https://doi.org/10.1002/ccr3.1007.

Gadhave, D., Khot, S., Tupe, S., Shinde, M., Tagalpallewar, A., Gorain, B., Kokare, C. (2022). Nose-to-brain delivery of octreotide acetate in situ gel for pituitary adenoma: Pharmacological and in vitro cytotoxicity studies. International Journal of Pharmaceutics, 629, 122372. https://doi.org/10.1016/j.ijpharm.2022.122372.

Gheorghiu, M.L., Negreanu, F., Fleseriu, M. (2020). Updates in the medical treatment of pituitary adenomas. Hormone and Metabolic Research, 52(1), 8–24. https://doi.org/10.1055/a-1066-4592.

Glezer, A., Bronstein, M.D. (2015). Pituitary apoplexy: pathophysiology, diagnosis and management. Archives of Endocrinology and Metabolism, 59(3), 259–264. https://doi.org/10.1590/2359-3997000000047.

Ilie, M.D., Vasiljevic, A., Bertolino, P., Raverot, G. (2023). Biological and therapeutic implications of the tumor microenvironment in pituitary adenomas. Endocrine Reviews, 44(2), 297–311. https://doi.org/10.1210/endrev/bnac024.

Inder, W.J., Jang, C. (2022). Treatment of prolactinoma. Medicina (Kaunas), 58(8), 1095. https://doi.org/10.3390/medicina58081095.

Kluczyński, Ł., Gilis-Januszewska, A., Rogoziński, D., Pantofliński, J., Hubalewska-Dydejczyk, A. (2019). Hypophysitis - new insights into diagnosis and treatment. Endokrynologia Polska, 70(3), 260–269. https://doi.org/10.5603/EP.a2019.0015.

Laway, B.A., Baba, M.S. (2021). Sheehan syndrome. Journal of the Pakistan Medical Association, 71(4), 1282–12568.

Laway, B.A., Baba, M.S. (2023). Sheehan syndrome: Cardiovascular and metabolic comorbidities. Frontiers in Endocrinology, 14, 1086731. https://doi.org/10.3389/fendo.2023.1086731.

Lopes, M.B. (2010). Growth hormone-secreting adenomas: Pathology and cell biology. Neurosurgical Focus [Electronic Resource], 29(4), E2. https://doi.org/10.3171/2010.7.FOCUS10169.

Lu, M., Wang, Y., Zhan, X. (2019). The MAPK pathway-based drug therapeutic targets in pituitary adenomas. Frontiers in Endocrinology, 10, 330. https://doi.org/10.3389/fendo.2019.00330.

Mannan, A., Singh, T.G., Singh, V., Garg, N., Kaur, A., Singh, M. (2022). Insights into the mechanism of the therapeutic potential of herbal monoamine oxidase inhibitors in neurological diseases. Current Drug Targets, 23(3), 286–310. https://doi.org/10.2174/1389450122666210707120256.

Marcus, H.J., Borg, A., Hussein, Z., Jaunmuktane, Z., Baldeweg, S.E., Grieve, J., Dorward, N.L. (2020). Rathke's cleft cysts following transsphenoidal surgery: Long-term outcomes and development of an optimal follow-up strategy. Acta Neurochir (Wien), 162(4), 853–861. https://doi.org/10.1007/s00701-020-04237-5.

Melmed, S. (2008). Update in pituitary disease. Journal of Clinical Endocrinology and Metabolism, 93(2), 331–338. https://doi.org/10.1210/jc.2007-1409.

Molitch, M.E. (2017). Diagnosis and treatment of pituitary adenomas: A review. JAMA, 317(5), 516–524. https://doi.org/10.1001/jama.2016.19699.

Naran, J., Can, A.S. (2023). Lymphocytic hypophysitis. In: *StatPearls*. Treasure Island (FL): StatPearls Publishing, 2024 Jan–.

Oki, Y. (2014). Medical management of functioning pituitary adenoma: An update. Neurologia Medico-Chirurgica, 54(12), 958–965. https://doi.org/10.2176/nmc.ra.2014-0239.

Ozoner, B., Aydin, S., Akgun, M.Y., Durmaz, E.S., Sahin, S., Gazioglu, N., Kizilkilic, O., Kadioglu, P., Tanriover, N. (2019). Predictive factors for Rathke's cleft cyst consistency. World Neurosurgery, 128, e522–e530. https://doi.org/10.1016/j.wneu.2019.04.188.

Petersson, M., Berinder, K., Eden Engström, B., Tsatsaris, E., Ekman, B., Wahlberg, J., Burman, P., Borg, H., Siesjö, P., Dahlqvist, P., Åkerman, A.K., Ragnarsson, O., Olsson, M., Förander, P., Bensing, S., Höybye, C. (2022). Natural history and surgical outcome of Rathke's cleft cysts-A study from the Swedish Pituitary Registry. Clinical Endocrinology, 96(1), 54–61. https://doi.org/10.1111/cen.14622.

Pivonello, R., De Leo, M., Cozzolino, A., Colao, A. (2015). The treatment of Cushing's disease. Endocrine Reviews, 36(4), 385–486. https://doi.org/10.1210/er.2013-1048.

Pivonello, R., Ferrigno, R., De Martino, M.C., Simeoli, C., Di Paola, N., Pivonello, C., Barba, L., Negri, M., De Angelis, C., Colao, A. (2020). Medical treatment of Cushing's disease: An overview of the current and recent clinical trials. Frontiers in Endocrinology, 11, 648. https://doi.org/10.3389/fendo.2020.00648.

Reglodi, D., Atlasz, T., Jungling, A., Szabo, E., Kovari, P., Manavalan, S., Tamas, A. (2018). Alternative routes of administration of the neuroprotective pituitary adenylate cyclase activating polypeptide. Current Pharmaceutical Design, 24(33), 3892–3904. https://doi.org/10.2174/1381612824666181112110934.

Samarasinghe, S., Emanuele, M.A., Mazhari, A. (2014). Neurology of the pituitary. Handbook of Clinical Neurology, 120, 685–701. https://doi.org/10.1016/B978-0-7020-4087-0.00047-4.

Samperi, I., Lithgow, K., Karavitaki, N. (2019). Hyperprolactinaemia. Journal of Clinical Medicine, 8(12), 2203. https://doi.org/10.3390/jcm8122203.

Sibal, L., Ball, S.G., Connolly, V., James, R.A., Kane, P., Kelly, W.F., Kendall-Taylor, P., Mathias, D., Perros, P., Quinton, R., Vaidya, B. (2004). Pituitary apoplexy: A review of clinical presentation, management and outcome in 45 cases. Pituitary, 7(3), 157–163. https://doi.org/10.1007/s11102-005-1050-3.

Simander, G., Dahlqvist, P., Oja, L., Eriksson, P.O., Lindvall, P., Koskinen, L.D. (2023). Intrasellar pressure is related to endocrine disturbances in patients with pituitary tumors. World Neurosurgery, 175, e344–e351. https://doi.org/10.1016/j.wneu.2023.03.085.

Simões Corrêa Galendi, J., Correa Neto, A.N.S., Demetres, M., Boguszewski, C.L., Nogueira, V. (2021). Effectiveness of medical treatment of Cushing's disease: A systematic review and meta-analysis. Frontiers in Endocrinology, 12, 732240. https://doi.org/10.3389/fendo.2021.732240.

Singh, V., Kaur, K., Kaur, S., Shri, R., Singh, T.G., Singh, M. (2022). Trimethoxyflavones from Ocimum basilicum L. leaves improve long term memory in mice by modulating multiple pathways. Journal of Ethnopharmacology, 295, 115438. https://doi.org/10.1016/j.jep.2022.115438.

Solari, D., Pivonello, R., Caggiano, C., Guadagno, E., Chiaramonte, C., Miccoli, G., Cavallo, L.M., Del Basso De Caro, M., Colao, A., Cappabianca, P. (2019). Pituitary adenomas: What are the key features? what are the current treatments? Where is the future taking us? World Neurosurg, 127, 695–709. https://doi.org/10.1016/j.wneu.2019.03.049.

Störmann, S., Schopohl, J. (2018). New and emerging drug therapies for Cushing's disease. Expert Opinion on Pharmacotherapy, 19(11), 1187–1200. https://doi.org/10.1080/14656566.2018.1504021.

Tang, T., Huang, X., Zhang, G., Hong, Z., Bai, X., Liang, T. (2021). Advantages of targeting the tumor immune microenvironment over blocking immune checkpoint in cancer immunotherapy. Signal Transduction and Targeted Therapy, 6(1), 72. https://doi.org/10.1038/s41392-020-00449-4.

Theodoropoulou, M., Reincke, M. (2019). Tumor-directed therapeutic targets in cushing disease. Journal of Clinical Endocrinology and Metabolism, 104(3), 925–933. https://doi.org/10.1210/jc.2018-02080.

Torres, A., Sanmillan, J.L., Lau, R., Gabarros, A. (2021). Final outcome in growth hormone-secreting adenomas after combination of maximal tumor resection and medical treatment. World Neurosurgery, 154, e292–e301. https://doi.org/10.1016/j.wneu.2021.07.018.

Tritos, N.A., Miller, K.K. (2023). Diagnosis and management of pituitary adenomas: A review. JAMA, 329(16), 1386–1398. https://doi.org/10.1001/jama.2023.5444.

Vilar, L., Naves, L.A., Machado, M.C., Bronstein, M.D. (2015). Medical combination therapies in Cushing's disease. Pituitary, 18(2), 253–262. https://doi.org/10.1007/s11102-015-0641-x.

Voellger, B., Zhang, Z., Benzel, J., Wang, J., Lei, T., Nimsky, C., Bartsch, J.W. (2021). Targeting aggressive pituitary adenomas at the molecular level-A review. Journal of Clinical Medicine, 11(1), 124. https://doi.org/10.3390/jcm11010124.

Zamanipoor Najafabadi, A.H., Zandbergen, I.M., de Vries, F., Broersen, L.H.A., van den Akker-van Marle, M.E., Pereira, A.M., Peul, W.C., Dekkers, O.M., van Furth, W.R., Biermasz, N.R. (2020). Surgery as a viable alternative first-line treatment for prolactinoma patients. A systematic review and meta-analysis. Journal of Clinical Endocrinology and Metabolism, 105(3), e32–41. https://doi.org/10.1210/clinem/dgz144.

CHAPTER 5

Age-Related Metabolic Skeletal Disorders: Therapeutical Approach

SANCHIT DHANKHAR[1*], HIMANSHU SHARMA[1], NITIKA GARG[1], POOJA MITTAL[1*], SAMRAT CHAUHAN[1], MONIKA SAINI[2], THAKUR GURJEET SINGH[1], SANJANA MEHTA[1], VISHNU MITTAL[3], DIVYA KANWAR[1], BHAVESH DHARMANI[1], and VENKATA SITA RAMA RAJU ALLAM[4]

[1]*Chitkara College of Pharmacy, Chitkara University, Rajpura, Punjab, India*

[2]*MM College of Pharmacy, Maharishi Markandeshwar (Deemed to be University), Mullana, Ambala, India*

[3]*Guru Gobind Singh College of Pharmacy, Yamuna Nagar, Haryana, India*

[4]*Department of Medical Biochemistry and Microbiology, Biomedical Centre (BMC), Uppsala University, Uppsala, Sweden*

*Corresponding author

ABSTRACT

Because of the continuous aging of the population, the frequency of age-related metabolic skeletal illnesses presents a severe issue for healthcare systems. This chapter delves into the intricate relationship between aging and complex metabolism, exploring its impact on skeletal muscles. Recognizing the complicated connections among these elements, a therapeutic strategy is presented here to mitigate the effects of aging on skeletal diseases associated with aging metabolism. Specialized methods that can

Pharmacotherapy Approaches Toward Endocrine and Metabolic Diseases.
Thakur Gurjeet Singh and Sanjana Mehta (Eds.)

DOI: 10.1201/9781779640154-5

stop aging's impact on metabolism and hence support the health of skeletal muscles are the main emphasis. The proposed therapeutic paradigm incorporates pharmacological, lifestyle, and nutritional considerations, emphasizing a comprehensive strategy for treating metabolic skeletal diseases associated with aging. Additionally, the treatments and advances in this field are being discussed in this chapter. The therapy strategy described tries to enhance the quality of life for the elderly population by addressing the complex character of these illnesses.

5.1 INTRODUCTION

Recently, there has been a notable increase in the prevalence of metabolic bone disorders (MBDs), primarily attributed to dietary inadequacies resulting from a significant decline in calcium, phosphorus, and vitamin D consumption (Rihal et al., 2022). As a consequence, MBDs have advanced, affecting over 200 million people globally and overtaking thyroid problems and diabetes to become the third-most prevalent illness in humans. In India alone, over half a million individuals are believed to be impacted by MBDs (Rihal et al., 2023). The spectrum of multiple bone disorders (MBDs) includes well-known conditions such as fluorosis disease, tumor-induced osteomalacia, primary hyperparathyroidism (PHPT), and osteoporosis. Older women face the highest likelihood of developing these disorders, followed by older men (Thapa et al., 2021). Unfortunately, many individuals remain unaware of the potential problems associated with MBDs and often ignore symptoms until they become apparent. Poor nutritional conditions during pregnancy have been identified as contributing to MBD development (Singh et al., 2020). MBDs in children can result in nontraumatic fractures, anomalies of the skeleton, difficulties with sequential development, and limits on motor growth and function. Early identification and treatment of lifestyle factors can significantly improve bone health. The treatment approach for MBDs is tailored to address their underlying causes (Dressler and Kaufman, n.d.).

Maintaining a healthy metabolism of bone minerals necessitates engaging in moderate physical activity, adhering to a calcium and vitamin-rich diet, and keeping an overall balanced meal plan. It is encouraging to know that particular osteoporosis medications and a healthy diet can effectively stop and even reverse the effects of bone loss (Rehni and Singh, 2011). Calcium, phosphorus, and vitamin D shortages are common in people with these illnesses; food supplements can compensate for these deficiencies. Regarding MBDs, this review sheds light on the existing situation and the progress in creating novel, potent treatments for these neurological conditions (Kant et al., 2020). Recognizing the significance, this process highlights the importance of early interventions to promote bone health and prevent the onset of MBDs (Natesan and Kim, 2022; Mehta et al., 2022). Peak bone density is typically achieved during adolescence and remains stable for approximately a decade. By 22, most adults have completed most of their skeletal growth. This emphasizes the importance of promoting and maintaining optimal bone density during the formative years to establish a foundation for long-term skeletal health (States, n.d.). Osteoporosis during menstruation leads to an annual loss of 2–3% in trabecular bone and 1–2% in cortical bone (Garg et al., 2021; Mehta et al., 2022). Previously, MBDs were perceived as unnoticed illnesses and considered a natural part of aging. The development of skeletal densitometry has provided a precise and experimental means to identify patients at high risk for osteoporosis.

This advancement has facilitated the implementation of effective treatment and prevention strategies, reducing the incidence of fractures (Nuti et al., 2019). More and more people realize how vital osteoclasts are to the body as a functioning unit. Additionally, the parathyroid glands, FGF23, and vitamin D work together to support the stability of calcium and phosphate homeostatic mechanisms (Indian Academy of Pediatrics 'Guideline for Vitamin D and Calcium in Children' Committee et al., 2017). The regular functioning of these systems is essential for three critical functions—bone creation, metabolic activity, and repair. These conditions highlight the intricate interplay between various factors in maintaining bone health Hannan (Hannan et al., 2019). This highlights the complex interplay between genetic factors and environmental influences in the development of MBDs (Farrow et al., 2024). Six inheritance patterns are associated with monogenic diseases: non-Mendelian mitochondrial abnormalities, which can also cause monogenic MBDs; autosomal recessive, autosomal dominant, X-linked recessive, and Y-linked (Alquorain, 2021).

An example of this would be a mutation in the SLC34A1 gene, which results in renal sodium phosphate cotransporters type 2a in a family with familial hypophosphataemic rickets with hypercalciuria. A second mutation in the SLC34A3 gene that results in a different orientation for the same protein results in hypercalciuria and rickets (HHRH). Another unusual variant is osteoporosis, which has an early start caused by heterozygous mutations in the Plastin 3 (PLS3) gene. These instances highlight the wide range of genetic variations that lead to metabolic bone diseases (Mäkitie and Zillikens, 2022).

5.2 COMMON SKELETAL DISORDERS ASSOCIATED WITH METABOLIC AGE

5.2.1 OSTEOPOROSIS

Osteoporosis-induced bone fractures occur approximately every 3 s, contributing to over 8.9 million fractures annually worldwide. According to the WHO, impacts of osteoporosis 21.2% of women and 6.3% of men aged 50 and above globally. Considering the total male and female populations worldwide, these statistics suggest that approximately 500 million people are affected by osteoporosis (Murray et al., 1994). In Europe, the United States, and Japan, 82 million people are affected by osteoporosis. In 2000, osteoporosis was a contributing factor in almost 9 million fractures. These included 1.6 million hip fractures, 1.7 million wrist fractures, and 1.4 million medical vertebral fractures. Five percent of all fractures are caused by the United States and Europe combined, with the remaining 50% coming from the Western Pacific and Southeast Asian nations. These figures underscore the significant impact of osteoporosis on the population in these regions (Barnsley et al., 2021). By 2050, hip fractures are expected to become more common in men and women, with a predicted increase of 31% and 24%, respectively, compared to the rates recorded in 1990. In 2010, osteoporosis posed a potential health concern for approximately 158 million individuals. However, projections suggest that this figure will more than quadruple by 2040 due to changing demographics. Unsettlingly, osteoporotic fractures are predicted to occur in three out of every five women over the age of 50, along with every five out of every 100 men. These predictions highlight the growing impact of osteoporosis and the associated risks of fractures in the coming decades (Ilic et al., 2023). Females account for 80%, 75%, 75%, and 58% of all fractures, primarily in the hip, humerus, arms, and spine. With a 1.6 to 1 female-to-male ratio, women account for 61% of all osteoporosis-related fracture cases. On the other hand, about 75% of hip, spine, and distal limb fractures occur in people 65 years of age or older. These statistics underscore the gender and age-related patterns in osteoporotic fractures, with women and older individuals being more susceptible to such fractures (Axelsson et al., 2023).

A disease known as "osteoporosis," which means "porous bone," occurs when the interior structure of bones thins down (Figure 5.1), and even minor impacts, such as contact with a vehicle door or the use of furniture, can lead to fractures. Although fractures can happen anywhere in the bones, the most prevalent forms seem to be those in the wrist, hip, and spine. This highlights how important it is to prevent and manage osteoporosis and the substantial influence that bone density has on fracture risk.

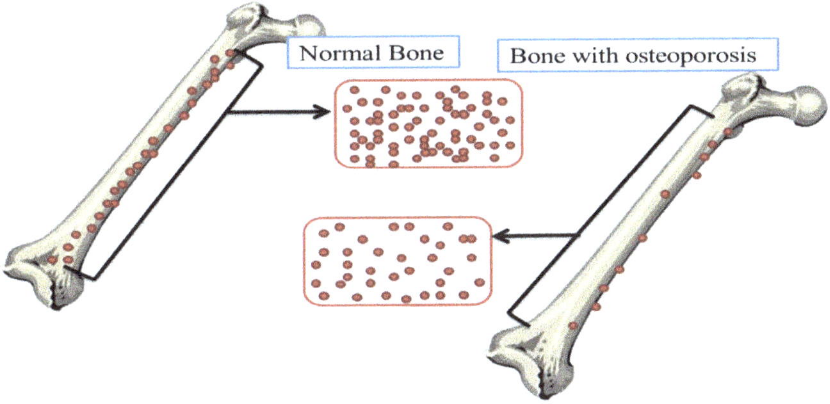

FIGURE 5.1 Occurrence of osteoporosis.

Despite this, the intricate structure of collagen, a specific protein, undergoes constant renewal by specialized cells, and minerals like calcium play a crucial role in maintaining robust bones throughout our lifetimes. New bone is constantly growing instead of the broken-down existing bone. The proportion of osteogenesis and osseous breakdown balances out to a generally consistent level in bone mass between the ages of 25 and 50. This mechanism preserves density by accumulating as many bone cells as it eliminates. After age 50, bone fractures become more prevalent, and osteoporosis often worsens, especially after menopause. Around this time, the body begins to develop more bone density. Historically, women's bones have been smaller and thinner than men's, leading to osteoporosis (fractures) and lower bone density in males (osteopenia). Men are also susceptible, although the danger is higher during menstruation when the hormones that create bones are less abundant (Iwaniec and Turner, 2016).

Having a family history of osteoporosis-related fractures is correlated with an increased risk of developing osteoporosis in both males and females. These factors highlight bone health's dynamic and gender-specific nature over the lifespan.

5.2.1.1 PATHOPHYSIOLOGY AND TYPES

Between the ages of 25 and 50, there is an equilibrium between bone cell addition (osteogenesis) and bone cell loss, resulting in a relatively constant bone mass (Wawrzyniak and Balawender, 2022). Bone density increases around 25, reaching its peak by approximately 30. However, this process slows down, and after the age of 50, the rate of bone fractures often surpasses that of bone development. Osteoporosis tends to deteriorate post-menopause, especially in women, and around age 50, the prevalence of bone fractures exceeds the rate of bone formation. Women experience more fractures (osteoporosis) and decreased bone density than men do because women's bones are frequently smaller and thinner than men's (osteopenia). This underscores the gender-specific considerations in understanding bone health and addressing the risks associated with osteoporosis, especially in postmenopausal women. The pathophysiological mechanism is shown in Figure 5.2.

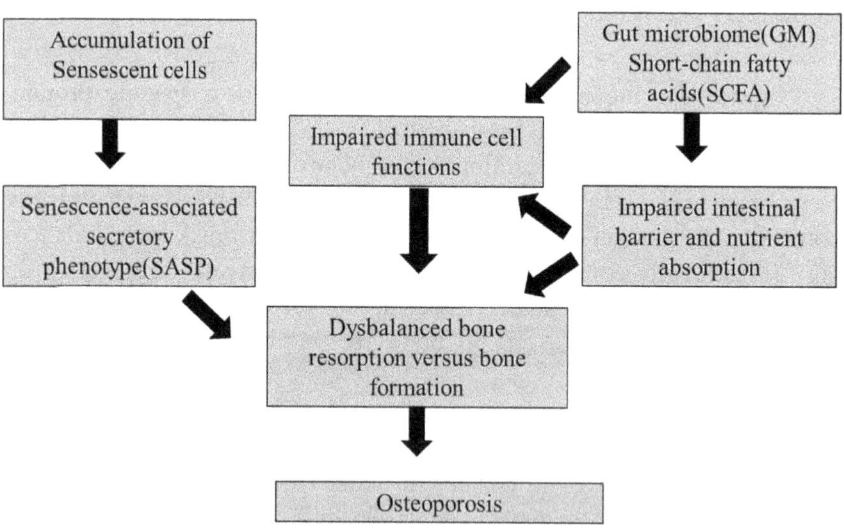

FIGURE 5.2 Pathophysiology behind osteoporosis.

5.2.1.2 THERAPEUTIC APPROACHES

The objectives of osteoporosis therapy include reducing the potential for bone loss and fractures, preventing disability, and controlling pain. A comprehensive preventative strategy includes minimizing fall-risk-inducing medicines (FRIDs), improving eyesight or hearing, building muscle, improving balance, and lowering the risk of falls (Rodrigues et al., 2023). You should ensure adequate protein, calcium, and vitamin D. You should also avoid smoking and drink alcohol in moderation. The best way to prevent osteoporosis is to exercise, participate in weight-bearing physical activity, keep good posture and balance, consume a diet rich in calcium and vitamin D, quit smoking, and use alcohol sparingly. The phrase "nonpharmacological treatment" encapsulates these actions. The second stage requires specific prescriptions for drugs (three primary categories of medications exist: anabolic, antiresorptive [anticatabolic], and their mixtures). Osteoblasts are becoming more exciting cells in this context, but osteoclasts are still the primary focus of medical intervention (Brent, 2023). Sclerostin and Dickkopf-1 are examples of Wnt signaling pathway inhibitors that have become exciting new targets for therapeutic intervention.

Only a tiny percentage of these therapy options are employed for eligible individuals. Population-based research revealed that just 21.8% of patients received adequate care. The undertreatment is caused by nonadherence, which is very problematic. Under "adherence," the subject covers the essential aspects of adherence. Remedy and action in bone metabolism with its side effects are explained in Table 5.1.

5.2.1.3 COMBINATION THERAPY

The usual way osteoporosis medicine is given is as monotherapy, in addition to calcium and vitamin D supplements. However, several clinical trials have explored combination therapy using both osteoanabolic and antiresorptive drugs to maximize the impact on bone production and reduce fracture risk. Although these trials observed improvements in bone mineral density with combination medications, for methodological reasons, they did not approve or recommend them. The omission of a monotherapy arm, the neglect of fracture risk assessment, and the achievement of comparable outcomes with monotherapy were among these shortcomings (Tonk et al., 2022).

TABLE 5.1 Remedy and Action in Bone Metabolism with Its Side Effects

Remedy	Action	Bone Metabolism	Selected Side Effects
Calcium	An endocrine feedback mechanism involving testosterone and vitamin D	Suppression of the resorption of bone	Gastrointestinal symptoms, urolithiasis, and hypercalcemia
Vitamin D	Modifications to the citrate metabolism	Stopping the resorption of bone	A blood level exceeding 150 mg/ml is known as vitamin intoxication
Alendronate	In osteoclasts, cell death occurs	Stopping the resorption of bone	Adverse gastrointestinal consequences, atypical femur fracture, and Whoa, osteonecrosis
Ibandronate	Osteoclast cell demise	Suppression of bone resorption	Yaw osteonecrosis, possible gastrointestinal problems, and uncommon femur fractures
Zoledronic acid	A decrease in the loss of bone. In osteoclasts, cell death	Less loss of bone	Yaw osteonecrosis, aberrant femur fracture, and gastrointestinal upset are possible side effects
Risedronate	Cell death of osteoclasts	Keeping bone mass from declining	Abnormal femur fracture, unfavorable effects on the gastrointestinal tract, and yaw osteonecrosis
Denosumab	A RANKL-specific antibody	Reduced resorption of bone	Atypical femur fracture and yaw osteonecrosis
Raloxifene	A bone-based estrogen agonist	A decrease in the loss of bone	There is an increased risk of stroke and thromboembolic consequences
Teriparatide	The activation of osteoblasts	Development of bones	Hypercalcemia and increased risk of osteosarcoma
Romosuzab	Control of Wnt signaling by gestures	Generating new bone and keeping existing bone from deteriorating	Events related to the heart

5.2.1.4 LONG-TERM TREATMENT AND MONITORING

After discontinuing teriparatide, Regaining lost bone mineral density is feasible through a series of antiresorptive therapies. While unusual femur fractures and mandibular osteonecrosis are uncommon adverse effects of antiresorptive medicines, they are time-dependent. As such, it is recommended that patients with osteoporosis receiving long-term therapy adjust their treatment plans and that they discontinue and reassess their condition after 3–5 years. A limitation of all research on combination treatments is the reliance on bone mineral density rather than treatment efficacy as a substitute measure for fracture risk (Leboff et al., 2022). Compared to alternative options, teriparatide with denosumab was the most successful combination for boosting bone mineral density. The antiresorptive drug regimen that is most often used, which is followed by osteoanabolic medicines, has little effect in this area. Denosumab therapy was more effective after teriparatide or antiresorptive medicine than when another antiresorptive substance was used sequentially (Leder, 2018). The most effective way to increase hip bone mineral density is to take an osteoanabolic therapy after taking an antiresorptive medicine, according to research on the best administration order for these drugs.

5.2.1.5 TREATMENT WITHOUT PHARMACEUTICALS

Based on an extensive review, nonpharmacologic therapy can be distilled into 14 points for therapeutic intervention.

5.2.2 BONE DISEASE: PAGET'S SYNDROME

Osteitis deformans, a common disorder that affects one or more bones, is another name for Paget's disease of the bone (PDB). While some people might not exhibit symptoms, others might have various adverse effects. Sir James Paget initially characterized the illness more than 130 years ago (Makaram and Ralston, 2021). The consequences of Paget's illness are primarily seen in the bones. While a significant portion of Paget's disease patients may not have any symptoms at all, a smaller proportion may experience grave complications such as neurologic diseases, secondary arthritis, bone discomfort, or bone lesions. Though calcitonin therapy has been accessible since the 1970s, more recent effective options are bisphosphonates.

PDB, or after osteoporosis, is a frequent condition affecting bone remodeling. A proportion of 1–2% of individuals with this condition are elderly white persons over 55. About 2.1% of individuals over 40 had PDB overall, according to a study done on skeletal remains from Northern England between 900 and 1850. The frequency was 3.1% after 1500, compared to 1.7% before that time. PDB is somewhat more common in men than in women as people age. PDB is rare in those under 25, and it is rare in those under 40. Eighty-six people in the research had an average age of 58 upon diagnosis (Shaker, 2009).

Different geographic and ethnic groupings have varying prevalence rates of Paget's disease (PDB), a bone illness. A more significant risk of catching the disease than native Britons and Western Europeans is experienced when emigrating to South Africa, Australia, New Zealand, and South America from the United Kingdom compared to black Africans, residents of China, Japan, Scandinavia, the Indian subcontinent, and Southeast Asia have a lower risk of contracting the illness. According to the United Kingdom and New Zealand data, PDB has decreased in incidence and severity during the past 25–30 years. Still, PDB does not appear to have become much less common in the United States or Spain. There may have been a recent increase in instances of highly severe illness in the southern area of Italy, even if the country's general incidence rate has remained relatively stable. First-degree relatives of people with PDB are more likely to get the disease, especially if the patient was diagnosed early or has a bone disease that deforms bones. A positive family history is present in 15–30% of PDB patients, and first-degree relatives of PDB patients are almost seven times more likely to develop Paget's disease. Furthermore, a more significant percentage of the skeleton is affected by familial PDB than sporadic disease, which is more prevalent in younger people.

5.2.2.1 PATHOPHYSIOLOGY AND CLINICAL FEATURES

Bone-related disorders such as bone-related Paget's disease (PDB) can affect one or more bones and are progressive and persistent. Its distinctive traits include enhanced bone vascularity, uneven bone growth, and accelerated osteoclastic bone resorption, which results in certain skeletal diseases. In PDB, there is an increase in the quantity and size of osteoclasts, potentially containing more nuclei than usual, and these nuclei may include inclusion bodies similar to virus particles. The initial lesion in PDB is believed to involve increased osteoclastic bone resorption in a specific area. Subsequently, bone production occurs at an accelerated rate. The faster turnover of bone results in the deposition of new collagen fibers in a chaotic, nonlinear fashion, creating a lamellar bone mosaic that is more prone to fracture or deformation and is mechanically insufficient.

PDB is widely recognized as an osteoclast-affecting disease. There is an increase in osteoclast precursors in circulation, and bone marrow shows increased sensitivity to stimuli that accelerate bone resorption. Factors contributing to this include 1,25-dihydroxyvitamin D and RANKL, the receptor activator of NF-kB ligand (Kim et al., 2019). Upregulation of interleukin-6 expression and signaling, specifically IL-6, is identified as a potential cause of increased osteoclastic activity. Recent studies indicate elevated levels of circulating RANKL in individuals with PDB, and the protein that promotes osteoclastic growth is expressed at greater concentrations in Pagetic marrow cells. While the number of osteoblasts increases in Pagetic sites, most experts do not consider these cells a major pathophysiologic component of PDB, as they exhibit a regular shape.

5.2.2.2 THERAPEUTIC APPROACHES

The medications that the United States Food and Drug Administration (FDA) authorized for treating PDB are listed in Table 5.2. Specific antiresorptive medications inhibit osteoclastic activity (Tsukamoto et al., 2021). Long available on the market, salmon calcitonin usually lowers serum alkaline phosphatase (SAP) by approximately 50% and relieves some symptoms when administered subcutaneously once a day at a dose of 100 IU. Improvements in bone pain reduction resolved neurologic issues, and improved healing of osteolytic lesions have all been reported. Once this is established, the maintenance dosage is often lowered to 50–100 IU, administered thrice weekly. However, calcitonin may become less effective due to the potential development of antibodies against it, and its efficacy is considered inferior to more potent bisphosphonates. Some patients may experience side effects such as flushing and nausea. Calcitonin is used less frequently than more potent bisphosphonates. However, it may be offered for individuals who cannot tolerate oral or intravenous (IV) bisphosphonate medication (Ralston and Medicine, 2020). The FDA has not approved calcitonin nasal spray for PDB.

TABLE 5.2 The Medications That the USFDA has Authorized for the Treatment of Paget's Disease of the Bone (PDB)

Calcitonin (Miacalcin)	Fifty to 100 units each day, three times per week, for 6–18 months
Etidronate (Didronel)	6–7 oz of water on an empty stomach and 200–400 mg taken orally once daily for six months; no liquids or food for at least two hours before and following the dosage. The maximum duration of the therapy regimen should be six months. After menstruation, extra dosages may be administered
Pamidronate (Ardica)	Provide 30 mg intravenously spaced four hours apart three times a week. Every 2–4 h, an intravenous dosage of 60 mg or 90 mg is typically administered; further doses are given as needed. Usually, one infusion is sufficient for a mild ailment; however, two or even three infusions may be required for a severe one
Alendronate (Fosamax)	Thirty milligrams every day for six months. Drink without a meal and a full glass of water in the morning, preferably 6–8 oz. Thirty minutes should pass before the patient takes food, nonwater-based drinks, or prescriptions. The patient should remain upright for at least 30 min
Tiludronate (Skelid)	400 mg administered once daily for three months. Take empty-handed, preferably with 6–8 oz of water, and wait 2 h or longer before and after taking any further prescription drugs
Risedronate (Acetonel)	30 mg administered once a day for 12 weeks. Take it first thing in the morning, without a meal, and ideally with a glass of juice or water. Patients should not eat, drink, or take any drugs for at least 30 min after the therapy. The patient must maintain consciousness for a minimum of 30 min
Zoledronic acid (Reclast)	Give yourself 5 mg intravenously over 15 min. The medicine shouldn't be taken if the creatinine clearance is 35 ml/min or less. To lower the risk of hypocalcemia, the patient has to consume adequate calcium and vitamin D

Synthetic forms of inorganic pyrophosphate resistant to environmental degradation are known as bisphosphonates. These drugs prevent osteoclastic bone resorption by adhering to mineralized surfaces and having remarkably extended skeletal half-lives. Simple bisphosphonates, like etidronate and tiludronate, and more powerful bisphosphonates that include nitrogen, such as zoledronic acid (ZA), pamidronate, alendronate, and risedronate, are among them. Etidronate is one of the simple bisphosphonates that prevents osteoclasts from doing their job by producing dangerous analogs of ATP. For a while now, etidronate has been marketed as a remedy for PDB. The usual dosage for PDB is 400 mg/day for six months, followed by a six-month break. About half of patients may return to normal SAP levels with this treatment, while around one in six may experience no change. Higher doses are not recommended due to the risk of mineralization deficiency. Tiludronate is another bisphosphonate considered "less potent." For three months, 400 mg once daily is the suggested dose. In one research, 72% of PDB patients saw a 50% or more drop in SAP with this medication, whereas 35% reached normal SAP levels. Etidronate appears to be slightly less effective than tiludronate when treating PDB.

Regarding nitrogen-containing bisphosphonates, the most popular and efficient ones are alendronate, pamidronate, risedronate, and ZA. Nitrogen-containing bisphosphonates can inhibit farnesyl diphosphate synthase, which may help reduce osteoclastic bone resorption. Elevate and descenderate are taken orally, while pamidronate and ZA are administered intravenously. For treating PDB, 40 mg of alendronate per day is recommended for six months. Alendronate was more effective than etidronate in treating PDB in 63% of patients, whereas etidronate was only effective in 17% of cases. The efficacy of two alendronate dosages—40 mg given once a day for six months and 280 mg orally thrice a week in a buffered solution was examined in recent trials (Koulouktsi et al., 2019). SAP levels were reduced comparably by both treatments; however, the 280-mg oral buffer solution caused more significant gastrointestinal adverse effects, including nausea, upset stomach, and diarrhea. A daily dosage of 30 mg of risedronate is administered for two months as part of the therapy for bone disease caused by PDB. In a significant study, 73% of PDB patients saw a normalization of SAP levels with risedronate, compared to 15% with etidronate. Compared to the etidronate group, the risedronate group experienced substantially less pain. SAP levels dropped by 77% following eight weeks of daily 30 mg risedronate treatment in a trial including 13 patients with severe PDB. In 10 participants, the average decrease in SAP levels following a second course of risedronate was 87%. While other regimens are more often employed, the FDA has authorized pazopanidate for PDB when it is injected intravenously for 4 h on three different days at a dosage of 30 mg. A single infusion of 60–90 mg could be adequate for people with mild illness; repeated infusions containing 90 mg might be required for those with severe disease (Konecki et al., 2021). An average of 63% was taken off the SAP levels of 80 people suffering from bone-related PDB due to intravenous pamidronate treatment, according to a prospective, nonrandomized controlled trial. The study's conclusion:

- SAP normalized in 86% of patients whose levels were less than three times the upper standard limit (UNL).
- SAP normalized in 38% of individuals whose levels were three to six times higher than the UNL.
- SAP normalization was achieved in 12% of individuals whose levels were more than six times the UNL.

Researchers looked at oral risedronate (30 mg daily for eight weeks) and intravenous pamidronate (30 mg three times) as chemotherapeutic medications for individuals resistant to intravenous clodronate; the former is the more popular alternative. About 80% of patients experienced remission with pamidronate, compared to 86% with risedronate. Different research discovered that 86% of patients experienced biochemical remission following oral alendronate, whereas 56% of patients experienced remission with intravenous pamidronate.

- The FDA authorized ZA for PDB in 2007. Five milligrams are given intravenously for 15–30 min (Hosking, 2007). In a trial where individuals with, for 60 days, patients with an average baseline SAP level that was around four times the normal range were given a single intravenous dose of either 5 mg of ZA or 30 mg of risedronate orally once daily.
- Six months after ZA initiation, 89% of patients had normalized SAP levels, compared to 58% of patients in the risedronate group.
- Compared to the risedronate group, the ZA group had superior physical performance at three months and overall health after six months, based on SF-36 data.
- In patients with a therapeutic response defined as SAP stabilization or throughout the 18-month extension, the ZA group's SAP levels remained constant with a reduction of 75% or more, indicating that ZA's biochemical impact was more long-lasting than risedronate.
- SAP levels increased from six to 24 months in the risedronate group.

Specific individuals have noted a biochemical response to pamidronate, clodronate, or etidronate. This reaction characterizes a shorter duration of remission after a new round of therapy, a rise in the nadir SAP with subsequent treatments, and the requirement for a higher dosage to elicit the same response (Review and Diseases, 2003). For those with these problems, looking into various bisphosphonates may be worthwhile because they could work better in certain situations.

Finally, when particular antipagetic therapy is needed, amino bisphosphonates such as ZA, alendronate, risedronate, and pamidronate are preferred. Both oral and injectable versions of these drugs are available. This treatment may be appropriate for those who have trouble swallowing, have neurological symptoms, are having emergency surgery on the Pagetic bone, or would rather have intravenous therapy. Intravenous injection may also be beneficial for patients with severe gastrointestinal or esophageal problems. With treatment benefits that persist for at least two years longer than those of rival medications, ZA seems to be the most successful therapy available.

Bisphosphonates may have unfavorable impacts, according to a recent assessment. When using oral amino bisphosphonates, there are frequently adverse effects on the gastrointestinal system and esophagus. An influenza-like sickness that usually appears a few days after commencing therapy is the most common adverse effect of intravenous pamidronate with ZA (Press, 2011). In pivotal osteoporosis research including ZA, following the first injection, acute phase responses happened in 31.6% of patients, 6.6% after the second, and 2.8% after the third. Oral bisphosphonates may have this uncommon but potential adverse effect. Acetaminophen could help lessen specific negative effects.

Several individuals have complained of ongoing musculoskeletal discomfort even after stopping their bisphosphonate medication. Every bisphosphonate prescription has information about this potential adverse effect, and in 2008, the FDA released a warning about it. But that seems to be an uncommon event.

5.2.3 RICKETS

The aberrant mineralization of the growth plate, which is usually seen in developing children, is the cause of rickets. In contrast, rickets can develop in individuals with osteomalacia, defined by aberrant prefabricated osteoid creation in adults and children. Globally, the leading causes of rickets and osteomalacia collectively known as nutritional rickets and osteomalacia—are deficiencies in sunshine exposure, calcium intake from diet, and vitamin D. The condition was once believed to be more severe when paired with calcium insufficiency, and vitamin D deficiency was the primary cause of nutritional rickets. Nevertheless, it was subsequently shown that rickets might occur without a vitamin D deficit due to a diet lacking calcium. Rickets symptoms can arise from specific calcium or vitamin D deficiencies or a combination. Asia and Africa have the highest rates of calcium insufficiency. Vitamin D-deficient rickets are becoming more common in affluent nations due to several causes. These elements include fewer hours spent in the sun, unfortified meals, insufficient supplementation plans, and international migration patterns (Joshi and Uday, 2023). While getting enough vitamin D through diet is relatively simple, getting enough calcium from the diet might be difficult since after being exposed to ultraviolet B (UVB) rays from the sun, the skin produces vitamin D. Living in high-latitude regions and having dark skin are two factors that might reduce the skin's capacity to synthesize vitamin D, dressing covertly, using a lot of sunscreen, and avoiding the sun. These reasons have made vitamin D deficiency more common, especially in countries with plenty of sunshine. However, those with dark complexion, immigrants, citizens of high-latitude countries, expectant mothers, and newborns are the groups most susceptible to these impairments.

5.2.3.1 PATHOPHYSIOLOGY OF RICKETS

Minerals comprise half and three-quarters of bone tissue, with calcium and phosphorus being the most common. Bone mineralization requires sufficient levels of calcitriol, phosphorus, and calcium (needed for intestinal mineral absorption). The primary cause of rickets determines the type: either calcipenic rickets, which is brought on by insufficient calcium and inefficient calcitriol, or phosphopenic rickets, which is brought on by an inadequate amount of phosphate. The growth plate undergoes a sequence of processes that culminate in the mineralization of bone upon the death of hypertrophic chondrocytes. The fundamental cause of both phosphopenic and calcipenic rickets is phosphopenia, which results from insufficient phosphate availability, which is necessary for apoptosis.

The causes and clinical signs of calcium shortage and hypophosphatemia result from inadequate vitamin D or calcium in the diet. The intestines need vitamin D to absorb calcium properly. Deficient calcium availability results from rickets regardless of whether the source is a diet deficient in calcium or vitamin D (Thandrayen and Pettifor, 2018). The outcome of decreased calcium availability is a drop in blood calcium levels instead of hypocalcemia. Increased parathyroid hormone (PTH) production happens when blood calcium levels fall below a person's genetically determined set point. Maximum intestinal calcium absorption is achieved by enhanced PTH-induced renal 1-hydroxylase activity and calcidiol-to-calcitriol conversion. Furthermore, by stimulating osteoclasts with PTH, secondary hyperparathyroidism releases stored calcium, replenishing serum calcium at the expense of bone loss. Renal calcium excretion is decreased by elevated PTH, although renal phosphate excretion is increased. Bent legs, swelling ankle and wrist joints, and a rachitic rosary are signs of osteomalacia and rickets brought on by hypophosphatemia and persistent phosphaturia (Haffner et al., 2022).

5.2.3.2 THERAPEUTIC APPROACHES

As part of the treatment for administering therapeutic doses of calcium and vitamin D rickets, it is possible to consistently take both vitamin D2 and D3 orally. Stoss therapy, a single high-dose treatment, is more appropriate for vitamin D3 because it has a longer half-life than vitamin D2. According to one research, there is more excellent safety and efficacy than a single high-dose intramuscular injection (600,000 IU) and weekly spaced oral dosages (60,000 IU for 10 weeks) (Wadia et al., 2018). However, because it may result in elevated blood calcium levels, patients with follow-up or compliance problems should be the only ones who can benefit from stoss treatment. Treatment should be given for at least 12 weeks, but the time patients receive their response should be determined. The various interventions in different age groups are shown in Table 5.3. Calcium is given intravenously or orally to children who have acute hypocalcemia issues, such as heart failure or seizures, to treat the illness. An intravenous calcium gluconate injection is recommended to treat acute problems, followed by an infusion until the blood calcium level returns to normal (Evaluation, n.d.). The youngster may begin taking calcium supplements orally if they have reached a suitable level of stability and normocalcemia.

TABLE 5.3 Intervention in Different Age Groups

Intervention	Infants	12 months to 12 years	More than 12 years
At least once a day, take your medicine (containing D2 or D3) (IU)	2000	3000–6000	6000
The Stoss approach (preferably combined with D3) (IU)	Just 50,000 babies are older than three months	150,000	300,000
Calcium from diet or supplements when required (milligrams daily)	200–300	500	500
A minimum of IU of vitamin D should be taken daily for prevention	400	600	600

5.3 CONCLUSION

Growing evidence of target molecules impacting bone regulation points to the possibility of novel and improved treatments. It is essential to investigate the efficacy of these medicines in treating different medical diseases; ideally, they should have few side effects. One possible strategy is examining the benefits and drawbacks of these medications separately, in combination, or the context of alternative or combinatorial therapies. Combining bone–anabolic pharmaceuticals with a "homing" molecule ensures that the therapies target the surface of the bone selectively, reducing their potential side effects on other organs. This is another promising approach. The function of specific proteins in the control of bone is still being investigated. For example, age-related osteoblast bone loss has been connected to decreased RICTOR, a protein in the mTOR complex. Activating the mTOR pathway regulates bone resorption, enhanced adipogenesis, and osteoclastogenesis. Sirt-3 is a critical protein in mitochondrial metabolism. Although medications like rapamycin and related mTOR inhibitors have demonstrated potential in mitigating age-associated diseases in rats, further research is necessary to fully understand their precise function as senolytic or xenomorphic medicines in the aging skeleton.

DNA damage response (DDR) protein PARP1 is an intriguing protein that regulates the NF-κB pathway, affecting inflammation and DDR. Age-related comorbidities may be exacerbated by elevated PARP1 levels above a certain threshold. It has been demonstrated that inhibiting PARP1 can restore alpha-synuclein breakdown and avert the neurodegeneration linked to Parkinson's disease. Finally, the chapter acknowledges that age-related metabolic skeletal disorders substantially influence healthcare systems in light of the aging population. It explores the intricate problems these conditions present and suggests a course of action to lessen their detrimental impact on the skeletal muscles. The proposed paradigm promotes a comprehensive strategy that considers lifestyle, nutrition, and medications to treat metabolic skeletal issues related to aging. Along with discussing new treatments and advancements in the industry, the chapter highlights how interventions are constantly changing. An older population that is healthier and more resilient may result from successfully applying an all-encompassing therapeutic strategy.

KEYWORDS

- **metabolic**
- **skeletal**
- **disorders**
- **treatment**
- **age-related metabolic**
- **skeletal illnesses**

REFERENCES

Alquorain, H. (2021). Phosphate supplement differentially affects the skeletal phenotypes in Hyp and FGF23 overexpression mice. McGill University (Canada)ProQuest Dissertations & Theses, 30548878.

Axelsson, K.F., Litsne, H., Lorentzon, M. (2023). Comparison of fractures among older adults who are ambulatory vs those who use wheelchairs in Sweden. JAMA Network Open, 6(2), e2255645. https://doi.org/10.1001/jamanetworkopen.2022.55645

Barnsley, J., Buckland, G., Chan, P.E., Ong, A., Ramos, A.S., Baxter, M., Laskou, F., Dennison, E.M., Cooper, C., Patel, H.P. (2021). Pathophysiology and treatment of osteoporosis: Challenges for clinical practice in older people. Aging Clinical and Experimental Research, 33(4), 759–773. https://doi.org/10.1007/s40520-021-01817-y

Brent M.B. (2023). Pharmaceutical treatment of bone loss: From animal models and drug development to future treatment strategies. Pharmacology & Therapeutics, 244, 108383. https://doi.org/10.1016/j.pharmthera.2023.108383

Dressler, W., Kaufman, S. (n.d.). Chronic Conditions, Fluid States.

Evaluation, D. (n.d.). Clinical review(s).

Farrow, S.L., Gokuladhas, S., Schilling, W., Perry, J.K., Cooper, A.A., Sullivan, J.M.O., Pudjihartono, M. (2024). *Identifying 27 Allele-specific Regulatory Variants in Parkinson's Disease Using a Massively Parallel Reporter Assay*. pp. 1–14. https://doi.org/10.1038/s41531-024-00659-5

From Indian Academy of Pediatrics 'Guideline for Vitamin D and Calcium in Children' Committee., Khadilkar, A., Khadilkar, V., Chinnappa, J., Rathi, N., Khadgawat, R., Balasubramanian, S., Parekh, B., Jog, P. (2017). Prevention and treatment of vitamin D and calcium deficiency in children and adolescents: Indian Academy of Pediatrics (IAP) guidelines. Indian Pediatrics, 54(7), 567–573. https://doi.org/10.1007/s13312-017-1070-x

Garg, N., Singh, T.G., Khan, H., Arora, S., Kaur, A., Mannan, A. (2021). Mechanistic interventions of selected Ocimum species in management of diabetes, obesity and liver disorders: Transformative developments from preclinical to clinical approaches. Biointerface Research in Applied Chemistry, 12(1), 1304-1323

Haffner, D., Leifheit-Nestler, M., Grund, A., Schnabel, D. (2022). Rickets guidance: Part I-diagnostic workup. Pediatric Nephrology (Berlin, Germany), 37(9), 2013–2036. https://doi.org/10.1007/s00467-021-05328-w

Hannan, F.M., Newey, P.J., Whyte, M.P., Thakker, R.V. (2019). Genetic approaches to metabolic bone diseases. British Journal of Clinical Pharmacology, 85(6), 1147–1160. https://doi.org/10.1111/bcp.13803

Hosking, D. (2007). Zoledronic acid in Paget's disease, Therapy, 4, 391–397.

Ilic, I., Ristic, B., Stojadinovic, I., Ilic, M. (2023). Epidemiology of hip fractures due to falls. Medicina (Kaunas, Lithuania), 59(9), 1528. https://doi.org/10.3390/medicina59091528

Iwaniec, U.T., Turner, R.T. (2016). Influence of body weight on bone mass, architecture and turnover. The Journal of Endocrinology, 230(3), R115–R130. https://doi.org/10.1530/JOE-16-0089

Joshi, M., Uday, S. (2023). Vitamin D deficiency in chronic childhood disorders: Importance of screening and prevention. Nutrients, 15(12), 2805. https://doi.org/10.3390/nu15122805

Kant, R., Singh, T.G., Singh, S. (2020). Mechanistic approach To herbal formulations used for urolithiasis treatment. Obesity Medicine. 2020, 100266

Kim, H.J., Kim, H.J., Choi, Y., Bae, M.K., Hwang, D.S., Shin, S.H., Lee, J.Y. (2019). Zoledronate enhances osteocyte-mediated osteoclast differentiation by IL-6/RANKL Axis. International Journal of Molecular Sciences, 20(6), 1467. https://doi.org/10.3390/ijms20061467

Konecki, C., Feliu, C., Cazaubon, Y., Giusti, D., Tonye-Libyh, M., Brixi, H., Cadiot, G., Biron, A., Djerada, Z. (2021). External evaluation of population pharmacokinetic models and bayes-based dosing of infliximab. Pharmaceutics, 13(8), 1191. https://doi.org/10.3390/pharmaceutics13081191

Koulouktsi, C., Nanaki, S., Barmpalexis, P., Kostoglou, M., Bikiaris, D. (2019). Preparation and characterization of Alendronate depot microspheres based on novel poly(-ε-caprolactone)/vitamin E TPGS copolymers. International Journal of Pharmaceutics: X, 1, 100014. https://doi.org/10.1016/j.ijpx.2019.100014

LeBoff, M.S., Greenspan, S.L., Insogna, K.L., Lewiecki, E.M., Saag, K.G., Singer, A.J., Siris, E.S. (2022). The clinician's guide to prevention and treatment of osteoporosis. Osteoporosis International, 33(10), 2049–2102. https://doi.org/10.1007/s00198-021-05900-y

Leder B.Z. (2018). Optimizing sequential and combined anabolic and antiresorptive osteoporosis therapy. JBMR Plus, 2(2), 62–68. https://doi.org/10.1002/jbm4.10041

Makaram, N.S., Ralston, S.H. (2021). Genetic determinants of Paget's disease of bone. Current Osteoporosis Reports, 19(3), 327–337. https://doi.org/10.1007/s11914-021-00676-w

Mäkitie, O., Zillikens, M.C. (2022). Early-onset osteoporosis. Calcified Tissue International, 110(5), 546–561. https://doi.org/10.1007/s00223-021-00885-6

Mehta, S., Nain, P., Agrawal, B.K., Singh, R.P. (2022). Vitamin D with calcium supplementation managing glycemic control with HbA1c and improve quality of life in patients with diabetes. Turkish Journal of Pharmaceutical Sciences, 19(2), 161–167. https://doi.org/10.4274/tjps.galenos.2021.62357

Murray, C.J., Lopez, A.D., Jamison, D.T. (1994). The global burden of disease in 1990: Summary results, sensitivity analysis and future directions. Bulletin of the World Health Organization, 72(3), 495–509.

Natesan, V., Kim, S.J. (2022). Metabolic bone diseases and new drug developments. Biomolecules & Therapeutics, 30(4), 309–319. https://doi.org/10.4062/biomolther.2022.007.

Nuti, R., Brandi, M.L., Checchia, G., Di Munno, O., Dominguez, L., Falaschi, P., Fiore, C.E., Iolascon, G., Maggi, S., Michieli, R., Migliaccio, S., Minisola, S., Rossini, M., Sessa, G., Tarantino, U., Toselli, A., Isaia, G.C. (2019). Guidelines for the management of osteoporosis and fragility fractures. Internal and Emergency Medicine, 14(1), 85–102. https://doi.org/10.1007/s11739-018-1874-2

Press, D. (2011). Role of zoledronic acid in the prevention and treatment of osteoporosis. Clinical Interventions in Aging, 6, 89–99. https://doi.org/10.2147/CIA.S7282

Ralston, S.H., Medicine, E. (2020). Diagnosis and management of Paget's disease of bone. Practitioner, 264(November), 11–15.

Rehni, A.K., Singh, T.G. (2011). Modulation of leukotriene D4 attenuates the development of seizures in mice. Prostaglandins, Leukotrienes, and Essential Fatty Acids, 85(2), 97–106. https://doi.org/10.1016/j.plefa.2011.04.003

Review, A.G.A.T., Diseases, G. (2003). AGA technical review on osteoporosis in gastrointestinal diseases. Gastroenterology, 124(3), 795–841. https://doi.org/10.1053/gast.2003.50106

Rihal, V., Khan, H., Kaur, A., Singh, T.G. (2023). Vitamin D as therapeutic modulator in cerebrovascular diseases: A mechanistic perspectives. Critical Reviews in Food Science and Nutrition, 63(25), 7772–7794. https://doi.org/10.1080/10408398.2022.2050349

Rihal, V., Khan, H., Kaur, A., Singh, T.G., Abdel-Daim, M.M. (2022). Therapeutic and mechanistic intervention of vitamin D in neuropsychiatric disorders. Psychiatry Research, 317, 114782. https://doi.org/10.1016/j.psychres.2022.114782

Rodrigues, D., Silvestre, S., Monteiro, C., Duarte, A.P. (2023). Medication and the risk of falls: An analysis of adverse drug reactions reported to the portuguese pharmacovigilance system. Journal of Clinical Medicine, 12(23), 7268. https://doi.org/10.3390/jcm12237268

Shaker J.L. (2009). Paget's disease of bone: A review of epidemiology, pathophysiology and management. Therapeutic Advances in Musculoskeletal Disease, 1(2), 107–125. https://doi.org/10.1177/1759720X09351779

Singh, R., Rao, H.K., Singh, T.G. (2020). Advanced glycated end products (ages) in diabetes and its complications: An insight. Plant Arch, 20(1), 3838–3841.

States, U. (n.d.). Skeletal Maturity of Children 6-11 Years (Issue 140).

Thandrayen, K., Pettifor, J.M. (2018). The roles of vitamin D and dietary calcium in nutritional rickets. Bone Reports, 8, 81–89. https://doi.org/10.1016/j.bonr.2018.01.005

Thapa, K., Singh, T.G., Kaur, A. (2021). Cyclic nucleotide phosphodiesterase inhibition as a potential therapeutic target in renal ischemia reperfusion injury. Life Sciences, 282, 119843. https://doi.org/10.1016/j.lfs.2021.119843

Tonk, C.H., Shoushrah, S.H., Babczyk, P., El Khaldi-Hansen, B., Schulze, M., Herten, M., Tobiasch, E. (2022). Therapeutic treatments for osteoporosis-which combination of pills is the best among the bad. International Journal of Molecular Sciences, 23(3), 1393. https://doi.org/10.3390/ijms23031393

Tsukamoto, S., Kido, A., Tanaka, Y., Facchini, G., Peta, G., Rossi, G., Mavrogenis, A.F. (2021). Current overview of treatment for metastatic bone disease. Current Oncology (Toronto, Ont.), 28(5), 3347–3372. https://doi.org/10.3390/curroncol28050290.

Wadia, U., Soon, W., Chivers, P., Thambiran, A., Burgner, D., Cherian, S., Siafarikas, A. (2018). Randomised controlled trial comparing daily versus depot vitamin D3 therapy in 0–16-year-old newly settled refugees in Western Australia over a period of 40 weeks. Nutrients, 10(3), 348. https://doi.org/10.3390/nu10030348

Wawrzyniak, A., Balawender, K. (2022). Structural and metabolic changes in bone. Animals, 12(15), 1946. https://doi.org/10.3390/ani12151946

CHAPTER 6

The Molecular Mechanisms Underlying Aging in Chronic Metabolic Disorders

BHAVANA SINGH[1*], AMRISH CHANDRA[1], VAIBHAV RASTOGI[2], DEEPIKA JOSHI[3], NIDHI SEMWAL[4], GAUREE KUKRETI[5], ANURAG VERMA[2], URVASHI SAXENA[2], ARVIND RAGHAV[2], DEEPANKAR AKOLIYA[6], VANDANA[1], HEMA ARYA[1], and GAUTAM KUMAR[1]

[1]*School of Pharmacy, Sharda University, Greater Noida, Uttar Pradesh, India*

[2]*TMCOP, Teerthanker Mahaveer University, Moradabad, Uttar Pradesh, India*

[3]*Siddhartha Institute of Pharmacy, Dehradun, Uttarakhand, India*

[4]*School of Pharmaceutical Science, Shri Guru Ram Rai University, Dehradun, Uttarakhand, India*

[5]*School of Pharmaceutical Sciences and Technology, Sardar Bhagwan Singh University, Dehradun, Uttarakhand, India*

[6]*Faculty of Medical and Health Sciences, Pharmacy, University of Auckland, Auckland, New Zealand*

*Corresponding author

ABSTRACT

Chronic metabolic disorders, including type 2 diabetes, obesity, and dyslipidemia, have been closely linked to accelerated aging. While aging is a multifactorial process influenced by genetic, environmental, and

Pharmacotherapy Approaches Toward Endocrine and Metabolic Diseases.
Thakur Gurjeet Singh and Sanjana Mehta (Eds.)

DOI: 10.1201/9781779640154-6

lifestyle factors, its intertwining with metabolic disorders highlights an intricate molecular landscape. A vital component of this interrelation is the dysregulation of the insulin/insulin-like growth factor-1 signaling pathway, which directly affects oxidative stress, mitochondrial function, and telomere length. This dysfunction is exacerbated by chronic low-grade inflammation, a hallmark of metabolic disorders. Such inflammation, primarily driven by the activation of the nuclear factor-kappa B pathway, induces DNA damage, promotes cellular senescence, and deteriorates tissue function. A perturbed autophagy system further intensifies this aging process by failing to clear cellular waste, compromising overall cell health. Moreover, the downregulation of sirtuins, proteins that play pivotal roles in lifespan extension, hinders their capacity to manage DNA repair, control inflammation, and regulate metabolic processes. Collectively, these molecular interactions elucidate the accelerated aging seen in individuals with chronic metabolic conditions. Future research aiming at untangling these mechanisms could offer therapeutic strategies to mitigate aging and metabolic disorders.

6.1 INTRODUCTION

As the global population continues to age, the prevalence of chronic metabolic disorders, such as diabetes and obesity, has reached alarming proportions. With this demographic shift, many complicated molecular mechanisms underlie the aging process within the context of these metabolic disorders (Accili, 2003). Once considered a predictable and passive biological phenomenon, aging is increasingly recognized as a dynamic and regulated process with profound implications for health and disease (States, 2014).

Chronic metabolic disorders significantly contribute to accelerated aging, forming a complex interplay between genetic predisposition, environmental factors, and lifestyle choices (Cantó and Auwerx, 2009). The mechanisms of this relationship are multifaceted, involving a spectrum of cellular and molecular processes that influence the rate of aging at the molecular level (Fontana et al., 2010). The mechanism revolves around intricate signaling pathways, genomic instability, mitochondrial dysfunction, and alterations in cellular metabolism (Ekta et al., 2020).

One essential facet of the molecular mechanisms of aging in chronic metabolic disorders is the role of oxidative stress (Thapa et al., 2021). Excessive production of reactive oxygen species (ROS) overwhelms cellular antioxidant defenses, damaging biomolecules, including proteins, lipids, and DNA. This oxidative stress contributes to cellular dysfunction and accelerates aging, creating a vicious cycle that exacerbates metabolic disorders (Galluzzi et al., 2014).

Another critical aspect involves the impact of chronic inflammation on aging in metabolic disorders. Persistent low-grade inflammation, often called "inflammaging," is a hallmark of aging and metabolic dysfunction (Gupta et al., 2021). Inflammatory mediators, such as cytokines and chemokines, perpetuate the metabolic imbalance and foster an environment favorable to accelerated aging (Guarente, 2013).

Understanding the molecular mechanisms underlying aging in chronic metabolic disorders is paramount for developing targeted interventions to mitigate both adverse effects (Singh et al., 2020a). This knowledge can potentially unveil novel therapeutic strategies to promote healthy aging and ease the burden of chronic metabolic disorders on individuals and healthcare systems. In exploring the intricate molecular landscape, researchers strive to uncover the molecular keys that unlock the mysteries of aging in the context of chronic metabolic disorders, paving the way for innovative and personalized approaches to promote longevity and well-being.

6.2 INSULIN/INSULIN-LIKE GROWTH FACTOR-1 (IGF-1) SIGNALING PATHWAY

6.2.1 OVERVIEW OF INSULIN/IGF-1 SIGNALING PATHWAY

The insulin/IGF-1 signaling pathway is a crucial regulatory system that controls cellular growth, metabolism, and survival. It involves a complex network of molecular events initiated by binding insulin or IGF-1 to their respective receptors. Activation of these receptors triggers a cascade of intracellular events, ultimately influencing glucose uptake, protein synthesis, and cell proliferation (Hotamisligil, 2006).

6.2.2 IMPORTANCE OF THE INSULIN/IGF-1 SIGNALING PATHWAY AND DYSREGULATION IN METABOLIC DISORDERS

Maintaining proper insulin/IGF-1 signaling is essential for metabolic homeostasis. Dysregulation of this pathway is a hallmark of various metabolic disorders, including diabetes and obesity. In insulin resistance, a common feature of type 2 diabetes, cells become less responsive to insulin, leading to elevated blood glucose levels (Singh et al., 2020b). Dysfunctional IGF-1 signaling has also been implicated in metabolic disturbances and the progression of metabolic disorders (Galizzi and Di Carlo, 2022).

6.2.3 IMPLICATIONS FOR AGING IN THE CONTEXT OF CHRONIC METABOLIC DISORDERS

The link between the insulin/IGF-1 signaling pathway, metabolic disorders, and aging is a subject of intense research. Dysregulation of this pathway contributes to metabolic dysfunction and has profound implications for aging. Chronic activation of insulin/IGF-1 signaling has been associated with accelerated aging and age-related diseases (Tiwari et al., 2022). This phenomenon is often called the "insulin/IGF-1 signaling pathway paradox," where its beneficial effects on growth and survival during formative years can transform into detrimental effects on aging and age-related pathologies (López-Otín et al., 2013).

The dysregulation of insulin/IGF-1 signaling in metabolic disorders may contribute to accelerated aging through several mechanisms (Garg et al., 2022). Excessive signaling can increase oxidative stress, inflammation, and cellular aging. Additionally, impaired insulin sensitivity can disrupt nutrient sensing and energy homeostasis, further exacerbating the aging phenotype in individuals with metabolic disorders.

To understand the complicated mechanism between insulin/IGF-1 signaling, metabolic disorders, and aging, it is critical to develop interventions that address chronic diseases' metabolic and aging aspects. Targeting this pathway may hold promise in promoting healthy aging and mitigating the impact of metabolic disorders on age-related complications. Researchers aim to unravel the molecular details of how dysregulation in insulin/IGF-1 signaling contributes to the aging process in chronic metabolic disorders, providing potential avenues for therapeutic strategies to enhance longevity and well-being (Medzhitov, 2010).

6.3 OXIDATIVE STRESS AND MITOCHONDRIAL DYSFUNCTION

Oxidative stress in metabolism arises from an imbalance between the production of ROS and the ability of the cellular antioxidant defense mechanisms to neutralize them (Thapa et al., 2022). Mitochondrial dysfunction significantly contributes to oxidative stress in the context of metabolism, and its impact on cellular aging is significant. Here are some sources of oxidative stress in metabolism and how mitochondrial dysfunction plays a crucial role (Nita and Grzybowski, 2016).

- **Mitochondrial electron transport chain (ETC):** The mitochondria are the primary sites for cellular energy production through oxidative phosphorylation. During this process, electrons leak from the ETC, generating ROS as byproducts. Mitochondrial ETC dysfunction, often associated with aging and metabolic disorders, increases ROS production, contributing to oxidative stress (Nolfi-Donegan et al., 2020; Rehni et al., 2012).
- **Metabolism of fatty acids:** Fat metabolism, particularly in excess lipid availability, can increase ROS production. The breakdown of fatty acids in mitochondria during beta-oxidation generates electrons that can leak from the ETC, promoting oxidative stress.
- **Glucose metabolism:** Dysregulated glucose metabolism, as observed in conditions like insulin resistance and diabetes, can contribute to oxidative stress. Hyperglycemia (elevated blood glucose levels) can increase ROS production through various pathways, including activating protein kinase C and the hexosamine pathway.
- **Inflammation:** Chronic inflammation, a common feature of metabolic disorders, can stimulate immune cells to produce ROS. Inflammatory cytokines and mediators can induce oxidative stress in metabolic tissues, further exacerbating mitochondrial dysfunction.
- **Endoplasmic reticulum (ER) stress:** Disruption of ER homeostasis, known as ER stress, is implicated in metabolic disorders. ER stress can induce ROS production, contributing to oxidative stress. The relation between ER stress and mitochondrial dysfunction amplifies the impact on cellular aging (Minamino and Komuro, 2007).

6.3.1 THE IMPACT OF MITOCHONDRIAL DYSFUNCTION ON CELLULAR AGING

Mitochondrial dysfunction contributes to oxidative stress and plays a central role in aging by the following mechanisms:

- **Accumulation of DNA damage:** Mitochondria have DNA, and oxidative stress can damage mitochondrial DNA (mtDNA). Accumulated mtDNA damage contributes to cellular dysfunction and is implicated in aging.
- **Induction of apoptosis:** Severe mitochondrial dysfunction can trigger apoptotic pathways, leading to cell death. The loss of functional cells contributes to tissue degeneration and aging.
- **Impaired cellular energetics:** Mitochondrial dysfunction compromises energy production, leading to decreased cellular function. This energy deficit contributes to cellular aging and the decline in tissue and organ function associated with aging.

6.4 CHRONIC LOW-GRADE INFLAMMATION

Chronic low-grade inflammation is a prominent feature of many chronic metabolic disorders, and it plays a crucial role in the molecular mechanisms underlying aging in these conditions. The NF-κB (nuclear factor-kappa B) pathway is a central mediator of inflammation, and inflammation-driven cellular senescence contributes to the progression of age-related complications in chronic metabolic disorders (Murphy, 2009). Here is an overview of the mechanisms and mediators involved.

6.4.1 MECHANISMS AND MEDIATORS OF CHRONIC LOW-GRADE INFLAMMATION

- **Adipose tissue inflammation:** In obesity, enlarged adipose tissue secretes pro-inflammatory cytokines, such as tumor necrosis factor-alpha (TNF-α) and interleukin-6. Adipocytes, as well as infiltrating immune cells like macrophages, contribute to the chronic inflammatory milieu.
- **Insulin resistance:** Dysfunctional adipose tissue and increased levels of circulating fatty acids can induce insulin resistance.

Insulin-resistant cells release inflammatory mediators, perpetuating a state of chronic low-grade inflammation.

- **Mitochondrial dysfunction:** Impaired mitochondrial function, a joint in metabolic disorders, contributes to releasing ROS and damage-associated molecular patterns, activating inflammatory pathways.
- **ER stress:** Disturbed ER homeostasis, seen in conditions like obesity and diabetes, activates the unfolded protein response, leading to inflammation. ER stress is interconnected with mitochondrial dysfunction and oxidative stress.
- **Gut microbiota dysbiosis:** Alterations in the gut microbiota composition can lead to increased intestinal permeability and the translocation of bacterial products. This triggers an inflammatory response and systemic inflammation.
- **Role of NF-κB pathway:** The NF-κB pathway is a crucial regulator of inflammation and is activated in response to various stimuli, including proinflammatory cytokines, pathogens, and cellular stress.
- **Cytokine activation:** Proinflammatory cytokines, such as TNF-α and IL-1β, activate the NF-κB pathway. This activation initiates a transcriptional program leading to the expression of inflammatory genes.
- **Adipose tissue activation:** NF-κB is activated in adipose tissue, promoting the release of inflammatory mediators. Adipocytes and infiltrating immune cells contribute to NF-κB-mediated inflammation.
- **Insulin signaling disruption:** Activation of NF-κB can interfere with insulin signaling, exacerbating insulin resistance and promoting inflammation in metabolic tissues (Ristow and Schmeisser, 2011).

6.4.2 INFLAMMATION-DRIVEN CELLULAR SENESCENCE

Chronic inflammation contributes to cellular senescence, a state of irreversible cell cycle arrest. In the context of chronic metabolic disorders:

- **Senescence-associated secretory phenotype (SASP):** Senescent cells secrete various pro-inflammatory cytokines, growth factors, and proteases, collectively known as SASP. This perpetuates inflammation and contributes to tissue dysfunction.
- **Impact on tissue homeostasis:** The accumulation of senescent cells compromises tissue integrity and function, contributing to aging. Senescence in metabolic tissues exacerbates metabolic dysfunction and insulin resistance (Salminen et al., 2012).

6.5 AUTOPHAGY IN METABOLIC DISORDERS

Autophagy, a cellular self-digestion process, is fundamental in maintaining cellular homeostasis, especially in metabolic disorders. Here are the basic principles of autophagy, its dysregulation in metabolic diseases, and its intricate relationship with the aging process.

6.5.1 BASIC PRINCIPLES OF AUTOPHAGY

- **Autophagosome formation:** Autophagy begins by forming a double-membraned autophagosome structure, which engulfs cellular components targeted for degradation.
- **Cargo recognition:** Autophagy selectively targets damaged organelles, misfolded proteins, and other cellular components for degradation. Specific receptors and adaptors mediate the recognition of these cargo materials.
- **Lysosomal fusion:** Autophagosomes fuse with lysosomes, forming autolysosomes. The acidic and enzymatic environment of the lysosome facilitates the degradation of the engulfed cargo (Satoh et al., 2010).
- **Release of building blocks:** Degradation within autolysosomes breaks cellular components into basic building blocks such as amino acids, fatty acids, and sugars. These building blocks are then recycled for new cellular structures and energy production.

6.5.2 DYSREGULATION IN METABOLIC DISEASES

- **Insulin resistance and autophagy:** Insulin resistance, a hallmark of metabolic disorders like type 2 diabetes, is associated with impaired autophagy. Dysregulation of autophagy contributes to the accumulation of dysfunctional mitochondria and ER, exacerbating metabolic dysfunction.
- **Obesity and lipid metabolism:** In obesity, autophagy is often dysregulated in adipose tissue and the liver. Impaired autophagy can lead to the accumulation of lipid droplets, promoting lipotoxicity and insulin resistance.
- **Mitochondrial dysfunction:** Dysfunctional mitochondria are targeted for degradation by autophagy in a process known as mitophagy. Impaired mitophagy contributes to the accumulation of damaged mitochondria, increasing oxidative stress and metabolic dysfunction.
- **ER stress:** ER stress, present daily in metabolic diseases, can influence autophagy. Dysregulation of autophagy contributes to the accumulation of misfolded proteins, exacerbating ER stress and insulin resistance (Schieber and Chandel, 2014).

6.5.3 RELATIONSHIP WITH AGING

- **Decline in autophagic activity with age:** Autophagic activity tends to decline with aging, leading to the accumulation of damaged cellular components. This decline is associated with various age-related diseases, including metabolic disorders.
- **Impact on cellular senescence:** Autophagy mitigates cellular senescence by clearing damaged cellular components. Impaired autophagy can contribute to the accumulation of senescent cells, promoting inflammation and tissue dysfunction associated with aging.
- **Longevity and healthspan:** Enhanced autophagy has been linked to increased longevity and improved health span. Maintaining robust autophagic activity may help mitigate the impact of age-related metabolic disorders and promote healthy aging.

6.6 ROLE OF SIRTUINS IN AGING AND METABOLISM

Sirtuins are a family of evolutionarily conserved proteins that play a critical role in regulating cellular processes related to aging and metabolism. These proteins maintain genomic stability, promote DNA repair, influence energy metabolism, and modulate stress responses. Sirtuins are nicotinamide adenine dinucleotide (NAD+)-dependent deacetylases, meaning they require NAD^+ as a cosubstrate to remove acetyl groups from target proteins. The sirtuin family consists of seven members in mammals, labeled SIRT1–SIRT7, each with distinct cellular functions (Sacramento et al., 2024).

6.6.1 DOWNREGULATION IN METABOLIC DISORDERS

Sirtuin activity is often downregulated or dysregulated in metabolic disorders, such as obesity, type 2 diabetes, and metabolic syndrome. A decrease in sirtuin levels or function is associated with developing insulin resistance, impaired glucose metabolism, and other metabolic abnormalities. Several factors contribute to the downregulation of sirtuins in metabolic disorders, including nutrient excess, oxidative stress, and inflammation.

- **Excess nutrient:** High levels of nutrients, especially fatty acids, can inhibit sirtuin activity. This is particularly relevant in conditions of overnutrition and obesity, where elevated circulating fatty acids are prevalent.
- **Oxidative stress:** Increased oxidative stress, a common feature of metabolic disorders, can negatively impact sirtuin function. Sirtuins are involved in antioxidant defense mechanisms, and their downregulation contributes to a vicious cycle of oxidative damage.
- **Inflammation:** Chronic low-grade inflammation, characteristic of metabolic disorders, is linked to reduced sirtuin expression. Inflammatory signals can interfere with sirtuin activity, exacerbating metabolic dysfunction (Hamed et al., 2024).
- **Protective mechanisms in aging:** Despite their downregulation in metabolic disorders, sirtuins are recognized for their protective

roles in aging. Several mechanisms underlie their beneficial effects.

- **Metabolic regulation:** Sirtuins, particularly SIRT1, influence energy metabolism by regulating key transcriptional coactivators such as peroxisome proliferator-activated receptor-γ coactivator 1-α and Forkhead box, subgroup O. This can enhance mitochondrial function, promote fatty acid oxidation, and improve insulin sensitivity (Niccoli and Partridge, 2012).
- **DNA repair and genomic stability:** Sirtuins contribute to DNA repair mechanisms, helping to maintain genomic stability and prevent the accumulation of DNA damage over time. This is crucial for preserving cellular function during aging.
- **Longevity pathways:** Sirtuins are implicated in various longevity pathways, such as regulating sirtuin-activating compounds like resveratrol. Activation of sirtuins has been associated with increased lifespan in several model organisms (Mei et al., 2016).
- **Autophagy promotion:** Sirtuins regulate autophagy, the cellular recycling process. Enhanced autophagy facilitated by sirtuins helps remove damaged cellular components and promotes cellular health (Kenyon, 2010).

6.7 CONCLUSION AND FUTURE DIRECTION

In conclusion, the intricate molecular mechanisms governing the aging process within chronic metabolic disorders constitute a complex interplay of factors with profound implications for human health. The convergence of oxidative stress, chronic inflammation, dysregulated insulin/IGF-1 signaling, and impaired autophagy contributes to an accelerated aging phenotype, disrupting delicate cellular homeostasis and instigating a cascade of events that compromise tissue function. Our deepening understanding of these mechanisms suggests several crucial implications and future directions. Targeted therapeutic approaches hold substantial potential, as interventions tailored to modulate molecular pathways implicated in aging within metabolic disorders could offer novel and effective treatments. Precision medicine, acknowledging the heterogeneity within metabolic disorders and their influence on aging, emphasizes the need for personalized interventions that consider individual genetic, epigenetic, and lifestyle factors. Integrating systems biology approaches, exploring novel biomarkers, and understanding the impact of lifestyle interventions provide avenues for a comprehensive understanding of the molecular dynamics underlying aging in metabolic disorders. As breakthroughs continue, ethical considerations related to genetic manipulation, longevity, and societal impact must be carefully addressed. Ongoing research and technological advancements are poised to illuminate the intricate molecular connections between aging and chronic metabolic disorders, offering transformative therapeutic strategies that manage diseases, promote healthy aging, and enhance the global quality of life. The convergence of multidisciplinary research, technological innovation, and a commitment to translating scientific insights into clinical practice will undoubtedly shape the future landscape of this critical field.

KEYWORDS

- **aging**
- **chronic metabolic disorder**
- **type 2 diabetes**
- **obesity**
- **chronic low-grade inflammation**

REFERENCES

Accili, D. (2003). Perspectives in Diabetes. 13, 1633–1642.

Cantó, C., Auwerx, J. (2009). PGC-1alpha, SIRT1 and AMPK, an energy sensing network that controls energy expenditure. Current Opinion in Lipidology, 20(2), 98–105. https://doi.org/10.1097/MOL.0b013e328328d0a4

Ekta, Gupta, M., Kaur, A., Singh, T.G., Bedi, O. (2020). Pathobiological and molecular connections involved in the high fructose and high fat diet induced diabetes associated nonalcoholic fatty liver disease. Inflammation Research, 69(9), 851–867. https://doi.org/10.1007/s00011-020-01373-7

Fontana, L., Partridge, L., Longo, V.D. (2010). Extending healthy life span—from yeast to humans. Science (New York, N.Y.), 328(5976), 321–326. https://doi.org/10.1126/science.1172539

Galizzi, G., Di Carlo, M. (2022). Insulin and its key role for mitochondrial function/dysfunction and quality control: A shared link between dysmetabolism and neurodegeneration. Biology, 11(6), 943. https://doi.org/10.3390/biology11060943

Galluzzi, L., Pietrocola, F., Levine, B., Kroemer, G. (2014). Metabolic control of autophagy. Cell, 159(6), 1263–1276. https://doi.org/10.1016/j.cell.2014.11.006

Garg, C., Khan, H., Kaur, A., Singh, T.G., Sharma, V.K., Singh, S.K. (2022). Therapeutic implications of sonic hedgehog pathway in metabolic disorders: Novel target for effective treatment. Pharmacological Research, 179, 106194. https://doi.org/10.1016/j.phrs.2022.106194

Guarente, L. (2013). Calorie restriction and sirtuins revisited. Genes & Development, 27(19), 2072–2085. https://doi.org/10.1101/gad.227439.113.Freely

Gupta, M., Krishan, P., Kaur, A., Arora, S., Trehanpati, N., Singh, T.G., Bedi, O. (2021). Mechanistic and physiological approaches of fecal microbiota transplantation in the management of NAFLD. Inflammation Research, 70(7), 765–776. https://doi.org/10.1007/s00011-021-01480-z

Hamed, Y.M.F., Ghosh, B., Marshall, K.L. (2024). PIEZO ion channels: Force sensors of the interoceptive nervous system. The Journal of Physiology, 602(19), 4777–4788, https://doi.org/10.1113/JP284077

Hotamisligil G.S. (2006). Inflammation and metabolic disorders. Nature, 444(7121), 860–867. https://doi.org/10.1038/nature05485

Kenyon C.J. (2010). The genetics of ageing. Nature, 464(7288), 504–512. https://doi.org/10.1038/nature08980

López-Otín, C., Blasco, M.A., Partridge, L., Serrano, M., Kroemer, G. (2013). The hallmarks of aging. Cell, 153(6), 1194–1217. https://doi.org/10.1016/j.cell.2013.05.039

Medzhitov R. (2010). Inflammation 2010: New adventures of an old flame. Cell, 140(6), 771–776. https://doi.org/10.1016/j.cell.2010.03.006

Mei, Z., Zhang, X., Yi, J., Huang, J., He, J., Tao, Y. (2016). Sirtuins in metabolism, DNA repair and cancer. Journal of Experimental & Clinical Cancer Research: CR, 35(1), 182. https://doi.org/10.1186/s13046-016-0461-5

Minamino, T., Komuro, I. (2007). Vascular Cell Senescence. 1–8. https://doi.org/10.1161/01.RES.0000256837.40544.4a

Murphy M.P. (2009). How mitochondria produce reactive oxygen species. The Biochemical Journal, 417(1), 1–13. https://doi.org/10.1042/BJ20081386

Niccoli, T., Partridge, L. (2012). Ageing as a risk factor for disease. Current Biology: CB, 22(17), R741–R752. https://doi.org/10.1016/j.cub.2012.07.024

Nita, M., Grzybowski, A. (2016). The role of the reactive oxygen species and oxidative stress in the pathomechanism of the age-related ocular diseases and other pathologies of the anterior and posterior eye segments in adults. Oxidative Medicine and Cellular Longevity, 2016, 3164734. https://doi.org/10.1155/2016/3164734

Nolfi-Donegan, D., Braganza, A., Shiva, S. (2020). Mitochondrial electron transport chain: Oxidative phosphorylation, oxidant production, and methods of measurement. Redox Biology, 37, 101674. https://doi.org/10.1016/j.redox.2020.101674

Rehni, A.K., Singh, T.G., Arora, S. (2012). SU-6656, a selective Src kinase inhibitor, attenuates mecamylamine-precipitated nicotine withdrawal syndrome in mice. Nicotine & Tobacco Research, 14(4), 407–414. https://doi.org/10.1093/ntr/ntr228

Ristow, M., Schmeisser, S. (2011). Extending life span by increasing oxidative stress. Free Radical Biology & Medicine, 51(2), 327–336. https://doi.org/10.1016/j.freeradbiomed.2011.05.010

Sacramento, K.B., Melbourne, V.M., Auckland, L.B., Zealand, N., Dublin, R.C., Nottingham, P.G., Hamilton, K.L., Collins, F., Nashville, B.K., Omaha, H.D.S., Ottawa, K.T., Bath, S.W., Okazaki, Y.K., Vancouver, P.A., Nottingham, M.B., Kaohsiung, J.C., Auckland, J.D., Zealand, N., Dundalk, B.D., … Birmingham, A.H. (2024). Editor-in-Chief Deputy Editor-in-Chief opinions editor statistics editor senior ethics editor alex stewart managing editor. The Journal of Physiology, 602(5), 761–987. https://doi.org/10.1113/tjp.15583

Salminen, A., Kaarniranta, K., Kauppinen, A. (2012). Inflammaging: Disturbed interplay between autophagy and inflammasomes. Aging, 4(3), 166–175. https://doi.org/10.18632/aging.100444

Satoh, A., Brace, C.S., Ben-Josef, G., West, T., Wozniak, D.F., Holtzman, D.M., Herzog, E.D., Imai, S. (2010). SIRT1 promotes the central adaptive response to diet restriction through activation of the dorsomedial and lateral nuclei of the hypothalamus. The Journal of Neuroscience, 30(30), 10220–10232. https://doi.org/10.1523/JNEUROSCI.1385-10.2010

Schieber, M., Chandel, N.S. (2014). ROS function in redox signaling and oxidative stress. Current Biology: CB, 24(10), R453–R462. https://doi.org/10.1016/j.cub.2014.03.034

Singh, R., Rao, H.K., Singh, T.G. (2020a). Advanced glycated end products (ages) in diabetes and its complications: An insight. Plant Arch, 20(1), 3838–3841

Singh, T.G., Sharma, R., Kaur, A., Dhiman, S., Singh, R. (2020b). Evaluation of renoprotective potential of Ficus religiosa in attenuation of diabetic nephropathy in rats. Obesity Medicine, 19, 100268

States, I. (2014). Insulin Receptor Signaling in Normal.

Thapa, K., Singh, T.G., Kaur, A. (2021). Cyclic nucleotide phosphodiesterase inhibition as a potential therapeutic target in renal ischemia reperfusion injury. Life Sciences, 282, 119843. https://doi.org/10.1016/j.lfs.2021.119843

Thapa, K., Singh, T.G., Kaur, A. (2022). Targeting ferroptosis in ischemia/reperfusion renal injury. Naunyn-Schmiedeberg's Archives of Pharmacology, 395(11), 1331–1341. https://doi.org/10.1007/s00210-022-02277-5

Tiwari, P., Khan, H., Singh, T.G., Grewal, A.K. (2022). Poly (ADP-ribose) polymerase: An overview of mechanistic approaches and therapeutic opportunities in the management of stroke. Neurochemical Research, 47(7), 1830–1852. https://doi.org/10.1007/s11064-022-03595-z

CHAPTER 7

Menkes Kinky Hair Syndrome

NAVJYOTI GOYAL[1], SUMEET GUPTA[1], SARITA SHARMA[1], RUBY BHATIA[2], NASIR A. SIDDIQUI[3], and SHEENAM SHARMA[1*]

[1]*M.M. College of Pharmacy, Maharishi Markandeshwar (Deemed to Be University), Mullana, Ambala, Haryana, India*

[2]*Maharishi Markandeshwar Institute of Medical Science and Research (MMIMSR), Mullana, Ambala, Haryana, India*

[3]*Department of Pharmacognosy, King Saud University, Riyadh, Saudi Arabia*

*Corresponding author

ABSTRACT

Menkes disease (MD), also called Menkes syndrome, kinky hair disease, or copper transport disease, is a rare, X-linked recessive disorder of copper (Cu) metabolism affecting primarily male infants. It is caused by mutations in the *ATP7A* gene, which disrupt copper transport and utilization, leading to deficiency in Cu-dependent enzymes vital for normal development. This impairment affects multiple systems, particularly the brain, bones, liver, arteries, and hair. Copper accumulates in tissues like the kidneys and intestinal lining, while being deficient in other areas, causing diverse clinical manifestations. Infants with MD often present with symptoms such as hypothermia, hypoglycemia, prolonged jaundice, hypotonia, seizures, and delayed development. Distinctive features include brittle, kinky hair, osteoporosis, and intellectual disability. The condition is usually fatal, with death commonly occurring before the age of three. The estimated prevalence ranges from 1 in 35,000 to 50,000 live male births.

Pharmacotherapy Approaches Toward Endocrine and Metabolic Diseases.
Thakur Gurjeet Singh and Sanjana Mehta (Eds.)

DOI: 10.1201/9781779640154-7

Early diagnosis is difficult due to vague clinical signs and nonspecific molecular markers, yet it is critical for genetic counseling and timely treatment. Although there is no definitive cure, early administration of parenteral copper histidine—within the first 28 days of life—can improve survival and neurological outcomes. Better understanding of MD is essential for effective clinical management.

7.1 INTRODUCTION

Menkes disease (MD) is a fatal disease of Cu metabolism in the body associated with an X-linked chromosome. Despite severe clinical courses prescribed to patients, several deaths in early childhood have been reported (Roach and Miller, 2004). Among various forms of this disease, occipital horn syndrome (OHS) is known to be less mild or moderate form. The faulty gene in MD is expected to encode ATPase Copper Transporting Alpha (ATP7A), which is involved in exporting excess Cu from cells and transporting Cu to the secreted Cu enzymes (Steinmann et al., 2002; Kaur et al., 2021).

Copper (Cu) is a crucial trace element needed to develop the nervous system properly. Several biological functions are necessary, such as myelin formation and synthesis of connective tissue in the body. It is requisite by cuproenzymes such as ceruloplasmin; it acts as a significant systemic protein transporter for Cu and lysyl oxidase, necessary for initializing the cross-linkage of connective tissues via oxidizing peptidyl lysine in elastin and collagen (Solomons, 1985; Rehni et al., 2010). Cu is necessary for cellular metabolism, and the Cu transporter CTR1 (copper transport protein 1) is recognized as a crucial regulator of cellular absorption of Cu in the intestinal and hepatic epithelium. Several chaperones circulate Cu to specific proteins or cell organelles, including antioxidant 1 (ATOX1), chaperone of Cu, and human cytochrome c oxidase Cu chaperone (hCOX17). While ATP7B circulates Cu in the liver and ceruloplasmin and controls biliary excretion, ATP7A carries Cu from enterocytes into the blood circulation (Kaler, 2011; Singh et al., 2019).

Several genes, including divalent metal transporter 1, another modulator of Cu uptake, and CTR1, a high-affinity Cu transporter, mediate Cu metabolism. ATOX1, a crucial gene in Cu transport, removes Cu from the cell's cytosol to the transporters (ATP7A and ATP7B). The Golgi network contains ATP7A and ATP7B. ATP7A moves Cu in the blood, whereas ATP7B oversees ceruloplasmin maturation. With 23 exons, ATP7A, found at chromosome Xq21.1, spans around 150 kb of genomic DNA (González et al., 2008; Kumar et al., 2023). ATP7A belongs to the P-type ATPase P1B-subfamily. The transmembrane P-type ATPase that transports Cu is encoded by this gene (Di Donato and Sarkar, 1997). Cu-transporting ATPases, or Cu-ATPases, mediate Cu transport, growth, development, and several physiological functions of Cu. Cu-ATPases move Cu from the cell's cytosol across the plasma membrane, reducing intracellular Cu levels and controlling the body's Cu homeostasis (Baeza et al., 2012).

Genetic anomalies in the Cu-ATPase encoding ATP7A gene are associated with X-linked distal spinal muscular atrophy, OHS, and a catastrophic neurological disorder termed MD. Given the widespread expression of ATP7A in extrahepatic organs and cells, MD or OHS patients' systemic abnormalities result from its deficiency or inactivation (De Bie et al., 2007; Singh et al., 2022). Two types of MD have been identified: mild MD and classic MD. Mild MD is a less severe form of MD based on its symptoms. Atypical "kinky" hair and neurological abnormalities are the hallmarks of classical MD (Beyens et al., 2019; Sharma and Singh, 2020). Mutations in the ATP7A gene alter intracellular Cu transport, severely compromising Cu absorption in MD. OHS patients are characterized by "occipital horns," a downward-pointing exostosis (benign outgrowth) arising from the occipital bone, as well as a few anomalies of the connective tissue, including cutis laxa (connective tissue disorder), hernias, joint hypermobility, and bladder diverticula (protrusions of the bladder) (Kennerson et al., 2010). Table 7.1 represents the clinical phenotype of ATP7A-linked disorders.

Depending on the demographic studied, incidence estimates for MD vary from 1/50,000 to 1/360,000 live births, making it a very uncommon condition. A dysfunctional ATP7A causes a systemic Cu shortage because it stops dietary Cu from being absorbed and is necessary for directed transport across polarized epithelial cells like intestinal enterocytes (Gohil, 2021). Children with MD often die in the triennial of life due to Cu deficiency, which causes distinctive kinky hair, unusual lack of skin color, abnormalities in connective tissue, convulsions, and progressive neurodegeneration. A milder type of MD called OHS has been linked to partial loss-of-function ATP7A mutations (Panichsillaphakit et al., 2022). OHS individuals are

TABLE 7.1 Clinical Phenotype of ATP7A-Linked Disorders

ATP7A-Linked Disorder	Age of Onset	Clinical Features
Menkes disease	0–8 months	Kinky hair; floppy infant; severe metabolic disorders of lysosomes, mitochondria, and peroxisomes; dysautonomia, osteoporosis, hemorrhages, bladder, and bowel diverticula; poor mobility; no head control; severe mental retardation; connective tissue abnormality; neurodegeneration
Mild MD	2–3 years	Coarse hair, dysautonomia; mild initial course; clinical diagnosis difficult; minimal to moderate connective tissue dysfunction; skeletal dysplasia; walk with difficulty; and, with the use of aid, moderately retarded; slow and dull
Classical MD	2–3 months	Coarse hair; dysautonomia; initial course milder; clinical diagnosis difficult; connective tissue dysfunction present; skeletal dysplasia may occur; wheelchair bound; cannot sit unsupported; mentally retarded
Occipital horn syndrome	Childhood	Coarse hair; X-linked family history; connective tissue problems; muscle affection; dysautonomia; exostoses on occipital bones; skeletal dysplasia; cutis laxa; hyperextensible joints; vascular complications: walking independently, appearing clumsy, slow, or dull to average IQ

associated with connective tissue and hair abnormalities like MD patients, although their neurological symptoms are less severe.

Moreover, it has been found that AP1S1 (σ1A subunit of adaptor protein complex I) mutations in MD patients affect intracellular trafficking of the Cu transporters ATP7A and ATP7B (Kaler, 2011). X-linked distal hereditary motor neuropathy has been connected to missense mutations in the carboxyl half of ATP7A. For these illnesses, there is currently no proven therapy. Nonetheless, some MD patients may benefit from early Cu-histidine treatment, primarily if the mutant ATP7A still functions somewhat (Kaler et al., 2008).

MD is a recessive X-linked disorder of Cu metabolism characterized by aberrant hair development, abnormalities in connective tissues, and progressive loss of both the structure and functions of neurons (Danks et al., 1972; Chelly et al., 1993). In Japan, the incidence of MD is one in 360,000 people, making it incredibly rare (Tümer and Møller, 2010). Mutations in the ATP7A gene, found on chromosome Xq13.3, result in ATP7A malfunction, which causes MD (Vulpe et al., 1993; Gu et al., 2005). ATP7A transports Cu from the cell's cytosol to the Golgi complex, which is integrated into enzymes that need Cu and then secreted by the cells. A mutation in ATP7A in intestinal cells causes Cu to build up in the intestines and prevents Cu from being absorbed, which causes Cu insufficiency throughout the body, including the brain. Most clinical features of multiple sclerosis are caused by reduced activity of Cu-dependent enzymes, including cytochrome c oxidase, dopamine β-hydroxylase, and lysyl oxidase, which are associated with Cu shortage (Mercer et al., 1993; Kodama et al., 1999). Neurological abnormalities manifest between two and three months of age if left untreated.

Due to vascular anomalies, many of these patients are immobile and experience persistent seizures, trouble eating, and cerebral hemorrhage (Kodama et al., 2012). Most MD patients who are not diagnosed or treated promptly die at the age of less than three years. Parenteral delivery of Cu-histidine injections is the current therapy for MD. While starting therapy after the newborn period does not help neurological problems, it can somewhat avoid neurological symptoms with a better clinical outcome if therapy is started during the neonatal period. As a result, therapy must begin as soon as possible (Sarkar et al., 1993). A family history of MD, such as older brothers, cousins, or uncles who have had the disease in the past, facilitates the identification of MD in pregnant or neonatal patients. However, these situations are uncommon. A diagnosis of MD is often given when the infant is two months old when neurological abnormalities such as seizures have started to manifest (Kaler et al., 2008).

7.1.1 CLASSICAL MD

Up to the age of two or three months, infants seem healthy. At that point, they start to fail to thrive, exhibit hypotonia and seizures, and lose early developmental milestones. When newborns have typical neurologic abnormalities and concurrent distinctive changes in their hair (short, sparse, coarse, twisted, frequently weakly colored) and facial jowls, classic MD is typically initially recognized. In newborns, nonspecific symptoms such as transient low blood glucose levels, extended physiologic jaundice, and constant temperature fluctuations may be observed. Cerebrovascular accidents and subdural hematomas are also prevalent. Classic MD develops into severe neurodegeneration and mortality, usually between the ages of seven months and 3.5 years, despite the early initiation of daily subcutaneous Cu injections. Pneumonia frequently triggers cardiorespiratory failure, which is a prevalent cause of mortality. Cerebellar and cerebral atrophy, ventriculomegaly, delayed myelination, and vascular tortuosity are all visible in brain imaging. Mild MD patients can learn to speak in formal language and walk independently. Some neurological symptoms include ataxia, tremors, weakness, and head bobbing. Seizures often begin in mid-to-late infancy, if at all; intellectual damage is negligible. Connective tissue disorder may be more prevalent than in traditional medicine (Kaler and DiStasio, 2021).

7.1.2 OCCIPITAL HORN SYNDROME

The main clinical characteristics of OHS, the mildest MD currently known, are connective tissue-related. The radiographic detection of distinctive occipital horns is the primary differentiator between OHS and the other types of MD. These are down-pointing, symmetrical exostoses that extend from the occipital bone. At birth, there may be loose, wrinkled skin and an inguinal or umbilical hernia. Hypotonia, jaundice, hypothermia, and feeding difficulties might appear in a few days. Clinical issues become evident gradually; persistent diarrhea or repeated urinary tract infections (UTIs) may be the initial symptoms that prompt a parent to take their kid to the doctor. Despite these issues, OHS is typically only diagnosed in children between the ages of five and 10. A delay in motor development brought on by muscular hypotonia is associated with unusual clumsiness. Height is frequently average despite the prevalence of mild disproportions, including a long trunk, narrow chest and shoulders, thoracolumbar kyphosis or scoliosis, and pectus deformity; the joints move freely. Unusual facial features include long, thin faces with large noses, high foreheads, down-slanting eyes, big ears, long philtrums, and high-arching palates. The inguinal hernia frequently recurs. In addition, arterial aneurysms have also been reported. One specific issue is orthostatic hypotension. The characteristics of the clinical history include elbow limitations, joint instability in the inferior extremities, orthostatic syncope, recurrent UTIs, bladder diverticula with intermittent spontaneous bladder ruptures, and chronic diarrhea. Surgery may be necessary in some instances due to insufficient mitral valve tissue, spontaneous retinal ablation, or severe progressive thoracolumbar kyphosis. OHS is expected to have a significantly longer life than MD (Tümer and Møller, 2010).

7.1.3 CELLULAR CU METABOLISM

An energy-independent membrane transporter (CTR1) is suspected to be used for Cu absorption across the cellular membrane (Lee et al., 2002). The cytoplasm contains Cu-specific chaperones, tiny proteins that bind to Cu to protect the cell from the harmful effects of free ions (Formigari et al., 2007; Speisky et al., 2009). The three identified Cu-chaperons, copper chaperone for superoxide dismutase, ATOX1, and cytochrome *c* oxidase copper chaperone (COX17), direct the Cu ion to different cell areas, facilitating efficient metal transport to the enzymes (Culotta et al., 2006). The proteins COX11, SCO1 (synthesis of cytochrome *c* oxidase), and SCO2 are among those involved in COX Cu metalation, while COX17 directs Cu to mitochondria, where it is integrated into COX (Turski and Thiele, 2009). ATOX1 carries Cu to the trans-Golgi network (TGN), which is incorporated into secretory-produced enzymes that need Cu. Two homologous membrane-bound, Cu-specific ATPases, ATP7A and ATP7B (defective in MD and Wilson disease, respectively), transport Cu over the membrane and into the TGN lumen. Cu is then supplied to secrete enzymes within the TGN lumen (Hamza et al., 2003). Accordingly, ATP7B in hepatocytes incorporates Cu into ceruloplasmin, whereas ATP7A is responsible for delivering Cu to tissue-specific enzymes (Camakaris et al., 1995). Apart from supplying Cu to enzymes via the secretory pathway, ATP7A (as well as ATP7B) manages the ATP-stimulated release of Cu from cells (Monty et al., 2005). ATP7A is localized to TGN at average physiological Cu concentrations and moves Cu to the Cu-dependent enzymes inside the lumen. When Cu concentrations rise, ATP7A translocate to vesicles or the plasma membrane (Petris et al., 1996) (Figure 7.1).

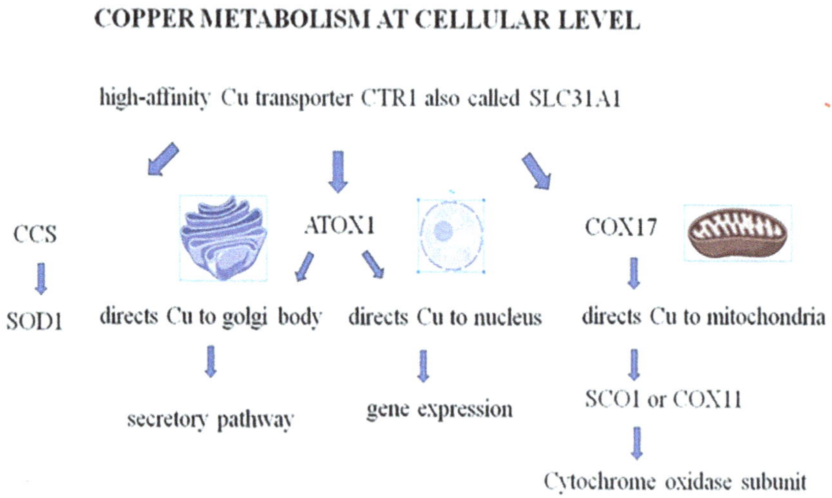

FIGURE 7.1 Cellular copper metabolism.

7.1.4 HOMEOSTASIS OF CU IN MD

The primary anomaly in MD is the removal of Cu from cells; almost every organ will accumulate Cu to excessively high levels, except for the liver and brain. This is caused by a combination of factors, including reduced intestinal absorption of Cu already present, impaired Cu transport from the epithelium of mucous membrane, and metallothionein scavenger function (Nishihara et al., 1998). The cause of the low Cu concentration in the livers of MD patients is different from that of normal livers, where ATP7B causes the low concentration of Cu as the primary Cu transporter but not ATP7A. The mammalian brain is one of the organs in the body with the highest concentration of Cu. While the exact mechanism regulating brain Cu levels is unknown, ATP7A must be involved because MD lowers Cu levels in the brain (Liu et al., 2005). In individuals with MD, Cu is probably trapped in the blood–cerebrospinal fluid and blood–brain barriers, depriving neurons and glial cells of Cu. This provides even more evidence for ATP7A's involvement in brain Cu absorption. Another sign of ATP7A inactivation in MD patients is neuronal demyelination. Apart from Cu-dependent enzyme deficit, ATP7A-related Cu release is mediated by stimulation of *N*-methyl-D-aspartate (NMDA) receptors, suggesting a new role for this protein in brain dysfunction. Thus, the dysfunction of NMDA receptors may lead to aberrant neuronal transmission, which in turn may correlate with seizures and neuronal degeneration in MD patients (Schlief et al., 2005) (Figure 7.2).

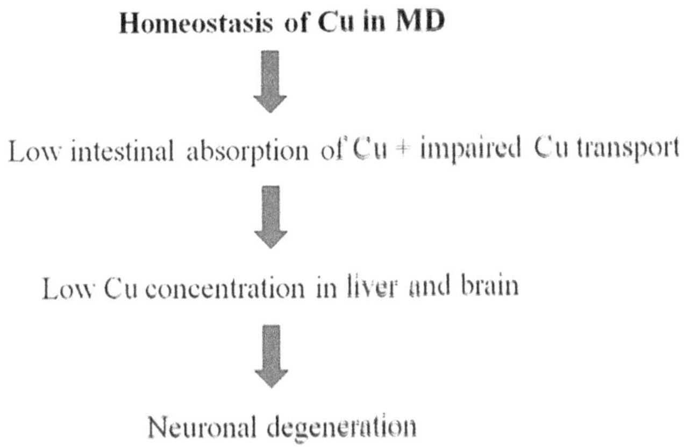

FIGURE 7.2 Homeostasis of copper in Menkes disease.

7.2 GENETIC BASIS OF STEELY HAIR DISEASE

Mutations in the X-linked ATP7A gene result in a lack of ATP7A activity, which causes MD, a rare and deadly genetic disorder of the Cu metabolism in humans (Kaler et al., 2008; Tümer, 2013). Both the export of extra Cu from the cells and the delivery of Cu to the secreted Cu-dependent enzymes are facilitated by the ATP7A protein (Møller et al., 2009). Duodenal enterocytes usually absorb dietary Cu in MD patients; nevertheless, the microelement's intracellular trafficking and bloodstream passage via the basolateral membrane are disrupted (Rehni et al., 2010; Lenartowicz et al., 2012a). Similarly, as ATP7A is known to participate in basolateral Cu transport recycling in healthy conditions, the amount of Cu recycled from the primary urine to the blood is decreased in these individuals due to ATP7A activity loss (Lenartowicz et al., 2012b). Cu, therefore, builds up in the renal cortex of the kidney and the epithelium of the small intestine. However, its concentration in the serum and other tissues—like the liver and brain—is deficient. Patients with MD have reduced cuproenzyme activity because of an internal Cu deficiency (Horn et al., 2019). This enzyme is required for multiple metabolic processes, such as the synthesis of tyrosinase pigment, peptidyl α-amidating monooxygenase neurotransmitter synthesis, superoxide dismutase 1 and 3 free radical detoxification, cytochrome *c* oxidase-mediated mitochondrial respiration, and lysyl oxidase connective tissue formation (La Fontaine and Mercer, 2007) (Figure 7.3).

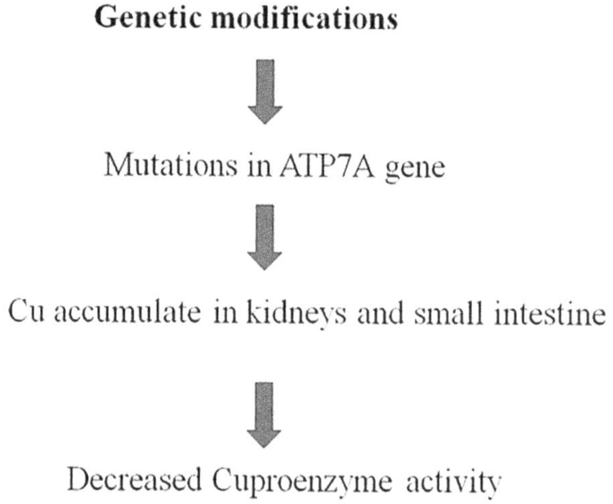

FIGURE 7.3 Genetic modifications in Menkes disease.

7.3 CLINICAL FEATURES OF TRICHOPOLIODYSTROPHY

Patients with classical MD frequently have a severe clinical history and pass away in their early years, usually by the age of three. The clinical picture of connective tissue dysfunction and increasing neurodegeneration are hallmarks of clinical MD (Chhabra et al., 2010; Yusoff et al., 2019). Most pregnancies and laborers are straightforward, and babies have standard anthropometry. The neonatal phase is characterized by clinical symptoms such as persistent jaundice, hypotonia, hypothermia, and feeding problems at birth. Cerebral hematoma and spontaneous fractures can occur from birth (Kim et al., 2019). The typical signs, which include distinctive skin and hair findings, often begin two months in advance. Although hair is normal at birth, it eventually becomes fine, thin, kinky, wiry, or steely. Notable facial traits include sagging, micrognathia, loose cutis, and blue iris. Other congenital disabilities include long arched palate, entropion, cerebellar hypoplasia, lung cystic alterations, and total atrioventricular block (Hicks et al., 2012).

MD in newborns is frequently overlooked due to its less-defined clinical and biochemical symptoms. Hypoglycemia, hypothermia, extended jaundice, cephalohematoma, and Pectus excavatum during delivery are possible presentations for the patient. Typical hair findings are frequently missing, and microscopic hair findings are not visible in the early stages of life. A more accurate and quicker test that diagnoses the patient before symptoms start is vital. It takes many weeks for the last diagnostic test, Cu egress in cultured fibroblast, to provide findings. Placental Cu concentrations and plasma catecholamine analysis are two of these recently approved assays (Verrotti et al., 2014).

Neurological symptoms most frequently characterize MD. Seizures and developmental regression often begin two to three months after each other. Infections or fevers bring on seizures. Additional manifestations of the condition include repeated bouts of apnea and nonconvulsive convulsions. There are three distinct phases in the development and progression of seizures in MD illness. The early stage often shows up between two and three months of age as focal clonic seizures that progress to status epilepticus, frequently accompanied by a fever. The reason might be a fluctuating disruption in the blood supply caused by a tortuosity in the vessels. At a mean age of 9.5 months, the intermediate stage usually begins as an uncontrollable infantile spasm. One possible cause might be neuronal degeneration in the subcortical regions, such as the thalamus and basal ganglia. Due to increasing cortical degeneration, late-stage patients exhibit multifocal myoclonic seizures and tonic spasms at a mean age of 24 months (Jain et al., 2014). Additional notable discoveries comprise neuroregression. The patient does not speak, but he or she does develop specific motor abilities. Growth limitation has also been linked to underwhelming outcomes.

MD is frequently associated with skeletal deformities and malfunction of the connective tissues. One of the most well-established causes of seizures is fluctuating blood flow, as well as tortuous blood arteries. Phlebectasia, or dilation of the internal jugular vein, and brachial artery aneurysms have been documented (Price et al., 2007). Another sign of poor connective tissue growth is loose, wrinkly skin. In addition, muscular hypotonia and other connective tissue abnormalities cause a delay in motor development. Bone abnormalities include lengthy bone fractures, Pectus excavatum or carinatum, Wormian bones in the head, and osteopenia. In these cases, fractures to the ribs, skull, and metaphysis are frequently misinterpreted as child abuse. Osteoporosis can be effectively managed, and bone mineral density increases with palidronate medication (Moon et al., 2017). Anomalies of the eyes include strabismus, abnormal eyelashes, iris stromal hypoplasia, blue iris, and hypopigmented peripheral retina (Gasch et al., 2002).

Patients with MD have dysautonomia symptoms, which are linked to aberrant catecholamine production because of dopamine beta-hydroxylase defects. Wide-ranging digestive symptoms include the possibility of colonic diverticula, reflux illness, gastric polyps, and developing hiatal hernias. Hepatomegaly in MD has been reported. A gastrostomy tube is frequently required for patients who have severe developmental failure and gastrointestinal issues. Urinary tract problems are a significant feature of MD, with bladder diverticula being the most prevalent presentation. There have been documented cases of cryptorchidism, vesicoureteral reflux, and renal rupture. According to reports, pneumonia and recurrent infections are two prominent causes of morbidity and death in MD (Kim et al., 2019).

7.4 DIAGNOSTIC APPROACH OF MD

The characteristics of MD and OHS include low quantities of Cu in some tissues due to reduced intestinal absorption and decreased activity of Cu-dependent enzymes, including lysyl oxidase and dopamine-beta-hydroxylase (DBH). Interestingly, healthy babies have low serum Cu and ceruloplasmin levels in the first few months of life; hence, these biomarkers are unsuitable for diagnostic tools in infants under two months of age (Mehta et al., 2022). *ATP7A*-associated, the most typical method of confirming Cu transport abnormalities, is to find a heterozygous *ATP7A* variant in a female with X inactivation or an X-autosome translocation or a hemizygous ATP7A variant in a man (the latter examples being exceedingly unusual). Approaches for molecular genetic testing include two panels as follows—using a multigene panel and testing single genes:

- Single-gene testing—Initially, the sequencing of *ATP7A* is conducted to detect splice site variations, missense, nonsense mutations, and minor intragenic deletions or insertions. This single-gene testing aims to identify any alterations or abnormalities within the *ATP7A* gene.
- A multigene panel—Other relevant genes, such as *ATP7B*, could also be considered (Kaler and DiStasio, 2021).

In cases where molecular genetic testing fails to detect a pathogenic variant in ATP7A, further biochemical investigations can be pursued to provide additional insights. These studies aim to shed light on the underlying biochemical mechanisms and offer a compelling presentation of the findings. Catecholamine analysis of plasma, cerebrospinal fluid. Males with OHS/or typical MD had distinctly aberrant plasma catechol concentrations at all ages. A partial lack of DBH, an enzyme that is reliant on Cu and essential to produce catecholamines, is indicated by abnormal levels (Manara et al., 2017). The diagnosis of MD is mainly based on neuroimaging. The two most often seen characteristics on a magnetic resonance imaging (MRI) are postponed myelination and brain atrophy. Additional features include leuko-encephalopathy, hematoma and hygroma, subdural effusion, anomalies in the basal ganglia signal, and intracranial vascular tortuosity (Rangarh and Kohli, 2018). Tumefactive demyelinating lesions on MRI are quite prevalent before 10 months. There have also been reports of hyperintense drop-shaped lesions with limited diffusion in the centrum semivalve (Loeffler, 2023). Thrombotic occlusion and artery-to-artery embolism, which result from irregular and chaotic circulation in a twisted blood vessel, can cause cerebral infarctions (Bindu et al., 2013). Apart from the previously mentioned results, a significant degree of vascular tortuosity strongly suggests MD Compared to standard MRI, these vascular alterations are more noticeable (White et al., 1993). As the illness progresses, MD electroencephalogram (EEG) exhibits three distinct phases. While interictal EEG displays multifocal polymorphic waves, ictal observations during the initial phase indicate sluggish spike waves and deceleration in the posterior region. In the intermediate phase, multifocal hyperarrhythmia is present, characterized by widespread irregular slow and spike waves. Mixed irregular slow waves and multifocal high-amplitude activity are characteristics of the late stage (Morris et al., 1999). The X-ray findings include metaphyseal flare, lengthy bone spurs, and widespread osteoporosis. Thickenings and periosteal diaphyseal responses are seen. Misdiagnoses of rib fractures due to child abuse are common. In the absence of retinal hemorrhage, babies with unexplained subdural hematomas should have MD ruled out as a differential diagnosis (Kreuder et al., 1993).

7.5 PHARMACOLOGICAL TREATMENT OF GENETIC DISEASE

In its severe forms, MD is a progressive condition that can cause mortality in early childhood; however, some people manage to live until the age of five. Nonetheless, life expectancy may be increased by up to 13 years or more with proper medical attention and perhaps Cu supplementation (Christodoulou et al., 1998). There have been several documented cases of MD patients with severe illness and extended life. Specific therapy for MD aims to increase Cu in the tissues and Cu-dependent enzymes. Since Cu becomes stuck in the intestines, oral delivery of Cu is inefficient; parenteral or subcutaneous Cu supplementation is preferable. Cu-histidine is the most successful Cu compound currently on the market (Kaler et al., 2008). At least partly functioning *ATP7A* and early commencement are prerequisites for a positive Cu–Cu-histidine supplementation result. Early subcutaneous Cu-histidine treatment has shown promising results in 12 younger children (Hui et al., 2021).

Replacing Cu results in minor therapeutic improvements, such as decreased seizure frequency and decreased irritability, but does not guarantee significant neurologic improvement in all patients with MD. Since Cu treatment offers relatively few advantages, parents should be involved in decision-making. In situations when the diagnosis is made prior to the onset of neurologic impairment, Cu replacement is unquestionably needed since, in certain circumstances, it may be feasible to stop further neurodegeneration (Ueki et al., 1985).

Overconsumption of Cu has been linked to proximal renal tubule damage. The underlying cause of this occurrence can be attributed to the inherent inclination of individuals with MD to accumulate Cu within their renal system. Nonetheless, the clinical significance of this side effect is usually negligible as renal losses rarely escalate to a point where oral bicarbonate supplementation is required (Donsante et al., 2011).

- The interaction between Cu and metallothionein may be limited by vitamin C.
- Diethyldithiocarbamate, a derivative of carbamic acid.
- Vitamin E and brain-directed viral gene therapy (Sato et al., 2009; Mehta et al., 2021).

The state of MD does not present an increased risk of anesthesia-related complications. However, various surgical scenarios may occur in MD that require careful consideration and management.

- Myringotomy tubes: used to treat persistent otitis media.
- Gastrostomy tube: used to address feeding issues.
- Repairing bladder diverticula (Ydemann et al., 2018).

According to Guthrie et al., the brain's levels of cytochrome c oxidase were elevated, and Cu was transported to the mitochondria via the tiny molecule elesclomol. Using this approach, elesclomol prevented negative changes in the neurological system and increased the lifespan of the mottled-brindled mouse. Consequently, elesclomol exhibits potential in treating MD and other associated disorders caused by inherited Cu deficiency. Their study demonstrated that the ES-Cu^{2+} (elesclomol–copper) complex's unique approach of selectively releasing mitochondrial Cu effectively addresses the malfunction of CTR1 and *ATP7A* membrane-Cu transport. This leads to a targeted and beneficial enhancement in mitochondrial cytochrome c oxidase metalation. Based on his research, ES or ES-Cu^{2+} exhibits potential as a feasible and efficient therapeutic agent for addressing inherited Cu-deficiency diseases in cardiac Ctr1 Knockout and mottled-brindled mice (Guthrie et al., 2020).

A model of MD was developed by Haberkiewicz et al. using mosaic mutant mice that showed functional failure of *ATP7A*. Despite renal Cu excess, which is improved by Cu treatment and essential for extending these mice's life span, the animals have systemic Cu insufficiency. The primary objective of this study was to investigate the expression of *Slc31a1* and *Slc31a2* genes, responsible for encoding CTR1/CTR2 proteins, along with the cellular localization of the CTR1 protein in nursing, juvenile, and adult mosaic mutants. The study results indicate that the CTR1 mRNA level in the kidney of both intact and Cu-injected 14-day-old mutants with high renal Cu content remains unaltered, unlike wild-type mice injected with Cu. Compared to intact wild-type animals, 45-day-old mice have considerably lower levels of *Slc31a1* gene expression. Cu-injected sucking and juvenile mutants exhibit resocialization of the CTR1 protein from the apical membrane to the cytoplasm of proximal tubule epithelial cells. Through this process, cells are protected from Cu toxicity, and Cu transport from the primary urine is inhibited (Haberkiewicz et al., 2022).

7.6 CASE REPORT ON CU TRANSPORT DISEASE

A four-year-old MD kid who experienced a burst ureter—an uncommon consequence of a ureteric stone—was the subject of a case study by Hui et al. UTI, retroperitoneal abscess, and sepsis are possible outcomes. Many instances that have been recorded are linked to ureteric stones; connective tissue abnormalities or blockage of the bladder outflow are less common. Therefore, in addition to other predisposing urological or systemic variables, the patient may have had a ureteric rupture due to urea-splitting organisms producing urinary tract stones as a result of recurrent UTIs. Additionally, the tubular dysfunction exhibited by the patient was marked by an involvement of both the proximal and distal tubules. Urinary anion gap data were complicated by the patient's persistent diarrhea, making interpretation challenging. Urinary electrolyte wasting, widespread aminoaciduria, and β-2-microglobulinuria in this patient supported tubular dysfunction. For children with MD, urinary β-2-microglobulin levels have been used as a diagnostic tool for proximal tubular dysfunction associated with Cu-histidine therapy. Patient's results, however, suggest that children with MD, especially those who have had Cu-histidine therapy, could require routine evaluations of their renal performance, tubular performance, and electrolyte profile (Hui et al., 2021).

According to Pawar et al., a four-month-old kid who had been healthy before suddenly developed an acute episode of protracted, recurring seizures. A decline followed this in neurodevelopment, fragility, and hypopigmentation of the hair shaft. A brain MRI revealed extensive intracranial tortuosity; an EEG revealed electrical status epilepticus; and a generalized subcortical white matter abnormality with low serum Cu and ceruloplasmin were also observed. Furthermore, sequencing of the whole genome genetic analysis that supported the diagnosis of MD identified a hemizygous pathogenic variant at 2179G>A p (Gly727Arg). Antiepileptic medication was used for symptomatic treatment in addition to an immediate referral to a state-of-the-art facility for interdisciplinary medical attention and treatment with Cu-histidine replacement (Pawar and Mir, 2022).

According to Bhat et al., a boy, two years old, showed up at eight months old with kinky hair, recurrent hypotonia, and developmental regression. Low blood levels of ceruloplasmin (18 mg/dl) and Cu (5 mg/dl) and deletion/duplication analysis, focused on specific genes performed by the reference lab, were the basis for diagnosing MD. An MRI of the brain revealed typical MD vascular tortuosity and moderate hypoplasia of the cerebellar vermis. Immediately, Cu chloride therapy was started. The infant started to walk purposefully and showed superb eye contact as they became more awake. The youngster was admitted to the hospital due to recurring respiratory infections, which multiplex polymerase chain reaction proved were caused by enterovirus. He hypothesized that the aberrant Fenton chemistry within phagosomes caused by inadequate Cu incorporation in the endoplasmic reticulum might account for the malfunction of natural killer cells in a typical MD (Bhat and Maertens, 2020).

7.7 PARENTAL EDUCATION AND COUNSELING

Preventing MD includes administering subcutaneous injections of Cu-histidine, which improves neurodevelopmental outcomes and increases survival starting at age 28 days (adjusted for preterm and gestational age).

- Classical MD—Seizure control under a neurologist; prompt action and a tailored plan for education under a developmental pediatrician; feeding therapy and insertion of a gastrostomy tube to increase energy intake; preventive use of antibiotics to avoid UTIs and bladder surgery for diverticulitis; vaccination against influenza, COVID, and respiratory syncytial virus because of the risk of recurrent pneumonia.
- OHS—A developmental pediatrician could advise early academic help, a personalized education plan, bladder diverticula surgery, and antibacterial prevention when necessary. Other potential therapies for dysautonomia include physical therapy, and for joint splints, consult a rheumatologist or orthopedist (Tussolini et al., 2023).

Prenatal screening for high-risk pregnancies, pre-implantation genetic analysis, and heterozygote testing for female relatives at risk can all be done when a family member with the condition has been discovered to have a harmful mutation. MD can be prevented primarily with genetic counseling and prenatal diagnosis. Parents may be taught physical and occupational therapy practices. The effects of MD are harsh on families, and psychological help is frequently beneficial and essential (Kaler and DiStasio, 2021).

MD is a multisystem illness that progresses over time and lacks a single therapeutic therapy. Furthermore, there are no newborn screening programs available now. The modest clinical characteristics and nonspecific molecular markers of MD make early identification extremely difficult from a clinical standpoint. Therefore, an infant with low body temperature, jaundice, and decreased muscle tone should be screened with an elevated level of suspicion if there are substantial anomalies in connective tissue or variables associated with family health, as early replacement of Cu reverses and prevents issues. A multidisciplinary team strategy involving a physiotherapist, occupational therapist, geneticist, neonatologist, pediatric neurologist, and dietician is more effective in managing MD. Genetic counselors are essential in prenatal diagnosis and parental reproductive risk counseling. Families affected by MD require financial and local resources for health, education, and emotional assistance (Tussolini et al., 2023).

KEYWORDS

- **Menkes syndrome**
- **ATP7A gene**
- **copper metabolism**
- **diagnosis**
- **treatment**

REFERENCES

Baeza, I., Wong, C., de León-García, C., Henrríquez-Esquíroz, J.M., Pérez-González, C., Villegas-Sepúlveda, N., León-García, G. (2012). The T1048I mutation in the ATP7A gene causes an unusual Menkes disease presentation. BMC Pediatrics, 12, 150, https://doi.org/10.1186/1471-2431-12-150

Beyens, A., Van Meensel, K., Pottie, L., De Rycke, R., De Bruyne, M., Baeke, F., Callewaert, B. (2019). Defining the clinical, molecular and ultrastructural characteristics in occipital horn syndrome: Two new cases and literature review. Genes, 10(7), 528. https://doi.org/10.3390/genes10070528

Bhat, J.N., Maertens, P. (2020). The low function of natural killer cells in treated classic Menkes disease. The Turkish Journal of Pediatrics, 62(3), 498–500. https://doi.org/10.24953/turkjped.2020.03.021

Bindu, P.S., Taly, A.B., Kothari, S., Christopher, R., Gayathri, N., Sinha, S., Bharath, R.D. (2013). Electro-clinical features and magnetic resonance imaging correlate in Menkes disease. Brain and Development, 35(5), 398–405. https://doi.org/10.1016/j.braindev.2012.07.016

Camakaris, J., Petris, M.J., Bailey, L., Shen, P., Lockhart, P., Glover, T. W., Mercer, J.F. (1995). Gene amplification of the Menkes (MNK; ATP7A) P-type ATPase gene of CHO cells is associated with Cu resistance and enhanced Cuefflux. Human Molecular Genetics, 4(11), 2117–2123. https://doi.org/10.1093/hmg/4.11.2117

Chelly, J., Tümer, Z., Tønnesen, T., Petterson, A., Ishikawa-Brush, Y., Tommerup, N., Monaco, A.P. (1993). Isolation of a candidate gene for Menkes disease that encodes a potential heavy metal binding protein. Nature Genetics, 3(1), 14–19. https://doi.org/10.1038/ng0193-14

Chhabra, V.K., Rehni, A.K., Singh, T.G., Arora, S. (2010). Tacrolimus modulates the passive avoidance test and apomorphine induced stereotypy in rats. Australasian Medical Journal, 3(8)

Christodoulou, J., Danks, D.M., Sarkar, B., Baerlocher, K.E., Casey, R., Horn, N., Clarke, J.T. (1998). Early treatment of Menkes disease with parenteral Cooper-Histidine: Long-term follow-up of four treated patients. American Journal of Medical Genetics, 76(2), 154–164. https://doi.org/10.1002/(sici)1096-8628(19980305)76:2%3C154::aid-ajmg9%3E3.3.co;2-c

Culotta, V.C., Yang, M., O'Halloran, T.V. (2006). Activation of superoxide dismutases: Putting the metal to the pedal. Biochimica et Biophysica Acta (BBA)-Molecular Cell Research, 1763(7), 747–758. https://doi.org/10.1016/j.bbamcr.2006.05.003

Danks, D.M., Campbell, P.E., Walker-Smith, J., Stevens, B.J., Gillespie, J.M., Blomfield, J., Turner, B. (1972). Menkes'kinky-hair syndrome. The Lancet, 299(7760), 1100–1103. https://doi.org/10.1016/s0140-6736(72)91433-x

De Bie, P., Muller, P., Wijmenga, C., Klomp, L.W. (2007). Molecular pathogenesis of Wilson and Menkes disease: Correlation of mutations with molecular defects and disease phenotypes. Journal of Medical Genetics, 44(11), 673–688. https://doi.org/10.1136/jmg.2007.052746

Di Donato, M., Sarkar, B. (1997). Cutransport and its alterations in Menkes and Wilson diseases. Biochimica et Biophysica Acta (BBA)-Molecular Basis of Disease, 1360(1), 3–16. https://doi.org/10.1016/s0925-4439(96)00064-6

Donsante, A., Yi, L., Zerfas, P.M., Brinster, L.R., Sullivan, P., Goldstein, D.S., Kaler, S.G. (2011). ATP7A gene addition to the choroid plexus results in long-term rescue of the lethal Cutransport defect in a Menkes disease mouse model. Molecular Therapy, 19(12), 2114–2123. https://doi.org/10.1038/mt.2011.143

Formigari, A., Irato, P., Santon, A. (2007). Zinc, antioxidant systems and metallothionein in metal mediated-apoptosis: Biochemical and cytochemical aspects. Comparative Biochemistry and Physiology Part C: Toxicology & Pharmacology, 146(4), 443–459. https://doi.org/10.1016/j.cbpc.2007.07.010

Gasch, A.T., Caruso, R.C., Kaler, S.G., Kaiser-Kupfer, M. (2002). Menkes' syndrome: Ophthalmic findings. Ophthalmology, 109(8), 1477–1483. https://doi.org/10.1016/s0161-6420(02)01095-3

Gohil, V.M. (2021). Repurposing elesclomol, an investigational drug for the treatment of Cumetabolism disorders. Expert Opinion on Investigational Drugs, 30(1), 1–4. https://doi.org/10.1080/13543784.2021.1840550

González, M., Reyes-Jara, A., Suazo, M., Jo, W.J., Vulpe, C. (2008). Expression of copper-related genes in response to Cuload. The American Journal of Clinical Nutrition, 88(3), 830S–834S. https://doi.org/10.1093/ajcn/88.3.830s

Gu, Y.H., Kodama, H., Shiga, K., Nakata, S., Yanagawa, Y., Ozawa, H. (2005). A survey of Japanese patients with Menkes disease from 1990 to 2003: Incidence and early signs before typical symptomatic onset, pointing the way to earlier diagnosis. Journal of Inherited Metabolic Disease, 28, 473–478. https://doi.org/10.1007/s10545-005-0473-3

Guthrie, L.M., Soma, S., Yuan, S., Silva, A., Zulkifli, M., Snavely, T.C., Sacchettini, J.C. (2020). Elesclomol alleviates Menkes pathology and mortality by escorting Cu to cuproenzymes in mice. Science, 368(6491), 620–625. https://doi.org/10.1126/science.aaz8899

Haberkiewicz, O., Lipiński, P., Starzyński, R.R., Jończy, A., Kurowska, P., Ogórek, M., Lenartowicz, M. (2022). Decreased expression of the Slc31a1 gene and cytoplasmic relocalization of membrane CTR1 protein in renal epithelial cells: A potent protective mechanism against Cu nephrotoxicity in a mouse model of menkes disease. International Journal of Molecular Sciences, 23(19), 11441. https://doi.org/10.3390/ijms231911441

Hamza, I., Prohaska, J., Gitlin, J.D. (2003). Essential role for Atox1 in the copper-mediated intracellular trafficking of the Menkes ATPase. Proceedings of the National Academy of Sciences, 100(3), 1215–1220. https://doi.org/10.1073/pnas.0336230100

Hicks, J.D., Donsante, A., Pierson, T.M., Gillespie, M.J., Chou, D.E., Kaler, S.G. (2012). Increased frequency of congenital heart defects in Menkes disease. Clinical Dysmorphology, 21(2), 59. https://doi.org/10.1097/mcd.0b013e32834ea52b

Horn, N., Møller, L.B., Nurchi, V.M., Aaseth, J. (2019). Chelating principles in Menkes and Wilson diseases: Choosing the suitable compounds in the right combinations at the time. Journal of Inorganic Biochemistry, 190, 98–112. https://doi.org/10.1016/j.jinorgbio.2018.10.009

Hui, W.F., Hon, K.L., Leung, A.K., Pang, K.K.Y., Leung, M.W.Y. (2021). Tubular dysfunction and ruptured ureter in a child with menkes syndrome. Case Reports in Pediatrics, 2021, 4398456. https://doi.org/10.1155/2021/4398456

Jain, P., Kannan, L., Chakrabarty, B., Kumar, A., Gupta, N., Kabra, M., Gulati, S. (2014). Menkes disease–An essential cause of early onset refractory seizures. Journal of Pediatric Neurosciences, 9(1), 11. https://doi.org/10.4103/1817-1745.131471

Kaler, S.G. (2011). ATP7A-related Cu transport diseases—emerging concepts and future trends. Nature Reviews Neurology, 7(1), 15–29. https://doi.org/10.1038/nrneurol.2010.180

Kaler, S.G., DiStasio, A.T. (2021). ATP7A-related Cu transport disorders. https://doi.org/10.1016/b978-0-12-810532-0.00043-4

Kaler, S.G., Holmes, C.S., Goldstein, D.S., Tang, J., Godwin, S.C., Donsante, A., Patronas, N. (2008). Neonatal diagnosis and treatment of Menkes disease. New England Journal of Medicine, 358(6), 605–614. https://doi.org/10.1056/nejmoa070613

Kaur, M., Nagpal, M., Singh, M., Singh, T.G., Aggarwal, G., Dhingra, G.A. (2021). Improved antibacterial activity of topical gel-based on nanosponge carrier of cinnamon oil. BioImpacts: BI, 11(1), 23

Kennerson, M.L., Nicholson, G.A., Kaler, S.G., Kowalski, B., Mercer, J.F., Tang, J., Garbern, J.Y. (2010). Missense mutations in the Cutransporter gene ATP7A cause X-linked distal hereditary motor neuropathy. The American Journal of Human Genetics, 86(3), 343–352. https://doi.org/10.1016/j.ajhg.2010.01.027

Kim, M.Y., Kim, J.H., Cho, M.H., Choi, Y.H., Kim, S.H., Im, Y.J., Cheong, H.I. (2019). Urological problems in patients with Menkes disease. Journal of Korean Medical Science, 34(1), e4. https://doi.org/10.3346/jkms.2019.34.e4

Kodama, H., Fujisawa, C., Bhadhprasit, W. (2012). Inherited Cu transport disorders: Biochemical mechanisms, diagnosis, and treatment. Current Drug Metabolism, 13(3), 237–250. https://doi.org/10.2174/138920012799320455

Kodama, H., Murata, Y., Kobayashi, M. (1999). Clinical manifestations and treatment of Menkes disease and its variants. Pediatrics International, 41(4), 423–429. https://doi.org/10.1046/j.1442-200x.1999.01095.x

Kreuder, J., Otten, A., Fuder, H., Tümer, Z., Tønnesen, T., Horn, N., Dralle, D. (1993). Clinical and biochemical consequences of copper-histidine therapy in Menkes disease. European Journal of Pediatrics, 152, 828–832. https://doi.org/10.1007/bf02073380

Kumar, M., Nguyen, T.N., Kaur, J., Singh, T.G., Soni, D., Singh, R., Kumar, P. (2023). Opportunities and challenges in application of artificial intelligence in pharmacology. Pharmacological Reports, 75(1), 3–18

La Fontaine, S., Mercer, J.F. (2007). Trafficking of the copper-ATPases, ATP7A and ATP7B: Role in Cu homeostasis. Archives of Biochemistry and Biophysics, 463(2), 149–167. https://doi.org/10.1016/j.abb.2007.04.021

Lee, J., Pena, M.M.O., Nose, Y., Thiele, D.J. (2002). Biochemical characterisation of the human Cutransporter Ctr1. Journal of Biological Chemistry, 277(6), 4380–4387. https://doi.org/10.1074/jbc.m104728200

Lenartowicz, M., Grzmil, P., Shoukier, M., Starzyński, R., Marciniak, M., Lipiński, P. (2012a). Mutation in the CPC motif-containing sixth transmembrane domain affects intracellular localisation, trafficking and Cu transport efficiency of ATP7A protein in mosaic mutant mice—an animal model of Menkes disease. Metallomics, 4(2), 197–204. https://doi.org/10.1039/c1mt00134e

Lenartowicz, M., Krzeptowski, W., Koteja, P., Chrzascik, K., Møller, L.B. (2012b). Prenatal treatment of mosaic mice (Atp7a mo-ms) mouse model for Menkes disease, with Cu combined by diethyldithiocarbamate (DMDTC). PLoS One, 7(7), e40400. https://doi.org/10.1371/journal.pone.0040400

Liu, P.C., Chen, Y.W., Centeno, J.A., Quezado, M., Lem, K., Kaler, S.G. (2005). Downregulation of myelination, energy, and translational genes in Menkes disease brain. Molecular Genetics and Metabolism, 85(4), 291–300. https://doi.org/10.1016/j.ymgme.2005.04.007

Loeffler, D.A. (2023). Experimental approaches for altering the expression of Abeta-degrading enzymes. Journal of Neurochemistry, 164(6), 725–763. https://doi.org/10.1111/jnc.15762

Manara, R., D'agata, L., Rocco, M.C., Cusmai, R., Freri, E., Pinelli, L., Sartori, S. (2017). Neuroimaging changes in Menkes disease, part 1. American Journal of Neuroradiology, 38(10), 1850–1857. https://doi.org/10.3174/ajnr.a5186

Mehta, S., Nain, P., Agrawal, B.K., Singh, R.P. (2022). Vitamin D with calcium supplementation managing glycemic control with HbA1c and improve quality of life in patients with diabetes. Turkish Journal of Pharmaceutical Sciences, 19(2), 161–167. https://doi.org/10.4274/tjps.galenos.2021.62357

Mehta, S., Nain, P., Agrawal, B.K., Singh, R.P., Kaur, J., Maity, S., Bhattacharjee, A., Peela, J., Nauhria, S., Nauhria, S. (2021). Effectiveness of Empagliflozin with vitamin D supplementation in peripheral neuropathy in type 2 diabetic patients. Cureus, 13(12), e20208. https://doi.org/10.7759/cureus.20208

Mercer, J.F., Livingston, J., Hall, B., Paynter, J.A., Begy, C., Chandrasekharappa, S., Glover, T.W. (1993). Isolation of a partial candidate gene for Menkes disease by positional cloning. Nature Genetics, 3(1), 20–25. https://doi.org/10.1038/ng0193-20

Møller, L.B., Mogensen, M., Horn, N. (2009). Molecular diagnosis of Menkes disease: Genotype–phenotype correlation. Biochimie, 91(10), 1273–1277. https://doi.org/10.1016/j.biochi.2009.05.011

Monty, J.F., Llanos, R.M., Mercer, J.F., Kramer, D.R. (2005). Cuexposure induces trafficking of the Menkes protein in the intestinal epithelium of ATP7A transgenic mice. The Journal of Nutrition, 135(12), 2762–2766. https://doi.org/10.1093/jn/135.12.2762

Moon, S.J., An, Y.M., Kim, S.K., Kwon, Y.S., Lee, J.E. (2017). The effect of low-dose intravenous bisphosphonate treatment on osteoporosis in children with quadriplegic cerebral palsy. Korean Journal of Pediatrics, 60(12), 403. https://doi.org/10.3345/kjp.2017.60.12.403

Morris, A.A.M., Hoffmann, G.F., Naughten, E.R., Monavari, A.A., Collins, J.E., Leonard, J.V. (1999). Glutaric aciduria and suspected child abuse. Archives of Disease in Childhood, 80(5), 404–405. https://doi.org/10.1136/adc.80.5.404

Nishihara, E., Furuyama, T., Yamashita, S., Mori, N. (1998). Expression of Cutrafficking genes in the mouse brain. Neuroreport, 9(14), 3259–3263. https://doi.org/10.1097/00001756-199810050-00023

Panichsillaphakit, E., Kwanbunbumpen, T., Chomtho, S., Visuthranukul, C. (2022). Copper-histidine therapy in an infant with a novel splice-site variant in the ATP7A gene of Menkes disease: The first experience in South East Asia and literature review. BMJ Case Reports CP, 15(4), e247937. https://doi.org/10.1136/bcr-2021-247937

Pawar, N.V., Mir, F.F. (2022). Infantile neurodegeneration and hair changes: A rare case of menkes disease. Dubai Medical Journal, 5(1), 70–73. https://doi.org/10.1159/000521155

Petris, M.J., Mercer, J.F., Culvenor, J.G., Lockhart, P., Gleeson, P.A., Camakaris, J. (1996). Ligand-regulated transport of the Menkes CuP-type ATPase efflux pump from the Golgi apparatus to the plasma membrane: A novel mechanism of regulated trafficking. The EMBO Journal, 15(22), 6084–6095. https://doi.org/10.1002/j.1460-2075.1996.tb00997.x

Price, D.J., Ravindranath, T., Kaler, S.G. (2007). Internal jugular phlebectasia in Menkes disease. International Journal of Pediatric Otorhinolaryngology, 71(7), 1145–1148. https://doi.org/10.1016/j.ijporl.2007.02.021

Rangarh, P., Kohli, N. (2018). Neuroimaging findings in Menkes disease: A rare neurodegenerative disorder. Case Reports, 2018, bcr-2017. https://doi.org/10.1136/bcr-2017-223858

Rehni, A.K., Singh, T.G., Singh, N. et al. (2010).Tramadol-induced seizurogenic effect: a possible role of opioid-dependent histamine (H_1) receptor activation-linked mechanism. Naunyn-Schmiedeberg's Archives of Pharmacology, 381, 11–19. https://doi.org/10.1007/s00210-009-0476-y

Roach, E.S., Miller, V.S., Eds., (2004). *Neurocutaneous Disorders*. Cambridge University Press. https://doi.org/10.1007/s00415-004-0631-9

Sarkar, B., Lingertat-Walsh, K., Clarke, J.T. (1993). Copper-histidine therapy for Menkes disease. The Journal of Pediatrics, 123(5), 828–830. https://doi.org/10.1016/s0022-3476(05)80870-4

Sato, R., Okutani, K., Higashi, T., Satou, M., Fujimoto, K., Okazaki, K. (2009). Case report: Respiratory care for anesthesia in Menkes syndrome and micrognathia patients. Masui. The Japanese Journal of Anesthesiology, 58(1), 103–105. https://doi.org/10.18535/jmscr/v6i4.190

Schlief, M.L., Craig, A.M., Gitlin, J.D. (2005). NMDA receptor activation mediates Cu homeostasis in hippocampal neurons. Journal of Neuroscience, 25(1), 239–246. https://doi.org/10.1523/jneurosci.3699-04.2005

Sharma, V.K., Singh, T.G. (2020). Chronic stress and diabetes mellitus: Interwoven pathologies. Current Diabetes Reviews, 16(6), 546–556

Singh, H., Satija, S., Kaur, H., Khurana, N., Sharma, N., Vyas, M., Singh,T.G., Mahajan, S., Mehta, M. (2019). Novel drug delivery approaches for guggul. Plant Arch, 19(2), 983–993

Singh, R., Farooq, S.A., Mannan, A., Singh, T.G., Najda, A., Grażyna, Z., Albadrani, G. M., Sayed, A. A., Abdel-Daim, M.M. (2022). Animal models of diabetic microvascular complications: Relevance to clinical features. Biomedicine & Pharmacotherapy, 145, 112305

Solomons, N.W. (1985). Biochemical, metabolic, and clinical role of Cu in human nutrition. Journal of the American College of Nutrition, 4(1), 83–105. https://doi.org/10.1080/07315724.1985.10720069

Speisky, H., Gómez, M., Burgos-Bravo, F., López-Alarcón, C., Jullian, C., Olea-Azar, C., Aliaga, M.E. (2009). Generation of superoxide radicals by copper–glutathione complexes: Redox-consequences associated with their interaction with reduced glutathione. Bioorganic & Medicinal Chemistry, 17(5), 1803–1810. https://doi.org/10.1016/j.bmc.2009.01.069

Steinmann, B., Royce, P.M., Superti-Furga, A. (2002). The Ehlers-Danlos syndrome. In: *Connective Tissue and its Heritable Disorders: Molecular, Genetic, and Medical Aspects*, pp. 431–523. https://doi.org/10.1002/0471221929.ch9

Tümer, Z. (2013). An overview and update of ATP7A mutations leading to Menkes disease and occipital horn syndrome. Human Mutation, 34(3), 417–429. https://doi.org/10.1002/humu.22266

Tümer, Z., Møller, L.B. (2010). Menkes disease. European Journal of Human Genetics, 18(5), 511–518. https://doi.org/10.1038/ejhg.2009.187

Turski, M.L., Thiele, D.J. (2009). New roles for Cu metabolism in cell proliferation, signalling, and disease. Journal of Biological Chemistry, 284(2), 717–721. https://doi.org/10.1074/jbc.r800055200

Tussolini, I.G.A., Tussolini, G.R., Tussolini, J.F., da Silva Pontes, L., Junior, M.T.R., da Silva, P.D. (2023). Doença de Menkes: Relato de um caso raro na Amazônia. Brazilian Journal of Health Review, 6(1), 4016–4026. https://doi.org/10.34119/bjhrv6n1-311

Ueki, Y., Narazaki, O., Hanai, T. (1985). Menkes disease: Is vitamin C treatment effective? Brain and Development, 7(5), 519–522. https://doi.org/10.1016/s0387-7604(85)80122-4

Verrotti, A., Cusmai, R., Darra, F., Martelli, P., Accorsi, P., Bergamo, S., Giordano, L. (2014). Epilepsy in Menkes disease: An electroclinical long-term study of 28 patients. Epilepsy Research, 108(9), 1597–1603. https://doi.org/10.1016/j.eplepsyres.2014.08.006

Vulpe, C., Levinson, B., Whitney, S., Packman, S., Gitschier, J. (1993). Isolation of a candidate gene for Menkes disease and evidence that it encodes a copper-transporting ATPase. Nature Genetics, 3(1), 7–13. https://doi.org/10.1038/ng0193-7

White, S.R., Reese, K., Sato, S., Kaler, S.G. (1993). Spectrum of EEG findings in Menkes disease. Electroencephalography and Clinical Neurophysiology, 87(1), 57–61. https://doi.org/10.1016/0013-4694(93)90175-u

Ydemann, M., Nielsen, B.N., Henneberg, S., Jakobsen, J.C., Wetterslev, J., Lauritsen, T., Reinhardt, S. (2018). Intraoperative clonidine for prevention of postoperative agitation in children anaesthetised with sevoflurane (PREVENT AGITATION): A randomised, placebo-controlled, double-masked trial. The Lancet Child & Adolescent Health, 2(1), 15–24. https://doi.org/10.1016/s2352-4642(17)30127-x

Yusoff, A.A.M., Abdullah, W.S.W., Khair, S.Z.N.M., Abd Radzak, S.M. (2019). A comprehensive overview of mitochondrial DNA 4977-bp deletion in cancer studies. Oncology Reviews, 13(1), 409. https://doi.org/10.4081/oncol.2019.409

CHAPTER 8

Clinical Perspective on Obesity

DANIA MUGHAL[1*] and SAKSHI MALIK[2]

[1]*Complications of Excess Weight, Cambridge University Hospitals, Cambridge, United Kingdom*

[2]*Acute and General Medicine, Hull University Teaching Hospitals NHS Trust, Hull, United Kingdom*

*Corresponding author

ABSTRACT

Obesity is now recognized as a chronic disease by the American Medical Association and similar authorities. It is defined as a body mass index (BMI) >30 in adults and >95th percentile in children. Although BMI is a simple diagnostic tool, it lacks accuracy as it does not differentiate between fat and lean mass. Despite growing awareness among healthcare professionals, obesity rates continue to rise due to underdiagnosis and undertreatment. Effective management requires a comprehensive assessment, including factors like age, dietary habits, physical activity, mental health, social environment, medical and family history, motivation, and obesity-related comorbidities. Modern treatment guidelines advocate for personalized therapy. Nonpharmacological approaches should consider the gut microbiome, while psychological, pharmacological, and surgical options may be used as adjuncts. A deeper understanding of obesity's complex causes enables better outcomes. Obesity significantly increases the risk of numerous health issues: cardiovascular (e.g., hypertension, heart failure), metabolic (e.g., diabetes, fatty liver), malignancies, reproductive (e.g., PCOS, infertility), pulmonary (e.g., sleep apnea), musculoskeletal, urogenital, and thromboembolic disorders. Its rising prevalence is driven

Pharmacotherapy Approaches Toward Endocrine and Metabolic Diseases.
Thakur Gurjeet Singh and Sanjana Mehta (Eds.)

DOI: 10.1201/9781779640154-8

by modern lifestyles and an obesogenic environment. This chapter highlights the multifactorial causes, risks, and systemic impact of obesity, stressing the importance of holistic, individualized treatment strategies.

8.1 INTRODUCTION

Obesity is a low-grade systematic inflammatory state of the body that affects many organs anatomically and metabolically, resulting in several clinical complications. Obesity is a disorder that is well recognized yet often receives inadequate treatment. It is primarily identified as an abundance of adipose tissue. Previously, adipose tissue was considered solely an energy storage organ. However, it is now recognized as an endocrine organ responsible for producing various hormones, including steroid and peptide hormones such as leptin, dipsin, visfatin, acylation-stimulating protein, angiotensinogen, plasminogen activator inhibitor, adiponectin, resistin, estrogen, pro-inflammatory adipokines (TNF-ALPHA, IL-6), and anti-inflammatory adipokines (TGF-BETA, IL-10, IL-4, IL-13, IL-1RALPHA, apelin) (Sharma et al., 2022). Hormones are mainly produced by white adipose tissue, which serves as a lipid storage and release reservoir. In obesity, WAT profoundly changes and expands, which leads to dysfunctional adipose tissue and imbalanced hormone secretion. There is another type of tissue known as brown adipose tissue (BAT), which oxidizes lipids to conduct thermogenesis, and the prevalence of BAT is lower in obese individuals (Aragón-Vela et al., 2022; Sharma et al., 2023). The pathology of obesity is characterized by a negative energy balance, where calorie intake exceeds calorie expenditure. This imbalance results in the accumulation of excess fatty tissue, the primary source of systematic inflammation. The contributing factors are an energy-dense diet and a sedentary lifestyle. While obesity is a reversible state, very minimum support and education provided by healthcare professionals in clinical settings serve as one of the most significant barriers among a few others (Lin and Li, 2021).

Obesity meets the medical definition of disease as a dysfunction in the body caused by environmental, behavioral, or genetic factors. It also leads to clinical problems. An environment that contributes to obesity by influencing individuals' or populations' nutritional and physical activities is known as an obesogenic environment (Safaei et al., 2021; Khan et al., 2022a; Prabhakar et al., 2022). A mix of factors from the surrounding environment, living conditions, and available opportunities causes obesity. Various organizations, including the World Health Organization, have classified obesity as a chronic disease. Nevertheless, it is not acknowledged as a disease in several nations, such as the United Kingdom, potentially because of its demanding influence on the economy (Safaei et al., 2021; Singh et al., 2022). The American Association of Clinical Endocrinologists (AACE) and the American College of Endocrinology (ACE) use the term adiposity-based chronic disease as an alternative name for obesity (Ashique et al., 2022). This is primarily done to highlight the importance of having standardized protocols and treatment, while also aiming to reduce the societal stigma associated with the condition (Frühbeck et al., 2019).

The global obesity epidemic has resulted in over one billion individuals being categorized as obese, with around 60% being adults, 35% being adolescents, and the remaining percentage consisting of children. The relentless pace can only be controlled by implementing a planned intervention targeting this persistent ailment. Implementing early stage obesity management will benefit patients and alleviate the overall healthcare burden. Significantly, the longer an individual experiences obesity, the more pronounced its effect on mortality, making it a crucial factor to address in young adults with obesity.

Despite a few drawbacks, body mass index (BMI) remains the most readily accessible and extensively utilized method for screening and diagnosing obesity. BMI is calculated by dividing weight in kilograms by the square of height in meters. It solely considers the height and weight without considering the individual's muscle mass. However, it is crucial to prioritize the prevention of lean mass depletion in managing obesity, as this aspect is often overlooked when solely focusing on changes in body weight. A safer utilization of BMI can be achieved when a healthcare expert physically examines an individual. By considering clinical judgment and patient history, the professional can determine whether the weight is primarily fat mass or fat-free mass. There is a lack of comprehension regarding muscle mass, which leads to a failure to recognize the importance of resistance exercise and a healthy diet with optimal protein in contrast to a short-lived approach. A more modern approach involves using four categories (mental, mechanical, metabolic, and monetary) to assist busy practitioners in conducting a comprehensive examination (Khan et al., 2022b; Grewal et al., 2019). The 4Ms (monitoring, measurement, management, and motivation) and standard anthropometric measurements, such as BMI and waist circumference (WC), are recommended. In the case of children and adolescents, the relationship between height and weight percentile is particularly emphasized. BMI is the most convenient, efficient, and quantitative method for assessing adult obesity. It also allows for the classification of obesity into three grades: Grade I (30.0–34.9), Grade II (35.0–39.9), and Grade III (>40). However, to assess the decreased risk related to obesity management therapies, it is essential to utilize clinical biomarkers to evaluate the response (Vishwas et al., 2021).

8.2 IMPACTS OF OBESITY ON OTHER ORGAN FUNCTIONS

Unusually high adipose tissue levels lead to several anatomical and physiological alterations in the body. Obesity impacts several clinically significant health aspects, including suppressed or deranged cardiovascular, metabolic, pulmonary, cell malignancy, reproductive, musculoskeletal, mental, coagulation, skin, or urogenital health (Guerreiro et al., 2022).

8.2.1 EFFECT OF OBESITY ON CARDIOVASCULAR HEALTH

The alterations in structure and function that obesity induces in the heart are also called "obesity cardiomyopathy." Studies indicate that a 10-kg gain in weight is associated with a 12% higher risk of coronary artery disease (CAD), a 3 mmHg increase in systolic blood pressure, and a 2.3-mmHg increase in diastolic blood pressure. It exhibits a more pronounced correlation with segment elevation myocardial infarction (STEMI) and nonsegment elevation myocardial infarction (NSTEMI) compared to smoking. Out of all the cases of heart failure, 50% were classified as obese, while 40% were categorized as overweight. Heart failure is strongly associated with the duration of morbid obesity; moreover, having morbid obesity for 30 years increases the risk of heart failure by 90% (Poirier et al., 2006).

Elevated blood pressure and cardiac output result from hemodynamic and circulating blood volume alterations. In addition, the activation of the renin-angiotensin-aldosterone system and the increased activity of the sympathetic nervous system not only lead to high blood pressure but also contribute to the development of cardiac fibrosis, platelet aggregation, and endothelial dysfunction. Elevated blood flow promotes venous reflux, raising ventricular preload and augmenting ventricular wall tension and dilation. This anatomical alteration, observed in obesity, leads to left ventricular hypertrophy and impaired ventricular function, serving as a fundamental factor in the development of heart failure. Modifications in the structure of the heart muscle also elevate the likelihood of developing atrial fibrillation and experiencing sudden cardiac death. Furthermore, the presence of elevated inflammatory cytokines (such as TNF-ALPHA, IL-1, IL-6, IL-8) in the bloodstream increases the likelihood of myocardial fibrosis and stiffness, ultimately resulting in heart failure (Sagris et al., 2021).

8.2.2 EFFECT OF OBESITY ON METABOLIC HEALTH

An expansion of the endocrine organ leads to a disruption in the secretion of hormones, which has a metabolic impact on the body and can result in complications such as diabetes, dyslipidemia, fatty liver, and gallstones (GDs).

- **Diabetes:** Approximately 85% of individuals diagnosed with diabetes have a body weight that exceeds the healthy range or falls into the category of obesity. Diabetes is caused by excess adipose tissue, which leads to low-grade systematic inflammation. This inflammation results from various mechanisms, including mitochondrial dysfunction, inflammation, disrupted gut microbiome, high insulin levels in the blood (hyperinsulinemia), insulin resistance due to lipotoxicity, and other factors such as oxidative stress and genetic background. Excessive activation of inflammatory signaling pathways can result in various problems, including malfunctioning organs and tissue harm. An excess of adipocytes also induces a rise in inflammatory cytokines, which, in consequence, triggers insulin resistance in the liver and throughout the body. The alterations in gut flora also function as catalysts for metabolic inflammation. Furthermore, a reduction in mitochondrial function promotes the abnormal build-up of fat in muscles and adipose tissue, leading to insulin resistance without any inflammatory disruption (Rohm et al., 2022).
- **Dyslipidemia:** Approximately 70% of those who are obese experience dyslipidemia. Excessive release of free fatty acids from the liver, visceral adiposity, insulin resistance, and a pro-inflammatory state results in abnormal lipid levels. A high amount of free fatty acid in the body is caused by consuming many calories from

dietary fat. This stimulates the overproduction of chylomicrons and hyperinsulinemia, suppressing the breakdown of triacylglyceride lipolysis. However, it also increases the breakdown of adipose tissue and the production of new fatty acids via de novo fatty acid hepatic lipogenesis due to the excess carbohydrates consumed. As an adaptive mechanism, the liver upregulates the production of triacyl glycerides, resulting in excessive secretion of very low-density lipoproteins. Furthermore, in the case of obesity, there is a decreased affinity for apo A-I and high-density lipoproteins (HDL), resulting in lowered levels of circulating HDL and impaired reversed cholesterol transport (Klop et al., 2013).

- **Hepatic steatosis:** The prevalence of obesity in patients diagnosed with nonalcoholic fatty liver disease (NAFLD) ranges from approximately 50% to 90%. Obese individuals with high levels of triglycerides stored in the liver (intrahepatic triglyceride content) are most likely to have various metabolic problems, including insulin resistance, changes in free fatty acid metabolism, and an increased rate of secretion of very low-density lipoprotein triglycerides. The primary factor contributing to NAFLD is the liver's heightened absorption of free fatty acids from adipose tissue and an increase in the liver's production of new fats. Accumulating more than 5% fat in hepatocytes is metabolic-associated fatty liver disease (MAFLD) (Fabbrini et al., 2010).
- **Cholelithiasis:** Obesity is a significant risk factor for GD formation. The coexistence of MAFLD and GD disease has been established primarily due to shared modifiable risk factors such as obesity, insulin resistance, and metabolic syndrome. GDs are caused by an excess of cholesterol in bile. Obesity often leads to elevated insulin levels in the bloodstream, which stimulates the activity of 3-hydroxy-3-methylglutaryl-coenzyme A (HMG-CoA) reductase. This stimulation results in an excessive production of cholesterol.

8.2.3 EFFECT OF OBESITY ON PULMONARY HEALTH

Obesity affects respiratory health through various factors, including physical compression of the diaphragm, lungs, and chest cavity, resulting in restricted lung function. Additionally, inflammatory cytokines have been found to damage pulmonary health. Excessive adipose tissue diminishes overall respiratory system compliance, augments pulmonary resistance, and reduces the strength of respiratory muscles. These triggers can lead to asthma, asthma-like symptoms, or sleep apnea by causing airway hyperresponsiveness, respiratory muscle stiffness, and lower tidal volume due to limited chest expansion. Excessive fat deposition in the chest and abdomen has been found to damage the respiratory system significantly. Decreased airflow and heightened hyperresponsiveness elevate the likelihood of developing pulmonary hypertension, pulmonary embolism, respiratory tract infections, obstructive sleep apnea, and obesity hypoventilation syndrome. Among all pulmonary diseases, obstructive sleep apnea is the most common in the obese population (Kwok et al., 2020).

8.2.4 EFFECT OF OBESITY ON CELLULAR MALIGNANCY

Obesity is responsible for approximately 4–8% of all cancer cases. Obesity intensifies the likelihood of cancer development by various pathways, including the overproduction of hormones caused by increased fat tissue, specifically estrogen, which is linked to breast, endometrial, and ovarian cancer. Improper hormone release in obese persons leads to elevated leptin levels, which promotes aberrant cell proliferation. This contrasts with adiponectin, which inhibits cell proliferation and safeguards tumor growth. Also, the presence of hyperinsulinemia, which is characterized by increased levels of insulin and insulin-like growth factor in the bloodstream, is mainly caused by insulin resistance and is closely linked to the development of colon, renal, prostate, and endometrial cancer. Furthermore, obesity can lead to chronic inflammatory disorders such as NAFLD and gallstones. These illnesses can result in oxidative stress, which in turn can cause DNA damage and increase the likelihood of developing biliary tract cancer (Pati et al., 2023).

8.2.5 EFFECT OF OBESITY ON REPRODUCTIVE HEALTH

The obstacle to conception is higher for those who are obese. Hormone dysregulation primarily arises from elevated levels of adipokines such as leptin, ghrelin, resistin, visfatin, chemerin, omentin, and adiponectin. These adipokines are associated with decreased fertility, insulin-related disorders, low levels of sex hormone-binding protein, excessive androgen levels, and impaired hypothalamic gonadotropin secretion. Consequently, this leads to a decrease in follicles and progesterone levels. The presence of elevated harmful adipokines and reduced beneficial adipokines exacerbate the symptoms of polycystic ovarian syndrome. In obese individuals, there is a concurrent decrease in follicle-stimulating hormone secretion and an increase in oocytes with elevated levels of polyunsaturated fatty acids, greatly diminishing fertility (Chen et al., 2022).

Obesity negatively impacts female fertility and seminal quality. It is caused by increased oxidative stress, alterations in sperm DNA, and an increase in the production of inflammatory cytokines in the reproductive tract. Insulin resistance, combined with decreased levels of testosterone in the bloodstream, can lead to erectile dysfunction due to both androgen insufficiency and endothelial dysfunction. Obese males frequently have oligospermia and azoospermia.

8.2.6 EFFECT OF OBESITY ON PSYCHOLOGICAL WELL-BEING

The presence of low self-esteem, dissatisfaction with one's body image, emotional neglect/abuse, stigma, discrimination, physical pain, and diminished quality of life associated with obesity significantly affect mental well-being. Nearly half of the individuals considered for bariatric surgery have a lifelong record of depression. Approximately 15% of candidates disclosed experiencing an eating disorder, predominantly characterized by binge eating. A small proportion also reported symptoms of bulimia nervosa and night eating syndrome. This pertains to food consumption as a reaction to emotions, food cues, and the inability to regulate the frequency and quantity of meals. It is suspected that only a small group of the obese population gets formally diagnosed with eating problems; finally, around 9% of those eligible for bariatric surgery experience social anxiety.

8.2.7 EFFECT OF OBESITY ON MUSCULOSKELETAL HEALTH

Elevated BMI is a distinct risk factor for the occurrence of musculoskeletal disorders. Obesity causes injury to soft tissues due to variables related to structure and mechanics, increased stress on joints, reduced muscular strength, changes in biomechanics, and metabolic factors such as hormone and cytokine dysregulation. Obesity is linked to osteoarthritis (OA) in weight-bearing and nonweight-bearing joints. The prevalence of OA and low back pain in obese adults is 34% and 22%, respectively. The accumulation of abdominal fat exerts excessive pressure on the spine, leading to a forward-slanting of the pelvis and lower back. This results in a permanent and rounded arch in the back, which in turn produces back discomfort (Walsh et al., 2018).

8.2.8 EFFECT OF OBESITY ON COAGULATION

Obesity is associated with an elevated risk of clotting. An investigation reveals that almost 60% of individuals diagnosed with thrombosis are obese or overweight. Excessive accumulation of fat tissue results in persistent inflammation and impaired fibrinolysis, both of which contribute to the formation of blood clots. In addition, hormonal imbalance leads to elevated levels of prothrombotic adipokines such as leptin, resistin, and visfatin while simultaneously suppressing the production of antithrombotic adipokines such as adiponectin and apelin (Darvall et al., 2007).

8.2.9 EFFECT OF OBESITY ON SKIN

Approximately 70% of individuals who are obese exhibit a diverse range of alterations in their skin. Obesity affects the skin through various mechanisms. These include forming a thicker subcutaneous fat layer, resulting in more prominent skin folds and increased sweating (hyperhidrosis). It also impairs collagen production, leading to poor wound healing. Additionally, obesity hampers lymphatic flow in the subcutaneous tissue, causing lymphedema. Furthermore, decreased sensitivity to pain occurs due to poor vascularization of nerve endings, which can lead to ulcers. Lastly, obesity is associated with a chronic inflammatory skin condition called psoriasis, which is twice as common in individuals with a higher BMI due to increased levels of pro-inflammatory cytokines and growth factors (Barros et al., 2022).

8.2.10 EFFECT OF OBESITY ON UROGENITAL HEALTH

Excessive body weight exerts additional strain on the pelvic organs, such as the uterus, bladder, and vagina, which impacts the sphincter mechanism and results in stress urine incontinence. A direct correlation exists between elevated BMI, WC, and urine incontinence, particularly in females.

8.3 OBESITY PARADOX

Obesity is a significant risk factor for various health conditions. However, in individuals with preexisting chronic conditions, the presence of excess fat stores can provide a protective effect and improve survival rates, particularly in cardiovascular disease (such as CAD, myocardial infarction, and atrial fibrillation), cancer, and post-surgery situations. This phenomenon is commonly referred to as the "obesity paradox." Chronic disease is a condition that requires a high level of metabolic activity. Obese individuals have more significant metabolic reserves, allowing them to fulfill their bodies' higher energy demands by breaking down fat from excess fatty tissue. In addition, regular screening results in early detection compared to the nonobese group. It is not permissible for us to promote obesity due to its negative repercussions and a wide variety of undesirable complications. However, once diagnosed with chronic diseases, a different approach to weight management is necessary (Khafagy and Dash, 2021).

8.4 MANAGEMENT OF OBESITY FOR SUSTAINABLE WEIGHT LOSS

Obesity is a multifaceted and challenging condition to control. The advice and treatment should consider various factors such as age, dietary history, physical activity, mental health, past medical history, family history, the patient's current level of motivation, and any comorbidity related to obesity. The goal is to create an individualized treatment plan that promotes greater adherence to treatment and helps achieve the long-term benefits of therapy, a minimum duration of six months, particularly in preventing weight regain (Smith et al., 2020).

The initial strategy should involve lifestyle therapy, encompassing a personalized healthy meal plan, regular physical exercise, and behavioral intervention. However, given that it is a chronic condition, it should be managed in conjunction with additional treatment techniques, including medication, metabolic interventions, or bariatric surgery. Comprehensive anti-obesity treatment should be administered by combining multiple therapies to achieve more significant and enduring weight reduction. An open and nonjudgmental connection between patients and all clinicians is also crucial for effectively managing obesity (Soleymani et al., 2016).

The American College of Cardiology (ACC), American Heart Association (AHA), The Obesity Society (TOS), AACE, and ACE urge that individuals in obesity stage 0 focus on achieving weight loss or preventing additional weight gain while prioritizing the prevention of problems. However, the suggestions for stages 1 or 2 vary slightly. The AACE/ACE recommends weight loss to control weight-related complications and advises setting precise treatment targets. However, the ACC/AHA/TOS suggests determining weight loss goals in partnership with the patient. It is recommended that a minimum of 5% of body weight be lost, while AACE/ACE further suggests losing at least 10% of body weight to achieve specified therapeutic outcomes. In addition, the AACE/ACE recommends aiming for a 2.5% reduction in weight within one month as an initial weight loss goal, and the ACC/AHA/TOS suggests reaching a weight loss of 5–10% within 6 months (Soleymani et al., 2016).

However, to accomplish the recommended intervention for obesity, a three-step approach should be implemented. Weight loss, weight stabilization, and weight maintenance, now commonly known as the "managed obesity phase," are essential components of long-term therapy as motivation declines after attaining the ultimate weight goal. Weight-related problems should be addressed concurrently with any treatment for overweight or obesity. Extra therapy may or may not be necessary for such management (Montesi et al., 2016).

8.4.1 LIFESTYLE THERAPY

A practical and thorough lifestyle intervention involves a well-organized and extensive approach encompassing a nutritious meal plan, a tailored physical activity regimen, and a behavioral lifestyle intervention. Each of these components should be customized to suit each patient's specific needs, considering all the criteria discussed previously.

However, the primary strategy for weight loss is to decrease calorie consumption. Nevertheless, the procedure requires the assistance of a skilled dietitian. Conventional weight loss advice is ineffective, as seen by the ongoing rise in obesity and associated health conditions. Recent dietary approaches such as intermittent and alternate-day fasting have demonstrated encouraging outcomes. In addition, they enable intervals of complimentary meals that do not adversely affect weight loss as long as the remaining portion of the dietary regimen is adhered to rigorously. In addition, it enhances the overall relationship with food and offers a chance to stick to long-term treatment. An effective strategy is incorporating more protein, particularly whey protein, into hypocaloric diets. Obesity can be influenced by the disruption of the gut flora and alterations in gut hormones caused by food consumption. The gut microbiota produces short-chain fatty acids, which suppress the breakdown of fats and stimulate the development of fat cells. Lipopolysaccharides, found in the gut microbiota, induce inflammation and the infiltration of immune cells into adipose tissue. An unhealthy gut microbiome, influenced significantly by nutrition, has a detrimental effect on both the amount of energy consumed and the amount of energy expended, ultimately resulting in obesity.

Physical activity reduces body fat, preserves muscle mass, and, crucially, prevents weight reacquisition by boosting energy expenditure. Guidelines advocate for prescription exercise and emphasize the importance of reducing inactivity while promoting active leisure activities (Islam et al., 2022).

Furthermore, lifestyle therapy should incorporate behavioral interventions to promote adherence to meal plans and prescribed physical activity. These interventions encompass cognitive behavioral treatment, dietary education, and other methods in a multidisciplinary approach that can be delivered in person or remotely. Given the significant impact of behavior on the development of obesity, the AACE and the ACE recommend increasing behavioral intervention if a weight loss of at least 2.5% is not achieved during the first month of treatment (Leske et al., 2024).

8.4.2 MEDICATION

The use of anti-obesity medication (AOM) in conjunction with lifestyle adjustment results in more significant and enduring weight loss, particularly in cases of long-term obesity, compared to relying solely on lifestyle improvements. Obesity is a persistent medical condition, although only 2% of obese patients are provided AOM. This highlights the necessity for a standardized and optimal drug prescription process, as the current approach relies only on the treating physician's discretion. Additionally, it is necessary to establish protocols for drug tapering methods. However, medication administration should be tailored to specific therapeutic objectives for weight loss, weight-related ailments, and pharmacological precautions/warnings (Abdi Beshir et al., 2023). Combining therapy, as long as there are no negative interactions, is more effective than using monotherapy to address multiple pathways or mechanisms that worsen obesity. This approach can assist in achieving a weight loss of 10%, especially in individuals with obesity classes II and III. According to the AACE guidelines, a combination of AOM is recommended for adults with a BMI of more than 27 when lifestyle therapy alone is not practical. Additionally, AOM is recommended for all individuals with stage 2 obesity (Tak and Lee, 2021).

The Food and Drug Administration has approved a few drugs for weight management. These include semaglutide injection and liraglutide injection, which are glucagon-like peptide 1 receptor agonists. Another approved medication is orlistat, which is a lipase inhibitor. Orlistat has shown positive results in weight loss, treating conditions such as nonalcoholic steatohepatitis (NASH), and improving glycemic control. Phentermine hydrochloric acid (HCl) and topiramate extended-release capsules are another approved medication, combining a sympathomimetic amine-anorectic and an anti-epileptic analogue. Lastly, there are naltrexone HCl and bupropion HCl extended-release tablets, which are a combination of an opioid antagonist and an aminoketone antidepressant. These medications are taken in addition to lifestyle therapy for the management of chronic weight in adults with a BMI of 30 or higher or a BMI of 27 or higher in the presence of one or more weight-related comorbidities. Additional pharmaceuticals that aid in weight reduction include metformin, which functions as a liver and muscle insulin sensitizer and is primarily used in cases of insulin resistance. Another medicine, testosterone, is mainly administered when both hypogonadism and obesity coexist (Bays et al., 2022).

8.4.3 SURGERY

Bariatric surgery has resulted in significant weight reduction, sustained weight loss, improved weight-related comorbidities, and reduced mortality. This surgery is recommended for individuals with a BMI of 40 or more with at least one severe weight-related ailment. It may also be considered for individuals with a BMI of 35 if lifestyle changes and medication have not been effective. In addition, the AACE and the ACE have suggested that individuals with a BMI of 30 or more who have poorly controlled type 2 diabetes after receiving lifestyle interventions and pharmaceuticals should be considered for bariatric surgery. Nevertheless, in countries with lower incomes, there is a more significant occurrence of moderate and severe obesity. Providing optimal surgery and follow-up care to the entire affected population is impractical. However, implementing an effective clinical intervention based on a multi-disciplinary, intensive, and long-term approach can yield outcomes comparable to surgical treatments (Gulinac et al., 2023).

The cost of an intense, systematic, long-term, multidisciplinary strategy is approximately one-fifth of the predicted increase in price resulting from obesity-related issues. There is a pressing need to establish a comprehensive and efficient clinical approach for addressing the escalating prevalence and severity of obesity.

KEYWORDS

- **obesity**
- **management**
- **clinical view of obesity**
- **risk and obesity**

REFERENCES

Abdi Beshir, S., Ahmed Elnour, A., Soorya, A., Parveen Mohamed, A., Sir Loon Goh, S., Hussain, N., Al Haddad, A.H.I., Hussain, F., Yousif Khidir, I., Abdelnassir, Z. (2023). A narrative review of approved and emerging anti-obesity medications. Saudi Pharmaceutical Journal, 31(10), 101757. https://doi.org/10.1016/j.jsps.2023.101757. Erratum in: Saudi Pharm J. (2024). 32(5):102047.

Aragón-Vela, J., Alcalá-Bejarano Carrillo, J., Moreno-Racero, A., Plaza-Diaz, J. (2022). The role of molecular and hormonal factors in obesity and the effects of physical activity in children. International Journal of Molecular Sciences,. 23(23), 15413. https://doi.org/10.3390/ijms232315413.

Ashique, S., De Rubis, G., Sirohi, E., Mishra, N., Rihan, M., Garg, A., Reyes, R.J., Manandhar, B., Bhatt, S., Jha, N.K., Singh, T.G., Gupta, G., Singh, S.K., Chellappan, D.K., Paudel, K.R., Hansbro, P.M., Oliver, B.G., Dua, K. (2022). Short chain fatty acids: Fundamental mediators of the gut-lung axis and their involvement in pulmonary diseases. Chemico-Biological Interactions, 368, 110231. https://doi.org/10.1016/j.cbi.2022.110231.

Barros, G., Duran, P., Vera, I., Bermúdez, V. (2022). Exploring the Links between obesity and psoriasis: A comprehensive review. International Journal of Molecular Sciences, 23(14), 7499. https://doi.org/10.3390/ijms23147499.

Bays, H.E., Fitch, A., Christensen, S., Burridge, K., Tondt, J. (2022). Anti-obesity medications and investigational agents: An Obesity Medicine Association (OMA) Clinical Practice Statement (CPS) 2022. Obesity Pillars, 2, 100018. https://doi.org/10.1016/j.obpill.2022.100018.

Chen, P., Jia, R., Liu, Y., Cao, M., Zhou, L., Zhao, Z. (2022). Progress of adipokines in the female reproductive system: A focus on polycystic ovary syndrome. Frontiers in Endocrinology (Lausanne), 13, 881684. https://doi.org/10.3389/fendo.2022.881684.

Darvall, K.A., Sam, R.C., Silverman, S.H., Bradbury, A.W., Adam, D.J. (2007). Obesity and thrombosis. European Journal of Vascular and Endovascular Surgery, 33(2), 223–233. https://doi.org/10.1016/j.ejvs.2006.10.006.

Fabbrini, E., Sullivan, S., Klein, S. (2010). Obesity and nonalcoholic fatty liver disease: Biochemical, metabolic, and clinical implications. Hepatology, 51(2), 679–689. https://doi.org/10.1002/hep.23280.

Frühbeck, G., Busetto, L., Dicker, D., Yumuk, V., Goossens, G.H., Hebebrand, J., Halford, J.G.C., Farpour-Lambert, N.J., Blaak, E.E., Woodward, E., Toplak, H. (2019). The ABCD of obesity: An EASO position statement on a diagnostic term with clinical and scientific implications. Obesity Facts, 12(2), 131–136. https://doi.org/10.1159/000497124.

Grewal, A.K., Singh, N., Singh, T.G. (2019). Effects of resveratrol postconditioning on cerebral ischemia in mice: Role of the sirtuin-1 pathway. Canadian Journal of Physiology and Pharmacology, 97(11), 1094–1101. https://doi.org/10.1139/cjpp-2019-0188.

Guerreiro, V.A., Carvalho, D., Freitas, P. (2022). Obesity, adipose tissue, and inflammation answered in questions. World Journal of Obesity, 2022, 2252516. https://doi.org/10.1155/2022/2252516.

Gulinac, M., Miteva, D.G., Peshevska-Sekulovska, M., Novakov, I.P., Antovic, S., Peruhova, M., Snegarova, V., Kabakchieva, P., Assyov, Y., Vasilev, G., Sekulovski, M., Lazova, S., Tomov, L., Velikova, T. (2023). Long-term effectiveness, outcomes and complications of bariatric surgery. World Journal of Clinical Cases, 11(19), 4504–4512. https://doi.org/10.12998/wjcc.v11.i19.4504.

Islam, M.R., Arthur, S., Haynes, J., Butts, M.R., Nepal, N., Sundaram, U. (2022). The role of gut microbiota and metabolites in obesity-associated chronic gastrointestinal disorders. Nutrients, 14(3), 624. https://doi.org/10.3390/nu14030624.

Khafagy, R., Dash, S. (2021). Obesity and cardiovascular disease: The emerging role of inflammation. Frontiers in Cardiovascular Medicine, 8, 768119. https://doi.org/10.3389/fcvm.2021.768119.

Khan, H., Bangar, A., Grewal, A.K., Bansal, P., Singh, T.G. (2022b). Caspase-mediated regulation of the distinct signaling pathways and mechanisms in neuronal survival. International Immunopharmacology, 110, 108951. https://doi.org/10.1016/j.intimp.2022.108951.

Khan, H., Singh, T.G., Dahiya, R.S. (2022a). Abdel-Daim MM. α-lipoic acid, an organosulfur biomolecule a novel therapeutic agent for neurodegenerative disorders: An mechanistic perspective. Neurochemical Research, 47(7), 1853–1864. https://doi.org/10.1007/s11064-022-03598-w.

Klop, B., Elte, J.W., Cabezas, M.C. (2013). Dyslipidemia in obesity: Mechanisms and potential targets. Nutrients, 5(4), 1218–1240. https://doi.org/10.3390/nu5041218.

Kwok, S., Adam, S., Ho, J.H., Iqbal, Z., Turkington, P., Razvi, S., Le Roux, C.W., Soran, H., Syed, A.A. (2020). Obesity: A critical risk factor in the COVID-19 pandemic. Clinical Obesity, 10(6), e12403. https://doi.org/10.1111/cob.12403.

Leske, M., Galanis, C., Koczwara, B., Beatty, L. (2024). A meta-analysis of healthy lifestyle interventions addressing quality of life of cancer survivors in the post treatment phase. Journal of Cancer Survivorship. https://doi.org/10.1007/s11764-023-01514-x.

Lin, X., Li, H. (2021). Obesity: Epidemiology, pathophysiology, and therapeutics. Frontiers in Endocrinology (Lausanne), 12, 706978. https://doi.org/10.3389/fendo.2021.706978.

Montesi, L., El Ghoch, M., Brodosi, L., Calugi, S., Marchesini, G., Dalle Grave, R. (2016). Long-term weight loss maintenance for obesity: A multidisciplinary approach. Diabetes, Metabolic Syndrome and Obesity, 9, 37–46. https://doi.org/10.2147/DMSO.S89836.

Pati, S., Irfan, W., Jameel, A., Ahmed, S., Shahid, R.K. (2023). Obesity and cancer: A current overview of epidemiology, pathogenesis, outcomes, and management. Cancers (Basel). 15(2), 485. https://doi.org/10.3390/cancers15020485.

Poirier, P., Giles, T.D., Bray, G.A., Hong, Y., Stern, J.S., Pi-Sunyer, F.X., Eckel, R.H.; American Heart Association; Obesity Committee of the Council on Nutrition, Physical Activity, and Metabolism. (2006). Obesity and cardiovascular disease: Pathophysiology, evaluation, and effect of weight loss: An update of the 1997 American Heart Association Scientific Statement on Obesity and Heart Disease from the Obesity Committee of the Council on Nutrition, Physical Activity, and Metabolism. Circulation, 113(6), 898–918. https://doi.org/10.1161/CIRCULATIONAHA.106.171016.

Prabhakar, N.K., Khan, H., Grewal, A.K., Singh, T.G. (2022). Intervention of neuroinflammation in the traumatic brain injury trajectory: In vivo and clinical approaches. International Immunopharmacology, 108, 108902. https://doi.org/10.1016/j.intimp.2022.108902.

Rohm, T.V., Meier, D.T., Olefsky, J.M., Donath, M.Y. (2022). Inflammation in obesity, diabetes, and related disorders. Immunity, 55(1), 31–55. https://doi.org/10.1016/j.immuni.2021.12.013.

Safaei, M., Sundararajan, E.A., Driss, M., Boulila, W., Shapi'i, A. (2021). A systematic literature review on obesity: Understanding the causes & consequences of obesity and reviewing various machine learning approaches used to predict obesity. Computers in Biology and Medicine, 136, 104754. https://doi.org/10.1016/j.compbiomed.2021.104754.

Sagris, M., Vardas, E.P., Theofilis, P., Antonopoulos, A.S., Oikonomou, E., Tousoulis, D. (2021). Atrial fibrillation: Pathogenesis, predisposing factors, and genetics. International Journal of Molecular Sciences, 23(1), 6. https://doi.org/10.3390/ijms23010006.

Sharma, V., Singh, T.G., Kaur, A., Mannan, A., Dhiman, S. (2023). Brain-derived neurotrophic factor: A novel dynamically regulated therapeutic modulator in neurological disorders. Neurochemical Research, 48(2), 317–339. https://doi.org/10.1007/s11064-022-03755-1.

Sharma, V.K., Singh, T.G., Prabhakar, N.K., Mannan, A. (2022). Kynurenine metabolism and Alzheimer's disease: The potential targets and approaches. Neurochemical Research, 47(6), 1459–1476. https://doi.org/10.1007/s11064-022-03546-8.

Singh, R., Farooq, S.A., Mannan, A., Singh, T.G., Najda, A., Grażyna, Z., Albadrani, G.M., Sayed, A.A., Abdel-Daim, M.M. (2022). Animal models of diabetic microvascular complications: Relevance to clinical features. Biomedicine & Pharmacotherapy, 145, 112305. https://doi.org/10.1016/j.biopha.2021.112305.

Smith, J.D., Fu, E., Kobayashi, M.A. (2020). Prevention and management of childhood obesity and its psychological and health comorbidities. Annual Review of Clinical Psychology, 16, 351–378. https://doi.org/10.1146/annurev-clinpsy-100219-060201.

Soleymani, T., Daniel, S., Garvey, W.T. (2016). Weight maintenance: Challenges, tools and strategies for primary care physicians. Obesity Reviews, 17(1), 81–93. https://doi.org/10.1111/obr.12322.

Tak, Y.J., Lee, S.Y. (2021). Long-term efficacy and safety of anti-obesity treatment: Where do we stand? Current Obesity Reports, 10(1), 14–30. https://doi.org/10.1007/s13679-020-00422-w.

Vishwas, S., Gulati, M., Kapoor, B., Gupta, S., Singh, S.K., Awasthi, A., Khan, A., Goyal, A., Bansal, A., Baishnab, S., Singh, T.G., Arora, S., Porwal, O., Kumar, A., Kumar, V. (2021). Expanding the arsenal against Huntington's disease-herbal drugs and their nanoformulations. Current Neuropharmacology, 19(7), 957–989. https://doi.org/10.2174/1570159×18666201109090824.

Walsh, T.P., Arnold, J.B., Evans, A.M., Yaxley, A., Damarell, R.A., Shanahan, E.M. (2018). The association between body fat and musculoskeletal pain: A systematic review and meta-analysis. BMC Musculoskeletal Disorders, 19(1), 233. https://doi.org/10.1186/s12891-018-2137-0.

CHAPTER 9

New Insights Into the Metabolic Syndrome–Cancer Nexus

TEESHYO BHATTACHARYA[1], SHUBHAM SINGH BARTWAL[2], INDRAJIT BHATTACHARYA[1], MURALI DHANASEKARAN[3], REMYA SREEDHAR[4], and SOMASUNDARAM ARUMUGAM[1*]

[1]*Department of Pharmacology and Toxicology, National Institute of Pharmaceutical Education and Research (NIPER), Kolkata, West Bengal, India*

[2]*National Institute of Pharmaceutical Education and Research (NIPER), Hyderabad, Telangana, India*

[3]*Auburn University, Harrison College of Pharmacy, Auburn, AL, USA*

[4]*School of Pharmacy, Sister Nivedita University, Newtown, Kolkata, West Bengal, India*

*Corresponding author

ABSTRACT

The prevalence of metabolic syndrome is rising in various geographical locations worldwide. The major components of metabolic syndrome include abdominal obesity, hypertension, dyslipidemia, and insulin resistance. Recent research has effectively linked metabolic syndrome to be a leading cause of malignancies, including colorectal, breast, and 11 other forms of cancer. In this chapter, we discuss how people across the globe who suffer from metabolic syndrome often end up having different types of cancers in brief by taking examples of various cohort studies carried out across the world. We also discuss in brief multiple factors (like food

Pharmacotherapy Approaches Toward Endocrine and Metabolic Diseases.
Thakur Gurjeet Singh and Sanjana Mehta (Eds.)

DOI: 10.1201/9781779640154-9

habits, sleeping patterns, and lack of exercise) that lead to the development of metabolic syndromes, ultimately paving the way for numerous types of cancers. We will also focus on the various physiological and biochemical mechanisms like visceral adiposity, hyperglycemia, insulin-like growth factor/insulin-like growth factor receptor axis, inflammatory responses, estrogen signaling, plasminogen activator inhibitor-1, and Wnt signaling pathways. Additionally, we will emphasize the pharmacotherapeutic approaches to treat various metabolic syndrome-related cancers, like using antidiabetics and monoclonal antibodies. We will also discuss recently FDA-approved drugs targeting metabolic syndrome. We will also discuss the difficulties in developing effective therapies, and the future directions necessary.

9.1 INTRODUCTION

Good metabolism is the key to a better life, and metabolic disorders start a vicious cycle, which becomes the tipping point for various diseases (Muddapu et al., 2020; Chaitanya et al., 2022). Metabolic syndrome is an inflammatory disease characterized by obesity, hyperglycemia, and cardiovascular problems (Harding et al., 2015). It is caused by a complex network of interrelated causes facilitating the start and disease progression (Dabke et al., 2019; Yanai et al., 2021). The latest studies provide evidence of an inflammatory environment in metabolic syndrome causing reactive oxygen species formation (Esposito and Giugliano, 2004; Sharma et al., 2021a, 2021b), which damages proteins, lipids, and nucleic acids within the cell, leading to impaired energy metabolism and altered cell signaling and cell cycle. These changes, in turn, lead to altered genetic expressions, cellular transport mechanisms, and immune and inflammatory responses (McCracken et al., 2018; Rius-Pérez et al., 2020). Some studies have shown that oxidative stress is promoted by daily dietary intake of a high-fat, high-carb diet, characterized by elevated lipid peroxidation, protein carbonylation, a weakened antioxidant system, and lowered glutathione levels (Goutzourelas et al., 2018; Sharma et al., 2021a, 2021b). Several chronic diseases result from inflammation (Amorim et al., 2022; Lim et al., 2021). Research indicates that oxidative stress and chronic inflammation are significant contributing factors to the development of carcinogenesis. Recent data also suggests that people who suffer from metabolic syndrome have a high probability of having cancers (Garay-Sevilla et al., 2021; Klöting and Blüher, 2014). According to US studies, the prevalence of metabolic syndrome rises with age, with a total frequency of 24% in the general population and 50% in individuals with ischemic cardiopathy and other cardiovascular disorders (Thapa et al., 2022). In Spain, the prevalence rises with age as well; in the general population, it ranges from 23% to 31%, and among those under 65, it affects more men than women. However, recent data indicate that metabolic syndrome and allied ailments show a steeper prevalence rate than in men (Fernández-Bergés et al., 2012; Kant et al., 2020). According to recent research, metabolic syndrome increases a person's risk of developing endometrial, pancreatic, colorectal, ovarian, and postmenopausal breast cancer in women and liver, colorectal, and bladder cancer in men. Research on metabolic syndrome and prostate cancer has yielded conflicting results, with some indicating a higher risk (Sharma et al., 2020). Additionally, a published meta-analysis discovered that metabolic syndrome patients had an increased risk of hematological malignancy. Specific research suggests that one or two elements of metabolic syndrome are independently linked to colorectal, breast, endometrial, bladder, kidney, lung, and thyroid cancers (López-Jiménez et al., 2022; Khan et al., 2022).

9.2 CANCERS RELATED TO METABOLIC SYNDROME

Several intriguing studies that have been published in recent years have demonstrated a correlation between the risk of cancer and the several elements that make up metabolic syndrome. The two aspects of metabolic syndrome positively linked to cancer risk are abdominal obesity and hyperglycemia (Park et al., 2014; Ramteke et al., 2019), and meta-analysis studies showing the extent to which their impact have been listed in Table 9.1. There is insufficient data to link carcinogenesis with either hypertension or dyslipidemia. Obese patients have abnormally expanded adipose tissue that generates a variety of pro-inflammatory cytokines and bioactive molecules such as TNF-α, IL-6, leptin, visfatin, resistin, MCP-1, PAI-1, and RBP-4. These biomolecules produce an inflammatory atmosphere and encourage the growth of cells, insulin resistance, and gluconeogenesis (Deng et al., 2016; Thapa et al., 2021). The lipolysis that comes with obesity increases the circulation of free fatty acids, which raises the generation of very low-density lipoproteins and liver glucose while decreasing the sensitivity of muscles to insulin (Avgerinos et al., 2019; Batiha et al., 2022). In hyperglycemia, due to various cellular mechanisms, insulin-like growth factor binding protein-3 (Brauna et al., 2011; Prabhakar et al., 2022) is reduced, which leads to an increase in free insulin, IGF-F2, and IGF-1. Increased growth factors lead to activation of the PI3K/AKT and MAPK pathways, leading to the overstimulation of IR-A and IGF-1RA, ultimately leading to cell proliferation while suppressing cellular death (Keshet and Seger, 2010).

TABLE 9.1 Various Meta-Analysis Reports Linking Risks of Components of Metabolic Syndrome to Cancer in Males and Females

Cancer Type	Risk Ratio*	References
Gastric	T2DM: 1.20 in both males and females Obesity: 1.52 in males and 1.51 in females	Ling et al. (2020), Renehan et al. (2008)
Prostate	T2DM: 1.19 in males Obesity: 1.03 in males	Crawley et al. (2014), Esposito et al. (2012), Renehan et al. (2008)
Ovarian	T2DM: 1.34 in females Obesity: 1.03 in females	Choi et al. (2020), Yang et al. (2014), Renehan et al. (2008)
Lung	T2DM: 0.97 in males and 0.76 in females Obesity: 0.76 in males and 0.80 in females	Renehan et al. (2008), Tsilidis et al. (2015)
Breast	T2DM: 1.09 in females Obesity: 1.19 in females	Chen et al. (2017), Ling et al. (2020)
Liver	T2DM: 2.31 in both males and females Obesity: 1.18 in both males and females	Yang et al. (2014), Renehan et al. (2008)
Pancreas	T2DM: 1.20 in males and 1.58 in females Obesity: 0.97 in males and 1.04 in females	Renehan et al. (2008), Tsilidis et al. (2015), Esposito et al. (2012)
Colorectal	T2DM: 1.35 in both males and females Obesity: 1.02 in both males and females	Abar et al. (2019), Crawley et al. (2014)
Leukaemia	T2DM: 1.28 in both males and females Obesity: 1.08 in males and 1.17 in females	Renehan et al. (2008), Tsilidis et al. (2015)

*A risk ratio of 1.00 or above indicates positive association of the risk with the cause.

9.3 PATHWAYS/MECHANISM

In the previous section, we saw that obesity and hyperglycemia are key factors driving the inflammatory environment in metabolic syndrome. Given those two elements, we will explore the intricate cellular pathways and mechanisms that create the inflammatory environment, which ultimately transforms into a tumor microenvironment. Figure 9.1 briefly describes the cellular mechanisms driving the transformation.

9.3.1 VISCERAL ADIPOSITY

Visceral adiposity or obesity is an ailment that leads to metabolic syndrome-related cancers (Mili et al., 2021). Adipose or fat tissues are mainly of two types: white adipose tissues (WAT) or brown adipose tissues (Key et al., 2010). Among the adipose tissues, the WAT has been recognized as a critical driver of carcinogenesis. Still, in normal physiological conditions, it performs mechanical functions like protecting essential organs and active secretion of systemic hormones like adiponectin and leptin and cytokines like TNF-α and interleukin-6. The secretions from WAT interact with the immune system and different growth factors such as TGF-β, IGF-1, and IGFBPs (Unamuno et al., 2018). The PPAR-γ of fat cells triggers the release of adiponectin that improves the liver and muscle's metabolism of glucose and fatty acids (lowering the levels of FFA) and raises insulin sensitivity. Adiponectin is thought to have anticancer properties owing to its anti-inflammatory actions and is a negative regulator of angiogenesis. A high level of obesity leads to the development of hypoxia, which is sensed by various ion channels present on the surface of the WAT cells. It leads to decreased PPAR-γ receptors, causing a decrease in adiponectin and decreased caspases—meanwhile, the expression of leptin increases, leading to neoplastic transformation of tissues and angiogenesis. The hypoxia also causes an increase in various tumorigenic factors such as VEGF, HIF-1a, MMP2, and MMP9, which lead to pro-oncogenic transformation such as cell proliferation, angiogenesis, and matrix modifications (Said et al., 2023; Ion et al., 2023). WAT is also a rich source of stem cells that can become cancer-forming cells like cancer-associated fibroblasts in the future and enhance cancer formation (Bunnell et al., 2022).

9.3.2 HYPERGLYCAEMIA

Hyperglycemia is a key clinical feature of metabolic syndrome. Systemic hyperglycemia creates the perfect metabolic environment for cancer cells to thrive and multiply (Cheng et al., 2021). Research has shown that high blood glucose can trigger pro-tumorigenic signaling and metabolic reprogramming in normal cells (Byrne et al., 2020). The Warburg effect primarily synthesizes ATP in cancer cells (Wu et al., 2019); besides producing quick energy, glycolysis provides intermediate products. These intermediates create the biological macromolecules, such as proteins, fatty acids, and nucleotides, that tumors need to proliferate. The high amount of blood glucose transport into the cells via GLUT transporters leads to excess glycolysis, forming lactic acid. Lactic acid has been implicated in epithelial–mesenchymal transition (EMT) via the expression of ERα/GLUT4 (Gu et al., 2018). High glucose levels can also stimulate vascular endothelial growth factor (VEGF)/VEGFR, leading to vasculogenesis (Zhang et al., 2022).

Increased glucose uptake and glycolysis may stimulate AMPK/mTOR/S6 MAPK and STAT3 signaling pathways and promote invasiveness (Wallbillich et al., 2017). PKM2 is a critical metabolic enzyme in glycolysis and, through the Warburg effect, plays a vital role in tumorigenesis. High glucose levels have been linked to the abnormal expression of PKM2, which may promote the accumulation of glycolysis intermediates like lactic acid (Bohn et al., 2018; Goswami et al., 2022), and previously, it has been described how lactic acid drives a tumor microenvironment formation. Further studies have revealed that the lactic acid generated by the glycolysis of cancer cells can trigger the conversion of anti-tumor type M1 macrophages into M2 macrophages, which creates an inflammatory environment leading to carcinogenesis (Wei et al., 2017).

9.3.3 IGF/IGF-R AXIS

IGF has been implicated in tumorigenesis, like factor PDGF and TGF. Metabolic syndrome is characterized by a high amount of release of IGF (Haywood et al., 2019). IGF axis is composed of two ligands (IGF-I, IGF-II) and their receptors (IGF-IR, IGF-IIR) and six IGF binding proteins

(IGFBP-I to IGFBP-VI) (Hua et al., 2020). The IGF-I binds with IGF-IR with the help of IGFBPs, stimulates proliferation, and inhibits apoptosis. After binding of IGF-I with IGF-IR, it activates phosphatidylinositol-3 kinase (PI3K)-Akt pathway/protein kinase B (PKB) and Ras-MAPK pathway and their downstream pathway (Wong et al., 2010). The Akt activates the mammalian target of rapamycin (mTOR) and Forkhead box O (FoxO) and inhibits glycogen synthase kinase 3β (GSK3β), which leads to β-catenin accumulation and activates its downstream targets. The mTOR regulates cell growth, proliferation, drug resistance, and survival (Memmott and Dennis, 2009).

9.3.4 INFLAMMATION

Inflammation is the link between metabolic syndrome and different types of cancer. Chronic inflammation related to metabolic syndrome is associated with insulin resistance, type 2 diabetes (T2D), and obesity. Inflammation associated with a metabolic syndrome is characterized by elevation of serum level of C-reactive protein (CRP), IL-6, TNF-α, and MCP-1 (Vendramini-Costa and Carvalho, 2012). Tumor microenvironments comprise innate and adaptive immune cells, fibroblasts, mast cells, and epithelial cells (Allavena et al., 2008; Gupta et al., 2018). The macrophages in the tumor microenvironment are the key drivers of the inflammatory response, which transform into M2 macrophages from M1 form owing to signaling from cancer cells and adipocytes. These macrophages release inflammatory mediators and initiate NF-κB-dependent pathways, which results in other mediators for cancer-related inflammation like cyclooxygenase-2 (COX-2), which catalyzes the synthesis of prostaglandin E_2, a lipid proinflammatory mediator. Overexpression of COX-2 indicates poor prognosis in different cancers (Koki et al., 2002).

9.3.5 ESTROGEN SIGNALING

Estrogens are steroid hormones having aromatic rings synthesized from cholesterol in the rough endoplasmic reticulum. There are four forms of estrogens: estrone (E1), estradiol (E2), estriol (E3), and estetrol (E4)

(Hamilton et al., 2017). E1 and E2 are synthesized in adipose tissue from testosterone by aromatase (CYP19A1). The estrogen receptor (ER) has three types: nuclear ER (nER), membrane-bound ER (mbER), and extracellular receptor, which is G-protein coupled (GPER1). The nER signaling is known as genomic signaling or classical signaling. In humans, two isoforms of nER are ERα and ERβ, which ESR1 and ESR2 code. The ERβ and ERα comprise 595 and 530 amino acids, respectively (Enmark et al., 1997). The N-terminal consists of the A/B domain, also known as the activation of function domain-1 (AF-1). The C-domain is known as the DNA binding domain, which is responsible for receptor dimerization and binds with the estrogen response element (ERE); the D-domain is known as the hinge region (H), which undergoes conformational change after ligand binding, the E-domain is known as ligand binding domain where ligands like E2 bind, C-terminal consists of the F-domain also known as activation of functional domain-2 (AF-2) which controls genetic transcription in response to particular ligands. In genomic signaling, E2 binds with ERα and ERβ_separately in the cytoplasm, resulting in receptor conformational change and formed receptor dimerization and complex (Le Dily and Beato, 2018). The heat shock protein 90 (HSP90) protects unbound ER in unbound conditions, whereas HSP90 dissociated from ER after binding with E. Then this complex translocates to the nucleus, where it induces a transcriptional change in estrogenic responsive genes (with or without ERE dependent). In the ERE-dependent manner, dimerized receptors bind with DNA by ERE, and in the ERE-independent manner, dimerized receptors bind with DNA by transcription factor (TFs) (Fuentes and Silveyra, 2019).

In nongenomic signaling, estrogen binds with mbER and activates MAPK and PI3K/AKT with the activation of mTOR (Garcia Dos Santos et al., 2002). However, when estrogen binds with extracellular GPER1, it activates PLC, which cleaves phosphatidylinositol 4,5-bisphosphate (PIP2) into DAG and remains in the membrane. PKC and the other form, IP3, diffuse into the cytoplasm and bind with the IP3 receptor in the endoplasmic reticulum, releasing Ca^{2+} that stimulates downstream signaling (Nilsson et al., 2001). One of the hallmarks of ovarian, uterine, and breast epithelial cell cancer is the deregulation of ERα expression (López-Reig and López-Guerrero, 2020).

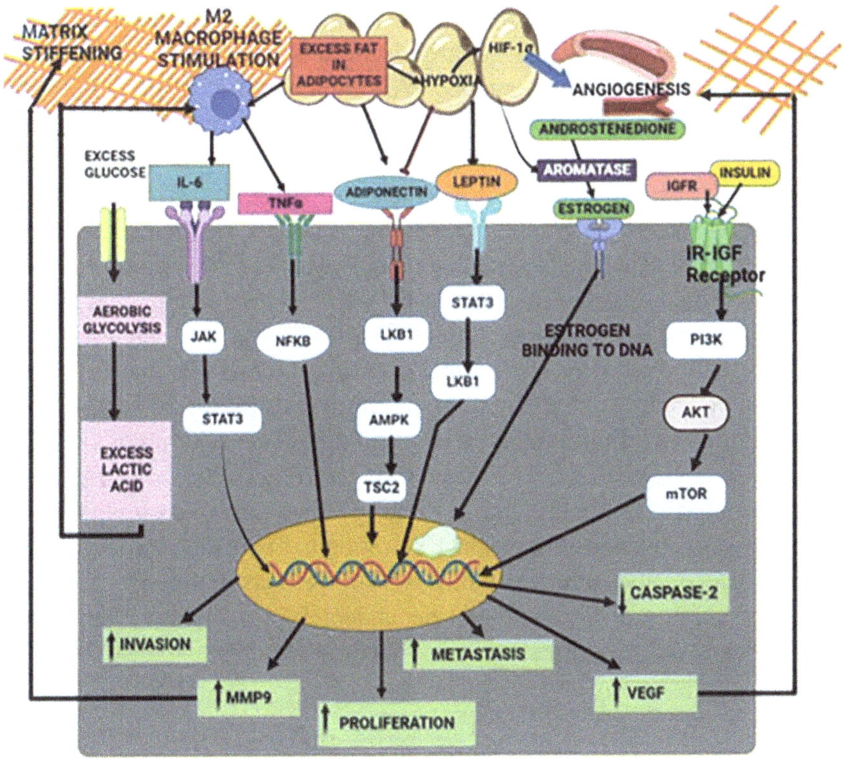

FIGURE 9.1 Tumor microenvironment due to metabolic syndrome.

9.3.6 PLASMINOGEN ACTIVATOR INHIBITOR-1 AND WNT SIGNALING PATHWAYS

Plasminogen activator inhibitor 1 (PAI-1) is a member of the serine protease inhibitor (Serpin) family that inhibits tissue-type plasminogen activator (tPA) and urokinase-type plasminogen activator (uPA). It has three domains: the first domain, known as the reactive center loop (RCL), binds with uPA; the second domain binds with vitronectin located in the flexible region, containing helix D (hD), helix E (hE), and helix F (hF); the third domain binds with low-density lipoprotein receptor-related protein (LRP1), located within hD and hE (Kubala and DeClerck, 2019). PAI-1 stimulates cancer cell proliferation, resisting cell apoptosis, angiogenesis, tumor progression, and inflammation (Jin et al., 2020). PAI-1 promotes cancer cell proliferation by upregulating cyclin D3/cdk4/6, which leads to cell cycle propagation from G1 to the S phase by maintaining thrombin activity (Giacoia et al., 2014). Thrombin binds with protease activation receptor (PAR), which upregulates PAI-1 transcription of PAI-1. PAI-1 decreases intrinsic apoptosis by inhibiting caspase three and induces anoikis by inhibiting cell adhesion to vitronectin, leading to cell migration and adhesion to fibronectin (Lademann and Rømer, 2008). PAI-1 stimulates angiogenesis by protecting endothelial cells (EC) from the Fas ligand (FasL)-dependent intrinsic apoptosis pathway, and PAI-1 also promotes fibrin deposition, leads to EC organization, and releases angiogenic protein like interleukin (IL)-8 (Bajou et al., 2008). PAI-1 promotes metastasis by detaching cells from vitronectin and preventing extracellular matrix protein degradation, leading to the migration of tumor cells (Maillard et al., 2008). PAI-1 stimulates inflammation by recruiting monocytes to tumor sites and activates p38/NFkB/Il-6/STAT3 signaling, leading to the polarization of M2 macrophages (Kubala et al., 2018). The Wnt pathway is classified into two pathways: β-catenin-dependent or canonical pathway and β-catenin-independent or noncanonical pathway. The primary hallmark of cancer is overexpression of the β-catenin-dependent Wnt pathway (Zhan et al., 2017). Figure 9.2 describes the pathway in detail.

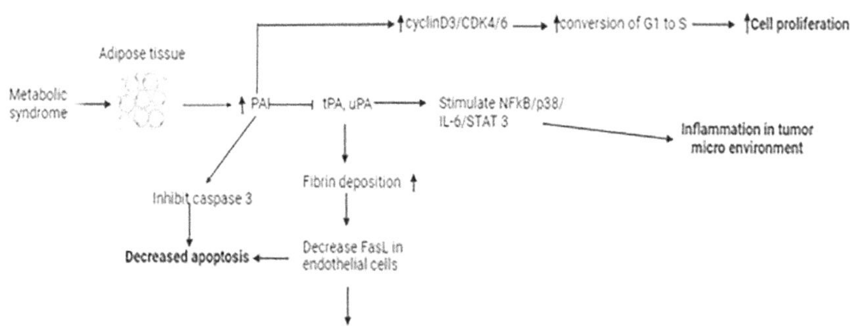

FIGURE 9.2 Depiction of plasminogen activator inhibitor-1 and Wnt-signaling pathways.

9.4 THERAPEUTIC APPROACHES AND LIFESTYLE MODIFICATION

Several intriguing studies have been published in recent years that demonstrate a correlation between various components of metabolic syndrome and cancer risk. There are, however, few epidemiologic studies that connect metabolic syndrome to cancer. A recent large-scale population-based study conducted in Milan, Italy, tracked 16,677 participants for up to 8 years while they were on medication for hypertension, diabetes, and hyperlipidemia. During the study period, 823 cases of cancer were reported, with men having a notably higher incidence of pancreatic cancer. The two significant elements of metabolic syndrome that have been positively linked to the risk of cancer are hyperglycemia and abdominal obesity (Mili et al., 2021). Different treatment modalities are employed to address cancer associated with metabolic syndrome. Among these are life-style modification, monoclonal antibody therapy, and antidiabetic therapy.

9.4.1 ANTIDIABETIC THERAPY IN CANCER

Since insulin resistance and hyperglycemia are critical factors in the processes underlying tumor formation, treating and preventing cancer by addressing these conditions with antidiabetic medication can be helpful (Zakikhani et al., 2006). Numerous studies have demonstrated that IGF-1 receptors are overexpressed in various malignancies. Insulin can increase the production of IGF-1 by upregulating growth hormone receptors in the liver, which serves as the principal stimulus for IGF-1 synthesis in the liver (Pollak, 2012; Quinn et al., 2013). There is an encouraging impact of antidiabetic and anti-hypertensive medications on cancer. Till March 2023, 52 clinical trials assessed the anticancer efficaciousness of antidiabetic medicines. It is interesting to note that most antidiabetic agents are in Phase II trials (67%) compared to Phase I (23%) and Phase III trials (10%) (Hijazi et al., 2023). Extracted from the legume *Galega officinalis*, Metformin (1,1-dimethyl-biguanide hydrochloride) is frequently utilized in trials [currently 37 trials (Phase I, II, III)] to evaluate and confirm its antitumorigenic properties (Hijazi et al., 2023). More than 50 clinical trials investigating the possible anticancer effect of Metformin against endometrial, prostate, pancreatic, lung, and breast cancer were initiated as a result of numerous *in vitro* and preclinical studies that confirmed the antineoplastic activity of the drug against various cancer types. A new meta-analysis of 67 trials with over 10 million type 2 diabetes patients and over 145,00 cancer cases demonstrated the preventive effect of Metformin. The overall risk of cancer was 30% lower for metformin users who had ever used the drug than for nonusers (Eibl and Rozengurt, 2021). Metformin exerts its anticancer activity by activating various pathways like the AMPK/mTOR pathway, which is a primary controller of the amount of energy inside the cells and with critical biological functions, including cell proliferation, autophagy, apoptosis, and the metabolism of lipids and glucose. Other antitumor effects of Metformin are AMPK independent (like redox shuttle enzyme mitochondrial glycerol-3-phosphate dehydrogenase (mGPDH) inhibition), which is known as the pleiotropic effect (Athreya et al., 2017; Janjetovic et al., 2011). In conjunction with imatinib mesylate, etoricoxib, and dexamethasone, pioglitazone is being studied in clinical Phase II for prostate cancer.

Regarding mechanism, pioglitazone reduces TNFα, TGF-β, and the chemokine monocyte chemoattractant protein-1 (MCP-1) levels (Miyazawa et al., 2018). Pioglitazone's most notable action is to trigger ferroptosis, a form of cell death in HNC cells (Kim et al., 2018). A Phase I clinical trial using the SGLT2 inhibitor dapagliflozin is currently being conducted to treat pediatric brain cancers. Acarbose, which blocks the breakdown of starch and other sugars, is a novel approach explored in Phase II clinical trials for its potential to enhance the effectiveness of conventional chemotherapy in treating renal sarcoma (Orlandella et al., 2020). An examination of retrospective cohort studies and meta-analyses shows that acarbose lowers the incidence of lung and colorectal cancer. Acarbose prolongs life and decreases tumors in mouse models of Apc+/Min mouse and APC knockout (Dodds et al., 2020).

9.4.2 MONOCLONAL ANTIBODY THERAPY

Since today's antibody medications are so selective, side effects are becoming less frequent. Consequently, therapeutic antibodies have emerged as the most common type of newly produced pharmaceuticals. In the last five years, antibodies have emerged as the pharmaceutical industry's bestselling medications; in 2018, biologics accounted for eight of the top ten bestselling medications globally (Lu et al., 2020). Anti-asprosin monoclonal antibodies (mAbs) are one of the relatively few advancements in Mab therapy for metabolic syndrome. Asprosin is a novel glucogenic and orexigenic hormone, and it is found in higher concentrations in the bloodstream of metabolic syndrome patients, mice, and rats (Mishra et al., 2021). Asprosin's ability to activate liver GPCR signaling and brain AgRP neurons explains its dual roles in glucose production and appetite stimulation (glucogenic and orexigenic functions). Anti-asprosin antibodies have a double whammy effect, not just by scavenging it from the bloodstream but also by inhibiting its downstream cAMP signaling cascade in the liver and AgRP hunger-controlling neurons of mice with metabolic syndrome. By aiding in the breakdown of the LDL receptor (LDL-R), proprotein convertase subtilisin/kexin type 9 (PCSK9) controls serum levels of LDL-C and is a desirable target for treating hypercholesterolemia. Anti-PCSK9, a novel fully human antibody, binds to hPCSK9 and elevates the hepatic LDL-R levels dose-dependently while diminishing serum LDL-C (Xu et al., 2021).

9.4.3 LIFESTYLE MODIFICATION

Life modification includes changes in diet, physical activity, and weight loss. The primary risk factors for obesity, belly fat, type 2 diabetes, dyslipidemia, and metabolic syndrome are a sedentary lifestyle without frequent exercise and an unhealthy diet high in fats and carbs. However, these risk factors are also reversible. A BMI of 25 or higher is considered overweight, while 30 or higher falls within the obese category. Consuming red and processed meat, which is prevalent in obese individuals, is closely linked to stomach, colon, and rectal cancer. Restoring a healthy BMI by exercise and eating a low-fat, low-carb diet rich in antioxidants may be the objectives. A diet rich in MUFAs, ω-3 PUFAs, antioxidants, and phytochemicals found in fruits, vegetables, whole grains, legumes, fish, and olive oil, combined with probiotic support, can optimize metabolic health by influencing gene expression, cellular pathways, and levels of stress, inflammation, and fat storage (Rani et al., 2016).

9.5 RECENTLY APPROVED DRUGS FOR METABOLIC SYNDROME

There are very few recently approved drugs that are used in metabolic syndrome. Tirzepatide, the active ingredient in *Mounjaro*, binds to the receptor of two hormones generated in the gut: glucagon-like peptide-1 (GLP-1) and glucose-dependent insulinotropic polypeptide (GIP). It increases the quantity of insulin the pancreas releases in response to meals, working like GIP and GLP-1 (Muzurović et al., 2022), aiding in regulating blood sugar levels. Participants in the clinical trial with obesity, 5 mg, 10 mg, or 15 mg of tripeptide once weekly provided substantial and sustained reductions in body weight (Jastreboff et al., 2022; Sinha et al., 2023).

9.6 FUTURE CHALLENGES

Metformin has the potential to treat cancer, and it can be administered safely with chemotherapy and radiation. Even if the data indicates that Metformin does not significantly improve cancer incidence or outcomes, future research should focus on particular genotypic or phenotypic subgroups that show promise (Yu and Suissa, 2023). Researchers need to identify the part played by the gut microbiota and how prebiotics and probiotics can influence it, which may shed light on the pathophysiology of metabolic syndrome and help create novel therapeutic strategies for the metabolic changes that cause the disease. Scientists are also working on wearable technology that detects sweat, which has great promise for collecting vital information on biomarkers linked to metabolic syndrome and related disorders. However, additional research is required to validate the reliability and efficacy of wearables based on sweat.

9.7 CONCLUSION

This chapter sheds light on metabolic syndrome and how some of its elements are intricately involved in carcinogenesis. This chapter also deeply discusses the possible therapeutic approaches and efforts to repurpose antidiabetics as anticancer drugs. Despite research progress, there is still a need to establish a mechanistic relationship between other elements of metabolic syndrome and carcinogenesis. Tirzepatide is a recently approved medication by the Food and Drug Administration that treats metabolic syndrome. However, more approvals are still required, and for that, there is a need for more studies at both preclinical and clinical levels.

KEYWORDS

- **metabolic syndrome**
- **hyperglycemia**
- **inflammation**
- **IGF/IGF-R axis**
- **estrogen**

REFERENCES

Abar, L., Sobiecki, J.G., Cariolou, M., Nanu, N., Vieira, A.R., Stevens, C., Aune, D., Greenwood, D.C., Chan, D.S., Norat T. (2019). Body size and obesity during adulthood, and risk of lympho-haematopoietic cancers: An update of the WCRF-AICR systematic review of published prospective studies. Annals of Oncology, 30(4), 528–541.

Allavena, P., Sica, A., Garlanda, C., Mantovani, A. (2008). The Yin-Yang of tumour-associated macrophages in neoplastic progression and immune surveillance. Immunological Reviews, 222(1), 155–161. https://doi.org/10.1111/J.1600-065X.2008.00607.X

Amorim, J.A., Coppotelli, G., Rolo, A.P., Palmeira, C.M., Ross, J.M., Sinclair, D.A. (2022). Mitochondrial and metabolic dysfunction in aging and age-related diseases. Nature Reviews Endocrinology, 18(4), 243–258. https://doi.org/10.1038/s41574-021-00626-7

Athreya, A.P., Kalari, K.R., Cairns, J., Gaglio, A.J., Wills, Q.F., Niu, N., Weinshilboum, R., Iyer, R.K., Wang, L. (2017). Model-based unsupervised learning informs metformin-induced cell-migration inhibition through an AMPK-independent mechanism in breast cancer. Oncotarget, 8(16), 27199. https://doi.org/10.18632/ONCOTARGET.16109

Avgerinos, K.I., Spyrou, N., Mantzoros, C.S., Dalamaga, M. (2019). Obesity and cancer risk: Emerging biological mechanisms and perspectives. Metabolism, 92, 121–135. https://doi.org/10.1016/J.METABOL.2018.11.001

Vendramini-Costa, D.B., Carvalho, J.E. (2012). Molecular link mechanisms between inflammation and cancer. Current Pharmaceutical Design, 18(26), 3831–3852. https://doi.org/10.2174/138161212802083707

Bajou, K., Peng, H., Laug, W.E., Maillard, C., Noel, A., Foidart, J.M., Martial, J.A., DeClerck, Y.A. (2008). Plasminogen activator inhibitor-1 protects endothelial cells from FasL-mediated apoptosis. Cancer Cell, 14(4), 324–334. https://doi.org/10.1016/J.CCR.2008.08.012

Batiha, G.E.S., Akhtar, N., Alsayegh, A.A., Abusudah, W.F., Almohmadi, N.H., Shaheen, H.M., Singh, T.G., De Waard, M. (2022). Bioactive compounds, pharmacological actions, and pharmacokinetics of genus Acacia. Molecules, 27(21), 7340

Bohn, T., Rapp, S., Luther, N., Klein, M., Bruehl, T.J., Kojima, N., Aranda Lopez, P., Hahlbrock, J., Muth, S., Endo, S., Pektor, S., Brand, A., Renner, K., Popp, V., Gerlach, K., Vogel, D., Lueckel, C., Arnold-Schild, D., Pouyssegur, J., Kreutz, M.,… Bopp, T. (2018). Tumour immunoevasion via acidosis-dependent induction of regulatory tumour-associated macrophages. Nature Immunology, 19(12), 1319–1329. https://doi.org/10.1038/s41590-018-0226-8

Brauna, S., Bitton-Worms, K., Roith, D. (2011). The link between the metabolic syndrome and cancer. International Journal of Biological Sciences, 7(7), 1003. https://doi.org/10.7150/IJBS.7.1003

Bunnell, B.A., Martin, E.C., Matossian, M.D., Brock, C.K., Nguyen, K., Collins-Burow, B., Burow, M.E. (2022). The effect of obesity on adipose-derived stromal cells and adipose tissue and their impact on cancer. Cancer and Metastasis Reviews, 41(3), 549–573. https://doi.org/10.1007/S10555-022-10063-1

Byrne, F.L., Martin, A.R., Kosasih, M., Caruana, B.T., Farrell, R. (2020). The role of hyperglycemia in endometrial cancer pathogenesis. Cancers, 12(5), 1191. https://doi.org/10.3390/CANCERS12051191

Chaitanya, M.V.N.L., Ramanunny, A.K., Babu, M.R., Gulati, M., Vishwas, S., Singh, T.G., Chellappan, D. K., Adams, J., Dua, K., Singh, S.K. (2022). Journey of rosmarinic acid as biomedicine to nano-biomedicine for treating cancer: Current strategies and future perspectives. Pharmaceutics, 14(11), 2401

Chen, Y., Wu, F., Saito, E., Lin, Y., Song, M., Luu, H.N., Gupta, P.C., Sawada, N., Tamakoshi, A., Shu, X.O., Koh, W.P. (2017). Association between type 2 diabetes and risk of cancer mortality: A pooled analysis of over 771,000 individuals in the Asia Cohort Consortium. Diabetologia, 60(6), 1022–1032.

Cheng, H.C., Chang, T.K., Su, W.C., Tsai, H.L., Wang, J.Y. (2021). A narrative review of the influence of diabetes mellitus and hyperglycemia on colorectal cancer risk and oncological outcomes. Translational Oncology, 14(7), 101089. https://doi.org/10.1016/J.TRANON.2021.101089

Choi, Y.J., Jeon, S.M., Shin, S. (2020). Impact of a ketogenic diet on metabolic parameters in patients with obesity or overweight and with or without type 2 diabetes: A meta-analysis of randomized controlled trials. Nutrients, 12(7), 2005.

Crawley, D.J., Holmberg, L., Melvin, J.C., Loda, M., Chowdhury, S., Rudman, S.M., Van Hemelrijck, M. (2014). Serum glucose and risk of cancer: A meta-analysis. BMC Cancer, 14, 1–1.

Dabke, K., Hendrick, G., Devkota, S. (2019). The gut microbiome and metabolic syndrome. The Journal of Clinical Investigation, 129(10), 4050–4057. https://doi.org/10.1172/JCI129194

Deng, T., Lyon, C.J., Bergin, S., Caligiuri, M.A., Hsueh, W.A. (2016). Obesity, Inflammation, and Cancer. Annual Review of Pathology, 11, 421–449. https://doi.org/10.1146/ANNUREV-PATHOL-012615-044359

Dodds, S.G., Parihar, M., Javors, M., Nie, J., Musi, N., Dave Sharp, Z., Hasty, P. (2020). Acarbose improved survival for Apc+/Min mice. Aging Cell, 19(2), e13088. https://doi.org/10.1111/ACEL.13088

Eibl, G., Rozengurt, E. (2021). Metformin: Review of epidemiology and mechanisms of action in pancreatic cancer. Cancer and Metastasis Reviews, 40(3), 865–878. https://doi.org/10.1007/S10555-021-09977-Z

Enmark, E., Pelto-Huikko, M., Grandien, K., Lagercrantz, S., Lagercrantz, J., Fried, G., Nordenskjöld, M., Gustafsson, J.Å. (1997). Human estrogen receptor beta-gene structure, chromosomal localisation, and expression pattern. The Journal of Clinical Endocrinology and Metabolism, 82(12), 4258–4265. https://doi.org/10.1210/JCEM.82.12.4470

Esposito, K., Giugliano, D. (2004). The Metabolic syndrome and inflammation: Association or causation? Nutrition, Metabolism and Cardiovascular Diseases, 14(5), 228–232. https://doi.org/10.1016/S0939-4753(04)80048-6

Esposito, K., Chiodini, P., Bellastella, G., Maiorino, M.I., Giugliano, D. (2012). Proportion of patients at HbA1c target <7% with eight classes of antidiabetic drugs in type 2 diabetes: Systematic review of 218 randomized controlled trials with 78,945 patients. Diabetes, Obesity and Metabolism, 14(3), 228–233.

Fernández-Bergés, D., Cabrera De León, A., Sanz, H., Elosua, R., Guembe, M.J., Alzamora, M., Vega-Alonso, T., Félix-Redondo, F.J., Ortiz-Marrón, H., Rigo, F., Lama, C., Gavrila, D., Segura-Fragoso, A., Lozano, L., Marrugat, J. (2012). Metabolic syndrome in Spain: Prevalence and coronary risk associated with the harmonised definition and

WHO proposal. DARIOS study. Revista Espanola de Cardiologia (English Ed.), 65(3), 241–248. https://doi.org/10.1016/J.RECESP.2011.10.015

Fuentes, N., Silveyra, P. (2019). Estrogen receptor signalling mechanisms. Advances in Protein Chemistry and Structural Biology, 116, 135–170. https://doi.org/10.1016/BS.APCSB.2019.01.001

Garay-Sevilla, M.E., Gomez-Ojeda, A., González, I., Luévano-Contreras, C., Rojas, A. (2021). Contribution of RAGE axis activation to the association between metabolic syndrome and cancer. Molecular and Cellular Biochemistry, 476(3), 1555–1573. https://doi.org/10.1007/S11010-020-04022-Z

Garcia Dos Santos, E., Dieudonne, M.N., Pecquery, R., Le Moal, V., Giudicelli, Y., Lacasa, D. (2002). Rapid nongenomic E2 effects on p42/p44 MAPK, activator protein-1, and cAMP response element binding protein in rat white adipocytes. Endocrinology, 143(3), 930–940. https://doi.org/10.1210/ENDO.143.3.8678

Giacoia, E.G., Miyake, M., Lawton, A., Goodison, S., Rosser, C.J. (2014). PAI-1 leads to G1-phase cell-cycle progression through cyclin D3/cdk4/6 upregulation. Molecular Cancer Research: MCR, 12(3), 322–334. https://doi.org/10.1158/1541-7786.MCR-13-0543

Goswami, K.K., Banerjee, S., Bose, A., Baral, R. (2022). The lactic acid in alternative polarisation and function of macrophages in the tumour microenvironment. Human Immunology, 83(5), 409–417. https://doi.org/10.1016/J.HUMIMM.2022.02.007

Goutzourelas, N., Orfanou, M., Charizanis, I., Leon, G., Spandidos, D.A., Kouretas, D. (2018). GSH levels affect weight loss in individuals with metabolic syndrome and obesity following dietary therapy. Experimental and Therapeutic Medicine, 16(2), 635–642. https://doi.org/10.3892/ETM.2018.6204

Gu, C.J., Xie, F., Zhang, B., Yang, H.L., Cheng, J., He, Y.Y., Zhu, X.Y., Li, D.J., Li, M.Q. (2018). High glucose promotes epithelial-mesenchymal transition of uterus endometrial cancer cells by increasing ER/GLUT4-mediated VEGF secretion. Cellular Physiology and Biochemistry, 50(2), 706–720. https://doi.org/10.1159/000494237

Gupta, S.C., Kunnumakkara, A.B., Aggarwal, S., Aggarwal, B.B. (2018). Inflammation, a double-edge sword for cancer and other age-related diseases. Frontiers in Immunology, 9, 2160. https://doi.org/10.3389/FIMMU.2018.02160

Hamilton, K.J., Hewitt, S.C., Arao, Y., Korach, K.S. (2017). Estrogen hormone biology. Current Topics in Developmental Biology, 125, 109–146. https://doi.org/10.1016/BS.CTDB.2016.12.005

Harding, J., Sooriyakumaran, M., Anstey, K.J., Adams, R., Balkau, B., Briffa, T., Davis, T.M.E., Davis, W.A., Dobson, A., Giles, G.G., Grant, J., Knuiman, M., Luszcz, M., Mitchell, P., Pasco, J.A., Reid, C., Simmons, D., Simons, L., Tonkin, A., Woodward, M.,… Magliano, D.J. (2015). The metabolic syndrome and cancer: Is the metabolic syndrome useful for predicting cancer risk above and beyond its components? Diabetes & Metabolism, 41(6), 463–469. https://doi.org/10.1016/J.DIABET.2015.04.006

Haywood, N.J., Slater, T.A., Matthews, C.J., Wheatcroft, S.B. (2019). The insulin-like growth factor and binding protein family: Novel therapeutic targets in obesity & diabetes. Molecular Metabolism, 19, 86–96. https://doi.org/10.1016/J.MOLMET.2018.10.008

Hijazi, M.A., Gessner, A., El-Najjar, N. (2023). Repurposing of chronically used drugs in cancer therapy: A chance to grasp. Cancers, 15(12), 3199. https://doi.org/10.3390/CANCERS15123199

Hua, H., Kong, Q., Yin, J., Zhang, J., Jiang, Y. (2020). Insulin-like growth factor receptor signalling in tumorigenesis and drug resistance: A challenge for cancer therapy. Journal of Hematology & Oncology, 13(1), 1–17. https://doi.org/10.1186/S13045-020-00904-3

Ion, R.M., Sibianu, M., Hutanu, A., Beresescu, F.G., Sala, D.T., Flavius, M., Rosca, A., Constantin, C., Scurtu, A., Moriczi, R., Muresan, M.G., Gabriel, P., Niculescu, R., Neagoe, R.M. (2023). A comprehensive summary of the current understanding of the relationship between severe obesity, metabolic syndrome, and inflammatory status. Journal of Clinical Medicine, 12(11), 3818. https://doi.org/10.3390/JCM12113818

Janjetovic, K., Vucicevic, L., Misirkic, M., Vilimanovich, U., Tovilovic, G., Zogovic, N., Nikolic, Z., Jovanovic, S., Bumbasirevic, V., Trajkovic, V., Harhaji-Trajkovic, L. (2011). Metformin reduces cisplatin-mediated apoptotic death of cancer cells through AMPK-independent activation of Akt. European Journal of Pharmacology, 651(1–3), 41–50. https://doi.org/10.1016/J.EJPHAR.2010.11.005

Jastreboff, A.M., Aronne, L.J., Ahmad, N.N., Wharton, S., Connery, L., Alves, B., Kiyosue, A., Zhang, S., Liu, B., Bunck, M.C., Stefanski, A. (2022). Tirzepatide once weekly for the treatment of obesity. New England Journal of Medicine, 387(3), 205–216. https://doi.org/10.1056/NEJMOA2206038/SUPPL_FILE/NEJMOA2206038_DATA-SHARING.PDF

Jin, Y., Liang, Z.Y., Zhou, W.X., Zhou, L. (2020). Expression, clinicopathologic and prognostic significance of plasminogen activator inhibitor 1 in hepatocellular carcinoma. Cancer Biomarkers, 27(3), 285–293. https://doi.org/10.3233/CBM-190560

Kant, R., Singh, T.G., Singh, S. (2020). Mechanistic approach to herbal formulations used for urolithiasis treatment. Obesity Medicine, 19, 100266

Keshet, Y., Seger, R. (2010). The MAP kinase signalling cascades: A system of hundreds of components regulates various physiological functions. Methods in Molecular Biology (Clifton, N.J.), 661, 3–38. https://doi.org/10.1007/978-1-60761-795-2_1/COVER

Key, T.J., Spencer, E.A., Reeves, G.K. (2010). Symposium 1: Overnutrition: Consequences and solutions obesity and cancer risk: Conference on 'Over- and undernutrition: Challenges and approaches.' Proceedings of the Nutrition Society, 69(1), 86–90. https://doi.org/10.1017/S0029665109991698

Khan, H., Sharma, K., Kumar, A., Kaur, A., Singh, T.G. (2022). Therapeutic implications of cyclooxygenase (COX) inhibitors in ischemic injury. Inflammation Research, 71(3), 277–292

Kim, E.H., Shin, D., Lee, J., Jung, A.R., Roh, J.L. (2018). CISD2 inhibition overcomes resistance to sulfasalazine-induced ferroptotic cell death in head and neck cancer. Cancer Letters, 432, 180–190. https://doi.org/10.1016/J.CANLET.2018.06.018

Klöting, N., Blüher, M. (2014). Adipocyte dysfunction, inflammation and metabolic syndrome. Reviews in Endocrine and Metabolic Disorders, 15(4), 277–287. https://doi.org/10.1007/S11154-014-9301-0/METRICS

Koki, A., Khan, N.K., Woerner, B.M., Dannenberg, A.J., Olson, L., Seibert, K., Edwards, D., Hardy, M., Isakson, P., Masferrer, J.L. (2002). Cyclooxygenase-2 in human pathological disease. Advances in Experimental Medicine and Biology, 507, 177–184. https://doi.org/10.1007/978-1-4615-0193-0_28

Kubala, M.H., DeClerck, Y.A. (2019). The plasminogen activator inhibitor-1 paradox in cancer: A mechanistic understanding. Cancer Metastasis Reviews, 38(3), 483–492. https://doi.org/10.1007/S10555-019-09806-4

Kubala, M.H., Punj, V., Placencio-Hickok, V.R., Fang, H., Fernandez, G.E., Sposto, R., DeClerck, Y.A. (2018). Plasminogen activator inhibitor-1 promotes the recruitment and polarization of macrophages in cancer. Cell Reports, 25(8), 2177–2191.e7. https://doi.org/10.1016/J.CELREP.2018.10.082

Lademann, U.A., Rømer, M.U. (2008). Regulation of programmed cell death by plasminogen activator inhibitor type 1 (PAI-1). Thrombosis and Haemostasis, 100(6), 1041–1046. https://doi.org/10.1160/TH08-04-0266/ID/JR10606-2/BIB

Le Dily, F., & Beato, M. (2018). Signalling by steroid hormones in the 3D nuclear space. International Journal of Molecular Sciences, 19(2), 306. https://doi.org/10.3390/IJMS19020306

Lim, S., Kim, J.W., Targher, G. (2021). Links between metabolic syndrome and metabolic dysfunction-associated fatty liver disease. Trends in Endocrinology & Metabolism, 32(7), 500–514. https://doi.org/10.1016/J.TEM.2021.04.008

Ling S, Brown K, Miksza JK, Howells L, Morrison A, Issa E, Yates T, Khunti K, Davies MJ, Zaccardi F. (2020). Association of type 2 diabetes with cancer: A meta-analysis with bias analysis for unmeasured confounding in 151 cohorts comprising 32 million people. Diabetes Care, 43(9), 2313–2322.

López-Jiménez, T., Duarte-Salles, T., Plana-Ripoll, O., Recalde, M., Xavier-Cos, F., Puente, D. (2022). Association between metabolic syndrome and 13 types of cancer in Catalonia: A matched case-control study. PloS One, 17(3). https://doi.org/10.1371/JOURNAL.PONE.0264634

López-Reig, R., López-Guerrero, J.A. (2020). The hallmarks of ovarian cancer: Proliferation and cell growth. EJC Supplements, 15, 27–37. https://doi.org/10.1016/J.EJCSUP.2019.12.001

Lu, R.M., Hwang, Y.C., Liu, I.J., Lee, C.C., Tsai, H.Z., Li, H.J., Wu, H.C. (2020). Development of therapeutic antibodies for the treatment of diseases. Journal of Biomedical Science, 27(1), 1–30. https://doi.org/10.1186/S12929-019-0592-Z

Maillard, C.M., Bouquet, C., Petitjean, M.M., Mestdagt, M., Frau, E., Jost, M., Masset, A.M., Opolon, P.H., Beermann, F., Abitbol, M.M., Foidart, J.M., Perricaudet, M.J., Noël, A.C. (2008). Reduction of brain metastases in plasminogen activator inhibitor-1-deficient mice with transgenic ocular tumours. Carcinogenesis, 29(11), 2236–2242. https://doi.org/10.1093/CARCIN/BGN204

McCracken, E., Monaghan, M., Sreenivasan, S. (2018). Pathophysiology of the metabolic syndrome. Clinics in Dermatology, 36(1), 14–20. https://doi.org/10.1016/J.CLINDERMATOL.2017.09.004

Memmott, R.M., Dennis, P.A. (2009). Akt-dependent and -independent mechanisms of mTOR regulation in cancer. Cellular Signalling, 21(5), 656–664. https://doi.org/10.1016/J.CELLSIG.2009.01.004

Mili, N., Paschou, S.A., Goulis, D.G., Dimopoulos, M.A., Lambrinoudaki, I., Psaltopoulou, T. (2021). Obesity, metabolic syndrome, and cancer: Pathophysiological and therapeutic associations. Endocrine, 74(3), 478–497. https://doi.org/10.1007/S12020-021-02884-X

Mishra, I., Duerrschmid, C., Ku, Z., He, Y., Xie, W., Silva, E.S., Hoffman, J., Xin, W., Zhang, N., Xu, Y., An, Z., Chopra, A.R. (2021). Asprosin-neutralizing antibodies as a treatment for metabolic syndrome. ELife, 10, e63784. https://doi.org/10.7554/eLife.63784

Miyazawa, M., Subbaramaiah, K., Bhardwaj, P., Zhou, X.K., Wang, H., Falcone, D.J., Giri, D.D., Dannenberg, A.J. (2018). Pioglitazone inhibits periprostatic white adipose tissue inflammation in obese mice. Cancer Prevention Research, 11(4), 215–226. https://doi.org/10.1158/1940-6207.CAPR-17-0296/36577/AM/PIOGLITAZONE-INHIBITS-PERIPROSTATIC-WHITE-ADIPOSE

Muddapu, V.R., Dharshini, S.A.P., Chakravarthy, V.S., Gromiha, M.M. (2020). Neurodegenerative diseases – is metabolic deficiency the root cause? Frontiers in Neuroscience, 14, 494659. https://doi.org/10.3389/FNINS.2020.00213/BIBTEX

Muzurović, E.M., Volčanšek, Š., Tomšić, K.Z., Janež, A., Mikhailidis, D.P., Rizzo, M., Mantzoros, C.S. (2022). Glucagon-like peptide-1 receptor agonists and dual glucose-dependent insulinotropic polypeptide/glucagon-like peptide-1 receptor agonists in the treatment of obesity/metabolic syndrome, prediabetes/diabetes and non-alcoholic fatty liver disease—current evidence. Journal of Cardiovascular Pharmacology and Therapeutics, 27, 10742484221146371. https://doi.org/10.1177/10742484221146371/ASSET/IMAGES/LARGE/10.1177_10742484221146371-FIG2.JPEG

Nilsson, S., Mäkelä, S., Treuter, E., Tujague, M., Thomsen, J., Andersson, G., Enmark, E., Pettersson, K., Warner, M., Gustafsson, J.Å. (2001). Mechanisms of estrogen action. Physiological Reviews, 81(4), 1535–1565. https://doi.org/10.1152/PHYSREV.2001.81.4.1535

Orlandella, R.M., Turbitt, W.J., Gibson, J.T., Boi, S.K., Li, P., Smith, D.L., Norian, L.A. (2020). The antidiabetic agent acarbose improves anti-PD-1 and rapamycin efficacy in preclinical renal cancer. Cancers, 12(10), 2872. https://doi.org/10.3390/CANCERS12102872

Park, J., Morley, T.S., Kim, M., Clegg, D.J., Scherer, P.E. (2014). Obesity and cancer—mechanisms underlying tumour progression and recurrence. Nature Reviews Endocrinology, 10(8), 455–465. https://doi.org/10.1038/nrendo.2014.94

Pollak, M.N. (2012). Investigating Metformin for cancer prevention and treatment: The end of the beginning. Cancer Discovery, 2(9), 778–790. https://doi.org/10.1158/2159-8290.CD-12-0263/32300/P/INVESTIGATING-METFORMIN-FOR-CANCER-PREVENTION-AND

Prabhakar, N.K., Khan, H., Grewal, A.K., Singh, T.G. (2022). Intervention of neuroinflammation in the traumatic brain injury trajectory: In vivo and clinical approaches. International Immunopharmacology, 108, 108902

Quinn, B.J., Kitagawa, H., Memmott, R.M., Gills, J.J., Dennis, P.A. (2013). Repositioning metformin for cancer prevention and treatment. Trends in Endocrinology & Metabolism, 24(9), 469–480. https://doi.org/10.1016/J.TEM.2013.05.004

Ramteke, P., Deb, A., Shepal, V., Bhat, M.K. (2019). Hyperglycemia associated metabolic and molecular alterations in cancer risk, progression, treatment, and mortality. Cancers, 11(9), 1402. https://doi.org/10.3390/CANCERS11091402

Rani, V., Deep, G., Singh, R.K., Palle, K., Yadav, U.C.S. (2016). Oxidative stress and metabolic disorders: Pathogenesis and therapeutic strategies. Life Sciences, 148, 183–193. https://doi.org/10.1016/j.lfs.2016.02.002

Renehan AG, Tyson M, Egger M, Heller RF, Zwahlen M. (2008). Body-mass index and incidence of cancer: A systematic review and meta-analysis of prospective observational studies. The Lancet, 371(9612), 569–578.

Rius-Pérez, S., Torres-Cuevas, I., Millán, I., Ortega, Á.L., Pérez, S., Sandhu, M.A. (2020). PGC-1 α, inflammation, and oxidative stress: An integrative view in metabolism. Oxidative Medicine and Cellular Longevity, 2020, 1452696. https://doi.org/10.1155/2020/1452696

Said, M.A., Nafeh, N.Y., Abdallah, H.A. (2023). Spexin alleviates hypertension, hyperuricaemia, dyslipidemia and insulin resistance in high fructose diet-induced metabolic syndrome in rats via enhancing PPAR-γ and AMPK and inhibiting IL-6 and TNF-α. Archives of Physiology and Biochemistry, 129(5), 1111–1116. https://doi.org/10.1080/13813455.2021.1899242

Sharma, A., Khan, H., Singh, T.G., Grewal, A.K., Najda, A., Kawecka-Radomska, M., Kamel, M., Altyar, A.E., Abdel-Daim, M.M. (2021a). Pharmacological modulation of ubiquitin-proteasome pathways in oncogenic signaling. International Journal of Molecular Sciences, 22(21), 11971

Sharma, V.K., Singh, T.G., Garg, N., Dhiman, S., Gupta, S., Rahman, M.H., Najda, A., Walasek-Janusz, M., Kamel, M., Albadrani, G.M., Akhtar, M.F., Saleem, A., Altyar, A.E., Abdel-Daim, M.M. (2021b). Dysbiosis and Alzheimer's disease: A role for chronic stress. Biomolecules, 11(05), 678.

Sharma, V., Kaur, A., Singh, T.G. (2020). Counteracting role of nuclear factor erythroid 2-related factor 2 pathway in Alzheimer's disease. Biomedicine & Pharmacotherapy, 129, 110373

Sinha, R., Papamargaritis, D., Sargeant, J.A., Davies, M.J. (2023). Efficacy and safety of tirzepatide in type 2 diabetes and obesity management. Journal of Obesity & Metabolic Syndrome, 32(1), 25–45. https://doi.org/10.7570/JOMES22067

Thapa, K., Khan, H., Kanojia, N., Singh, T.G., Kaur, A., Kaur, G. (2022). Therapeutic insights on ferroptosis in Parkinson's disease. European Journal of Pharmacology, 930, 175133

Thapa, K., Khan, H., Sharma, U., Grewal, A.K., Singh, T.G. (2021). Poly (ADP-ribose) polymerase-1 as a promising drug target for neurodegenerative diseases. Life Sciences, 267, 118975

Tsilidis, K.K., Kasimis, J.C., Lopez, D.S., Ntzani, E.E., Ioannidis, J.P. (2015). Type 2 diabetes and cancer: Umbrella review of meta-analyses of observational studies. BMJ, 350.

Unamuno, X., Gómez-Ambrosi, J., Rodríguez, A., Becerril, S., Frühbeck, G., Catalán, V. (2018). Adipokine dysregulation and adipose tissue inflammation in human obesity. European Journal of Clinical Investigation, 48(9), e12997. https://doi.org/10.1111/ECI.12997

Wallbillich, J.J., Josyula, S., Saini, U., Zingarelli, R.A., Dorayappan, K.D.P., Riley, M.K., Wanner, R.A., Cohn, D.E., Selvendiran, K. (2017). Metformin inhibits high glucose-mediated STAT3 activation in endometrial cancer: Therapeutic implications for endometrial cancer. PLOS ONE, 12(1), e0170318. https://doi.org/10.1371/JOURNAL.PONE.0170318

Wei, Y., Wang, D., Jin, F., Bian, Z., Li, L., Liang, H., Li, M., Shi, L., Pan, C., Zhu, D., Chen, X., Hu, G., Liu, Y., Zhang, C.Y., Zen, K. (2017). Pyruvate kinase type M2 promotes tumour cell exosome release via phosphorylating synaptosome-associated protein 23. Nature Communications, 8(1), 1–12. https://doi.org/10.1038/ncomms14041

Wong, K.K., Engelman, J.A., Cantley, L.C. (2010). Targeting the PI3K signalling pathway in cancer. Current Opinion in Genetics & Development, 20(1), 87–90. https://doi.org/10.1016/J.GDE.2009.11.002

Wu, Z., Wu, J., Zhao, Q., Fu, S., Jin, J. (2019). Emerging roles of aerobic glycolysis in breast cancer. Clinical and Translational Oncology, 22(5), 631–646. https://doi.org/10.1007/S12094-019-02187-8

Xu, M., Lei, G., Chen, M., Wang, K., Lv, W., Zhang, P., Hu, T., Gao, J., Lu, C., Mei, Y., Xu, Z., Bai, Z., Hu, H., Jiang, Y., Tan, S. (2021). Development of a novel, fully human, anti-PCSK9 antibody with potent hypolipidemic activity by utilising a phage display-based strategy. EBioMedicine, 65, 103250. https://doi.org/10.1016/j.ebiom.2021.103250

Yanai, H., Adachi, H., Hakoshima, M., Katsuyama, H. (2021). Molecular biological and clinical understanding of the pathophysiology and treatments of hyperuricemia and its association with metabolic syndrome, cardiovascular diseases and chronic kidney disease. International Journal of Molecular Sciences, 22(17), 9221. https://doi.org/10.3390/IJMS22179221

Yang, X.P., Lai, D., Zhong, X.Y., Shen, H.P., Huang, Y.L. (2014). Efficacy and safety of canagliflozin in subjects with type 2 diabetes: Systematic review and meta-analysis. European Journal of Clinical Pharmacology, 70, 1149–1158.

Yu, O.H.Y., Suissa, S. (2023). Metformin and cancer: Solutions to a real-world evidence failure. Diabetes Care, 46(5), 904–912. https://doi.org/10.2337/dci22-0047

Zakikhani, M., Dowling, R., Fantus, I.G., Sonenberg, N., Pollak, M. (2006). Metformin is an AMP kinase-dependent growth inhibitor for breast cancer cells. Cancer Research, 66(21), 10269–10273. https://doi.org/10.1158/0008-5472.CAN-06-1500/654451/P/METFORMIN-IS-AN-AMP-KINASE-DEPENDENT-GROWTH

Zhan, T., Rindtorff, N., Boutros, M. (2017). Wnt signaling in cancer. Oncogene, 36(11), 1461–1473. https://doi.org/10.1038/ONC.2016.304

Zhang, X., Lu, J.J., Abudukeyoumu, A., Hou, D.Y., Dong, J., Wu, J.N., Liu, L.B., Li, M.Q., Xie, F. (2022). Glucose transporters: Important regulators of endometrial cancer therapy sensitivity. Frontiers in Oncology, 12, 933827. https://doi.org/10.3389/FONC.2022.933827/BIBTEX

CHAPTER 10

Pathophysiology and Clinical Therapeutic Aspects of Diabetes

SOUMARSHI DAS[1], SONIA DHIMAN[1*], ASHI MANNAN[1], THAKUR GURJEET SINGH[1], and SANJANA MEHTA[1], and BEY HING GOH[2,3]

[1]*Chitkara College of Pharmacy, Chitkara University, Rajpura, Punjab, India*

[2]*College of Pharmaceutical Sciences, Zhejiang University, Hangzhou, China*

[3]*School of Medical and Life Sciences, Sunway University, Sunway City, Malaysia*

*Corresponding author

ABSTRACT

Diabetes mellitus is a long term and degenerative metabolic disorder that is characterized by the high levels of sugar in the blood as a result of either inappropriate insulin production or the failure of the body's cells to respond adequately to insulin. It mainly manifests in two forms—Type 1 diabetes mellitus (T1DM) which is caused by an autoimmune destruction of pancreatic beta-cells, resulting in absolute insulin deficiency, and Type 2 diabetes (T2DM)—characterized by insulin resistance, which is frequently associated with obesity, lack of physical exercise, and genetic predisposition. This chapter discusses the basic pathophysiology of diabetes, with a focus on the normal control of glucose metabolism by insulin and glucagon. It describes the clinical presentations of diabetes, including polyuria, polydipsia, and weight loss, and covers both acute

Pharmacotherapy Approaches Toward Endocrine and Metabolic Diseases.
Thakur Gurjeet Singh and Sanjana Mehta (Eds.)

DOI: 10.1201/9781779640154-10

complications such as diabetic ketoacidosis and hypoglycemia, as well as chronic complications, including nephropathy, retinopathy, neuropathy, and cardiovascular diseases. Diagnostic methods of the disease such as fasting blood glucose, HbA1c and oral glucose tolerance tests are discussed. Treatment options are based on lifestyle changes, drug intervention, insulin treatment, and patient education. We also detail diabetes care by population group, including children, Type 1 and Type 2 diabetes, pregnant women, the elderly and people with diabetes in resource-poor regions of the world. In summary, the chapter gives a comprehensive overview of diabetes mellitus, and stresses the importance of early diagnosis, holistic management and prevention of complications to enhance patient care.

10.1 INTRODUCTION TO DIABETES MELLITUS (DM)

"DM" originates from the Latin "mellitus," meaning sweet, and the Greek "diabetes," meaning syphon. Apollonius of Memphis coined "diabetes" around 250–300 BC. Ancient cultures like Greece, India, and Egypt first associated "DM" with sugary urine. Mering and Minkowski discovered the pancreas's role in diabetes development in 1889. An improperly increased blood glucose level is a metabolic illness known as DM. In addition to providing care and education, nurses are critical in monitoring and supporting their loved ones (Sapra and Bhandari, 2023; Khan et al., 2022). The diverse etiopathology includes impairments in insulin production action or both and abnormalities in the metabolism of proteins, lipids, and carbohydrates. The specific long-term impacts of diabetes include, among others, retinopathy, nephropathy, and neuropathy (WHO, 2019). Diagnosis circumstances determine diabetes types. Many defy a single classification. The main categories are type 1 (insulin insufficiency), type 2 (insulin resistance + insufficient secretion), and gestational diabetes in pregnancy. Rare types and genetic abnormalities are categorized separately (Solis-Herrera et al., 2018; Sharma and Singh, 2020).

PreDM: 12.0% prevalence (men 13.2%, women 11.1%). Increases with age, family history of diabetes mellitus (FHDM), hypertension, and obesity correlated. Diabetes: 10.2% prevalence (males 7.9%, females 10.8%). 1.9% undiagnosed. DM diagnoses: 10.6% educated, 15.1% illiterate. Type 1: 5.6%, Type 2: 91.2%. Type 2 is more common in older, non-Hispanic

Asians with lower education and higher BMI. Type 1 is more prevalent in younger, non-Hispanic Whites, higher education, and lower BMI (Xu et al., 2018). Patients with uncontrollable hyperglycemia were most common in the 18–54 age group (30.9%), 65–74 age group (22.9%), and ≥75 age group (20.6%). A higher total cholesterol to high-density lipoproteins ratio correlated strongly with uncorrected hyperglycemia. T1DM incidence was 4.45 per 100,000 in women, rising from 3.70 to 4.77 in males, with juvenile onset from 2009 to 2016 ($P = 0.002$). In men, T1DM incidence increased from 3.07 in 2008 to 4.89 in 2016 ($P < 0.001$). Incidence remained stable in females (4.39 in 2008, 4.64 in 2016), despite rising in boys aged 5–9 and 10–14 years (Chae et al., 2020).

Prediabetes risk factors: alcohol, smoking, sex, age, BMI, central obesity, lipoprotein ratios (CHOL/HDL, LDL/HDL, TG/HDL, ApoB/A1), hs-CRP. Logistic regression: smoking, central adiposity = I-IFG; female sex = I-IGT; male sex, hypertension, hs-CRP = C-IFG/IGT. T1DM is linked to infant weight gain (Chaitanya et al., 2022). Children with diabetes taller than 6–18 months. Diet and environment impact T1DM (Rewers et al., 2018). Type 2 diabetes arises from a complex interplay of metabolic, environmental, and genetic factors. Significant risk factors include age, obesity, physical inactivity, and a family history of diabetes. Women with a history of gestational diabetes in their infants are at higher risk of developing type 2 diabetes (Fletcher et al., 2002).

10.2 PATHOPHYSIOLOGY OF DM

DM is a complex metabolic disorder characterized by high blood sugar and hypertension. It is caused by insulin production or action issues. Hyperglycemia impairs insulin secretion, β-cell function, and metabolic performance. Insulin resistance is fueled by inflammation and excess fatty acids, hindering glucose delivery. Elevated glucagon worsens the condition (Sapra and Bhandari, 2023).

10.2.1 NORMAL GLUCOSE HOMEOSTASIS

Insulin and glucagon are mainly responsible for preserving normal glucose homeostasis. After Banting and Best (1921) discovered insulin and showed that it could reduce blood glucose levels in both healthy and diabetic conditions, Kimball and Murlin (1923) discovered another pancreatic factor glucagon that could raise animal blood glucose levels. Therefore, glucagon counteracts insulin's regulatory effects on blood glucose levels. Understanding the bioactive interaction between these two hormones is crucial for comprehending glucose homeostasis in healthy and diabetic conditions. The pancreas regulates glucagon and insulin, maintaining glucose balance. GLUT2 transports glucose into the pancreas, where glucokinase converts it to glucose-6-phosphate (GP6) (Sharabi et al., 2015). Glucokinase, a glucose sensor, controls insulin release from pancreatic β-cells and other cells involved in glucose balance. These include α- and γ-cells in the adrenal gland, entero-endocrine cells, glucose-sensitive neurons, anterior pituitary cells, and the endocrine pancreas (Matschinsky and Wilson, 2019).

Diabetes delays glucose control due to complex insulin production, secretion, and function changes. Pancreatic β-cells release insulin to regulate blood sugar. Disruption from lifestyle, environment, and genetics. Type 2: insulin resistance, tissues less sensitive to insulin. Types 1 and 2: β-cell dysfunction, reduced insulin output, or inadequate response to resistance (Defronzo, 2009). This dysfunction can be brought on by autoimmune β-cell death in type 1 diabetes and ongoing exposure to excessive glucose and metabolic stress in type 2 diabetes (Yoon and Jun, 2001). A diagnosis of type 2 diabetes leads to ongoing oxidative stress due to elevated glucose levels, increasing reactive oxygen species. Islets naturally lack antioxidants, but boosting antioxidant enzymes can shield β-cells from glucose-induced damage (Robertson et al., 2004; Singh et al., 2020).

10.2.2 INSULIN AND GLUCAGON

Glucose fuels energy production by the breakdown of carbohydrates, lipids, and proteins. It is the final substrate taken up by cells undergoing metabolic conversion into adenosine triphosphate (ATP) for energy. Insulin, a peptide hormone from pancreatic islets, regulates blood glucose levels by increasing cell growth, glucose absorption, and metabolism of proteins, lipids, and carbohydrates (Nakrani et al., 2023; Garg et al., 2022). Insulin comprises two chains, A chain (21 residues) and B chain (30 residues) and is a tiny, globular protein. The hormones enter the circulation as a Zn^{2+}

free monomer when they break loose from their Zn^{2+} stabilized hexamer state in the β-cell (Weiss, 2009; Singh et al., 2022). Preproinsulin is the precursor to proinsulin. Proinsulin is then converted into C-peptide and insulin, stored in secretory granules until needed. Insulin synthesis is regulated by transcription and translation. β-Cells fuse the plasma membrane with secretory granules for insulin release. Glucose is the major stimulus for insulin secretion. Other nutrients, including amino acids (e.g., arginine) and fatty acids, as well as hormones such as glucagon-like peptide-1 (GLP-1), leptin, growth hormone, melatonin, and estrogen, also regulate insulin release. Pancreatic β-cells are metabolic hubs that integrate nutrient metabolism signals with endocrine signals (Fu et al., 2013; Rohilla et al., 2023). The first phase of glucose-mediated insulin secretion starts with elevated glucose levels, triggering insulin release from β-cell secretory granules. Glucokinase in β-cells phosphorylates glucose upon entry, forming (GP6), which generates ATP. Closure of K+ ATP-dependent channels raises intracellular calcium, activating voltage-dependent calcium channels and membrane depolarization. This leads to fluctuating insulin release. K^+ ATP channel-dependent Ca^{2+} pathways and K^+ ATP channel-independent routes enhance this process (Singh et al., 2020).

Diabetes pathophysiology linked to glucagon: High glucagon levels drive liver glucose production, causing hyperglycemia. Glucagon, from pancreatic α-cells, regulates glucose levels. Hypoglycemia triggers glucagon release, affecting liver metabolism. Proglucagon, its precursor, generates related hormones. Proglucagon is expressed in various tissues. Convertases PC1/3 and PC2 process proglucagon, yielding glucagon, and related peptides (Rix et al., 2019).

10.2.3 TYPE 1 DIABETES MELLITUS

Type 1 diabetes is an autoimmune condition where insulin-producing pancreatic β-cells are destroyed, necessitating personalized treatment. Variation is a metabolic, genetic, and immunogenetic factor, and age-related differences require tailored approaches. It can result in a rapid or gradual decline in insulin secretion (Lucier and Weinstock, 2023). The destruction of the insulin-producing pancreatic β-cells by the immune system is one of the characteristics of type 1 diabetes, an autoimmune disease. Environmental causes and genetic predisposition work together in this complex process. Genetic variables are essential in determining the likelihood of developing a disease, especially variation in the human leukocyte antigen (HLA) area (Pociot and Lernmark, 2016). Genetic markers disrupt immunological tolerance, leading to an immune response targeting β-cells. Activated T-cells attack β-cell antigens, producing autoantibodies against proteins like insulin. Viral infection and other environmental variables can start or worsen this inflammatory process (Burrack et al., 2017). If β-cells are continuously destroyed, there is an insulin shortage, leading to persistent hyperglycemia and type 1 diabetes symptoms (Chen et al., 2017).

10.2.4 TYPE 2 DIABETES MELLITUS

T2DM is a metabolic disorder characterized by insulin resistance, β-cell dysfunction, and high blood sugar levels. Pro-inflammatory cytokines and adipokines secreted by adipose tissue exacerbate systemic inflammation and interfere with insulin signaling pathways in peripheral tissues, contributing significantly to insulin resistance. As a result, reduced insulin secretion in the liver, adipose tissue, and skeletal muscle leads to decreased glucose absorption and increased hepatic glucose synthesis. Prolonged hyperglycemia and increased demand on these cells lead to β-cell dysfunction in insulin production (Shoelson et al., 2006). Oxidative stress, endoplasmic reticulum (ER) stress, and inflammation worsen β-cell failure via insulin signaling and mitochondrial dysfunction. Gut dysbiosis (imbalance in bacteria, reduced diversity) is linked to insulin resistance and metabolic disorders. Gut microbiota affects energy balance, inflammation, and glucose metabolism. Epigenetic factors (histone modification, DNA methylation) influence gene expression in DM. Oxidative stress, inflammation, and hyperglycemia alter gene expression via epigenetic changes. Environmental factors and starvation also impact gene expression via chromatin modification (Singh et al., 2020).

10.3 CLINICAL PRESENTATION OF DM

The clinical presentation of DM is explained in Figure 10.1.

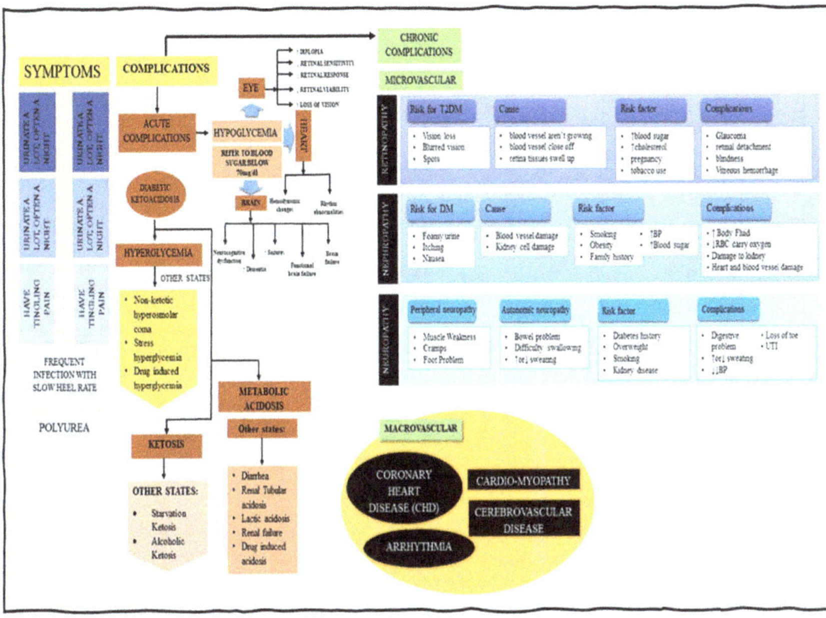

FIGURE 10.1 Clinical presentation of DM.

10.4 TREATMENT AND MANAGEMENT

10.4.1 LIFESTYLE MODIFICATIONS

Lifestyle modification under the treatment and management of DM is explained in Table 10.1.

10.4.2 PHARMACOLOGICAL THERAPY

10.4.2.1 INSULIN THERAPY

Insulin treats and manages type 1 and type 2 diabetes, reducing the risk of peripheral vascular disease, coronary artery disease, stroke, and other complications. Insulin, vital for cell division, metabolism, and glucose regulation, was isolated and purified by Dr. Frederick Banting in Toronto between 1921 and 1922 (Thota and Akbar, 2023). Ongoing research has aimed to enhance insulin quality since its discovery. Other hormones like glucagon were also discovered after insulin's identification. Insulin, a vital

TABLE 10.1 Lifestyle Modification of DM

Lifestyle Modification	*Description*	*Control Rate*
Diet	Dietary changes are crucial to diabetes prevention because they link to better glycemic control. When combined with more exercise, healthy eating practices can accelerate weight reduction, which is a successful diabetes preventive tactic	There was a range of 9–25% risk reduction, indicating that when this diet was started, the incidence of diabetes was decreased by 9–25%
Exercise	An organized, systemic, repeated, and intentional physical exercise where the goal is to maintain or enhance one or more aspects of physical fitness	Optimal physical activity levels lower risk by 8–30%
Weight management	Suggest using food and exercise in conjugation to reach and maintain a healthy weight. Losing weight can enhance glycemia management and insulin sensitivity	A yearly average increase in body weight of 7% was associated with a 58% reduction in the prevalence of diabetes
Stress management	Anxiety	People with diabetes had a 20% higher lifetime risk of having an anxiety disorder than persons without diabetes. Behavior and mental health include almost 200,000 adults. Adults under 30 years old and Hispanics reported having the highest rates of anxiousness
	Social burden	Diabetes has long been known to have significant effects on anxiety, depression, and relationships, in addition to possible disruption to social interaction. Though its full impact is unknown, social burdens and stigmatization significantly influence

TABLE 10.1 *(Continued)*

Lifestyle Modification	Description	Control Rate
Smoking cessation	While the impact of weight gain on glucose homeostasis may frequently obscure the effects of quitting smoking, at least one study has demonstrated that a brief cessation of smoking for 1–2 weeks is adequate to rectify impairments in insulin sensitivity and skeletal muscle insulin signaling, even in the absence of weight fluctuations (Maddatu et al., 2017)	Giving up smoking is linked to a roughly 30% drop in all-cause deaths (Driva et al., 2022)
Alcohol moderation	In the body mass index (BMI) <25 groups, moderate alcohol use was linked to significantly lower levels of insulin secretion capability and reduced fasting plasma glucose (Miyagi et al., 2021)	Moderate consumption was linked to a 30% lower risk of diabetes in both women and men (relative risk [RR] 0.68 [0.61–0.75] and 0.72 [95% CI 0.67–0.77])

anabolic hormone, impacts body metabolism extensively. β-Cell in the pancreas produces insulin. These cells monitor plasma levels of various substances like fatty acids, amino acids, ketones, and glucose to regulate insulin synthesis (Vargas et al., 2022).

10.4.2.1.1 Types of Insulin

Types of insulin used to treat DM are explained in a tabular form in Table 10.2.

Insulin, the first fully sequenced protein, consists of 51 amino acids forming two chains, A (21) and B (30), connected by two sulfide bonds. Proinsulin and its precursor undergo processing in the β-cell's Golgi apparatus and form granules. Proinsulin, an 86 amino acid peptide, splits into insulin and C-peptide, both released in equimolar amounts from the β-cell (Donnor and Sarkar, 2023).

Insulin is vital for T1DM treatment. The immune system attacks β-cells, reducing insulin—high blood sugar results. Exogenous insulin subcutaneously lowers glucose and prevents complications (American Diabetes Association, 2020a). A tailored insulin regimen is essential for optimal glycemic control and quality of life in type 1 diabetes. It addresses lifestyle, exercise, and diet to counter insulin deficiency, stabilize blood glucose, and prevent complications. Modern basal insulin analogs are preferred for lower hypoglycemia risk. Rapid-acting insulin can be added for persistent fasting or postprandial hyperglycemia, especially with increasing β-cell loss (Meneghini, 2013).

10.4.2.2 ORAL HYPOGLYCEMIC AGENTS

An interdisciplinary approach combining dietary adjustment, physical activity, and medication is essential for managing diabetes effectively. Lifestyle changes and oral medication should be combined for optimal glycemic control, particularly as type 2 diabetes progresses and insulin production declines. The approach assists healthcare providers in guiding patient therapy for the best outcomes in glycemic control and diabetes management.

Classification, mechanism of action, types, administration, adverse effects, and contraindications of oral hypoglycemic agents are explained in Table 10.3.

TABLE 10.2 Types of Insulin Used to Treat DM

Type	Insulin	Onset	Peak Effect	Duration	Indication
Rapid acting	Insulin Lispro	Insulin Lispro start to work within 15 min after being injected subcutaneously (Noble et al., 1998)	1–2 h (Donnor and Sarkar, 2023)	The action lasts for less than 5 h (Noble et al., 1998)	The FDA has approved the insulin analogue insulin lispro to control hyperglycemia in patients with type 1 and type 2 diabetes mellitus
	Insulin Aspart	It takes 15 min for Aspart insulin to start working (Rubin et al., 2022)	1–3 h (Donnor and Sarkar, 2023)	The activity lasts for 3–5 h (Rubin et al., 2022)	Insulin aspart controls how glucose is metabolized. It encourages the accumulation of fat, glucose, and amino acids while preventing breakdown (Rubin et al., 2022)
	Insulin Glulisine	Rapid onse	Peak effect at 1 h	Short action duration (around 4 h)	Insulin glargine, a recombinant human insulin analogue, binds to the receptor. The IR is classified as a tyrosine kinase receptor due to its two intracellular catalytic beta domains and two extracellular beta domains (Cunningham and Freeman, 2022)
Ultrarapid acting	FIAsp	Use of FIAsp insulin injection was linked to 4.9 min early onset of action (Dutta et al., 2023)	–	–	FIAsp has shown multiple daily injections to reduce postprandial glucose and HbA1c levels in individuals with type 1 diabetes
Short acting	Regular	Action in 30–40 min (Thota and Akbar; 2023)	Peak in 90–120 min (Thota and Akbar, 2023)	6–8 h (Thota and Akbar; 2023)	Like endogenous insulin found in the body, regular insulin is a synthetic protein hormone with a broad spectrum of physiological effects. It is a short-acting human insulin (Munguia and Correa, 2023)

TABLE 10.2 *(Continued)*

Type	Insulin	Onset	Peak Effect	Duration	Indication
Medium acting	NPH	1–4 h (Thota and Akbar, 2023)	4–8 h (Thota and Akbar, 2023)	14 h (Donnor and Sarkar, 2023)	It ↑ is the amount of glucose that is absorbed by the liver, adipose tissue, and skeletal muscles (Saleem and Sharma, 2023)
Long acting	Insulin Detemir	About 2 h (Donnor and Sarkar, 2023)	–	16–24 h (Donnor and Sarkar, 2023)	By administering insulin detemir, glycemic control in children and adults with diabetes mellitus can be improved (NCBI, 2023)
Ultralong acting	Insulin degludec	1 h (Donnor and Sarkar, 2023)	9 h (Donnor and Sarkar, 2023)	>40 h (Zhou et al., 2019)	Reduces postprandial glucose, FPG, and HbA1c while improving glycemic control and posing little risk of hypoglycemia (Kesavadev et al., 2022)

TABLE 10.3 Types of OHAs Used to Treat DM

Classification	Mechanism of Action	Types	Administration	Adverse Effects	Contraindications
Sulfonylureas	A group of chemicals called sulfonylureas can block the ATP-sensitive potassium channel (K) in pancreatic β cells. The β-cell membrane depolarizes, and potassium outflow slows down. When the membrane depolarizes, calcium channels open. This brings more calcium into the cell and causes the pancreatic β-cell to release insulin. Insulin is released by sulphonylureas independent of blood glucose level. K comprises two proteins, a sulfonyl receptor (SUR) and KIR6.2, which form the K channel's pore. A subtype of SUR includes SUR 1 and SUR 2 (Costello et al., 2023)	Glipizide	Start with 5 mg PO daily and work up to 5 mg, depending on how your blood glucose tolerance responds. The maintenance dosage range is PO every 12 h or 2.5–20 mg PO daily. 40 mg/day is maximum dose (Correa et al., 2023)	• Hypoglycemia • Weight gain • Nausea • Diarrhea • Cholesteric jaundice • Allergic reactions are rare • SIADH • Hyponatremia (Costello et al., 2023)	Contraindicated when GFR (>30 mL/min) (Mohan et al., 2022)
		Glyburide	Typically, people with type 2 diabetes do not require doses greater than 10 mg/day. Hence, the maximum dosage of 40 mg is rarely utilized. Glyburide is taken orally in beginning quantities of 2.5–5 mg. Moreover, clinical effects are negligible at levels higher than 10–15 mg/day	• Weight gain • Liver dysfunction • Cholesteric jaundice • Hepatitis • Liver failure	Limitations and possible hazards related to glyburide include kidney damage or a history of hypoglycemia
		Gliclazide	Two forms of gliclazide are available: an IR oral tablet and an MR oral tablet. Give gliclazide with immediate-release twice daily, half an hour before meals. There is an 80 mg pill of gliclazide IR available with a 320 mg daily maximum dosage. There are 30–60 mg tablets of Gliclazide MR available. Gliclazide MR should be taken once a day with a meal, up to a daily maximum dosage of 120 mg (Costello et al., 2023)	• Hypoglycemic events (Landman et al., 2014)	Gliclazide is not recommended for people who take metformin because it raises the risk of lactic acidosis, even when the drug is used correctly. People who have problems with their liver or kidneys should not be given the medicine (Azimova et al., 2014)
		Glimepiride	Glimepiride is usually started at 1–2 mg/day and taken orally before the first meal. Hypoglycemic people should start with 1 mg/day and slowly increase it until they reach the recommended dose. After starting treatment, the usual maintenance dose is 1–4 mg once a day. However, this can be increased to 8 mg once a day (Trerattanavong and Tadi, 2023).	• ↑ Endogenous insulin secretion • Weight gain • Vomiting • Abdominal pain • Diarrhea • Erythema multiforme • Exfoliative dermatitis (Trerattanavong and Tadi, 2023)	Diabetic ketoacidosis T1DM (Trerattanavong and Tadi, 2023)

TABLE 10.3 *(Continued)*

Classification	Mechanism of Action	Types	Administration	Adverse Effects	Contraindications
Meglitinides	Meglitinides lower blood glucose levels by promoting the body's natural insulin synthesis. Hemoglobin A1C levels are used to determine the current suggested beginning dose; individuals with a level of less than 8% (64 mmol/mol) are advised to begin with 0.5 mg preprandial, while those with a level above 8% should begin with 1–2 mg (Milner and Akhondi, 2023)	Repaglinide	When taken by mouth, repaglinide (0.5–4 mg) is taken two to three times a day, up to a maximum of 16 mg. It lowers blood sugar like other antihypertensive drugs. The drug should be taken about half an hour before a meal, and the dose should not be taken if a meal is missed. Dose modification has to be examined at least a week later (Milner and Akhondi, 2023)	• Hypoglycemia • Weight gain • ↑ Risk of cardiovascular • UTI • Sinusitis • Diarrhea • Joint pain • ↑ Risk of peripheral edema (Milner and Akhondi, 2023)	Hypersensitivity to any of the oral preparation's components Diabetic ketoacidosis and type 1 diabetes mellitus Profound hepatic dysfunction Use of gemfibrozil or clopidogrel concurrently Concurrent administration of NPH insulin (Milner and Akhondi, 2023)
		Nateglinide	Adults usually take 120 mg three times a day before meals as the first dose (LiverTox, 2019)	• Diarrhea • Nausea • Gastrointestinal upset • Hypoglycemia • Dizziness • Rash (LiverTox, 2019)	–
Biguanides	Biguanides block complex 1 of the mitochondria, causing energy stress and triggering energy sensor-mediated compensatory responses	Metformin	500–2550 mg is the typical daily dosage range for the oral medication metformin. Two formulations of metformin may be purchased: the extended-release form, which may be taken once daily, and the immediate-release version, which has to be taken twice daily. Weekly titration of metformin doses often occurs in increments of 500 or 850 mg (Corcoran and Jacobs, 2023)	• ↓ Blood sugar • Nausea • Vomiting • Chest discomfort • Headache • Diaphoresis • ↓ Vitamin B12 (Corcoran and Jacobs, 2023)	Contraindicated when GFR (>30 mL/min) (Corcoran and Jacobs, 2023)

TABLE 10.3 *(Continued)*

Classification	Mechanism of Action	Types	Administration	Adverse Effects	Contraindications
Thiazolidinediones	The primary function of Thiazolidinediones (TZDs) is activating the nuclear receptor known as peroxisome proliferator-activated receptor gamma or PPAR-γ. These receptors are primarily found in adipose tissue, although they are also found in muscle and liver. After binding to PPAR-γ, TZDs improve insulin sensitivity by controlling the transcription of genes involved in glucose and lipid metabolism. As a result, peripheral tissue, mainly muscle and adipose tissue, absorbs more glucose, lowering blood glucose. TZDs also control the formation of adipokines and the development of adipocytes, which affect the equilibrium of various metabolic processes (Lebovitz, 2019)	Rosiglitazone	Oral administration is used to provide rosiglitazone. There are pills containing 2 mg and 4 mg of it. Treatment of T2DM is one of its indications. The starting dosage is 4 mg taken orally/day, split into 12 h. After 8–12 weeks, if the glycemic response is still insufficient, the dosage can be ↑ 8 mg taken orally daily split every 12 hrs (Quintanilla Rodriguez and Mahdy, 2023)	• Edema • Hypertension • Heart failure • CHF • Myocardial ischemia • Diarrhea • Upper respiratory tract infection • Anemia • Back pain • Fatigue • Headache • Myalgia	Active liver disease Diabetic ketoacidosis (Quintanilla Rodriguez and Correa, 2023)
		Pioglitazone	Pioglitazone is taken orally, either with or without meals. Although it can be used as monotherapy, metformin/sulfonylurea or insulin treatment is typically used in conjugation with it. Adults should start with a daily oral dosage of 15 or 30 mg. When the patient's response is insufficient, a 15 mg medication dosage is recommended. The maximum amount that can be taken orally/day is 45 mg. The maximum amount administered: Adult: 45 mg/day Elder: 45 mg/day (Singh et al., 2023).	• Weight gain • Edema • Osteoporosis • CHF • (Singh et al., 2023)	Hypoglycemia Diabetic ketoacidosis Active liver disease Pregnancy Kidney failure (Singh et al., 2023)
α-Glucosidase inhibitor	α-Glucosidase inhibitors stop carbohydrates from being absorbed in the small intestine. They competitively inhibit the enzyme that changes complicated, nonabsorbable carbohydrates into simple, absorbable ones. This enzyme includes isomaltase, sucrase, maltase, and glucoamylase (Akmal and Wadhwa, 2022)	Acarbose	Oral tablets of 25 mg, 50 mg, or 100 mg of acarbose are available. It should be taken orally three times a day with the first bite of each meal. The recommended beginning dosage is 25 mg three times/day; however, GI side effects may be minimized by starting with a once-daily dose to achieve the required glycemic control while minimizing GI side effects. The dose can be titrated every 4–8 weeks, starting at 25 mg, and taken orally thrice daily. A maximum dosage of 100 mg is allowed (McIver et al., 2022)	• Malabsorption • Flatulence • Diarrhea • Abdominal boating • Skin rash • Pneumatosis intestinalis (LiverTox, 2021)	Diabetic ketoacidosis Liver cirrhosis Inflammatory bowel disease Colonic ulceration (McIver et al., 2022)

TABLE 10.3 *(Continued)*

Classification	Mechanism of Action	Types	Administration	Adverse Effects	Contraindications
		Miglitol	The highest dosage is 100 mg three times/day, while the starting dose is 25 mg three times/day (Akmal and Wadhwa, 2022)	• Malabsorption • Flatulence • Diarrhea • Abdominal boating • Rash • Pneumatosis cytokines (LiverTox, 2021)	Intestinal obstruction Diabetic ketoacidosis Chronic intestinal disease Colonic ulcer Inflammatory bowel disease (Akmal and Wadhwa, 2022)
		Voglibose	0.2 mg three times/day (starting dose); this can be raised to 0.3 mg three times a day (Akmal and Wadhwa, 2022)	• Diarrhea • Flatulence • Bloating • Abdominal discomfort • Nausea (Dabhi et al., 2013)	
DPP-4 inhibitor	DPP-4 is a ubiquitous enzyme that functions on incretin hormone, namely gastric inhibitory peptide (GIP) and glucagon-like-peptide-1 (GLP-1) that in order to preserve glucose homeostasis increase insulin synthesis and decrease glucagon secretion homeostasis (Kasina and Baradhi, 2023)	Sitagliptin	There are 25 mg, 50 mg,100 mg tablet. Adults usually take 100 mg of sitagliptin once daily (LiverTox, 2018)	• May include: • Headache • Nausea • Arthralgia • Rash (LiverTox, 2018)	Diabetic ketoacidosis History of pancreatitis (Kasina and Baradhi, 2023)
		Saxagliptin	For most people, a daily dosage of 5 mg is advised; for patients with moderate or several renal impairments (CrCl<50 mL/min), the recommended dose is 2.5 mg	• Hypoglycemia • Bullous pemphigoid • Severe arthralgias • Acute pancreatitis (LiverTox, 2018)	
		Vildagliptin	When provided once or twice daily, vildagliptin considerably decreases fasting and postprandial glucose levels. Doses higher than 50 mg twice a day do not appear to provide any appreciable further advantages	–	
		Linagliptin	One daily dose of 5 mg of linagliptin is the recommended dosage. You can take the pills with or without meals. Patients with hepatic or renal impairment do not require dose changes (Freeman, 2011)	• Headache • Nausea • Allergic reactions • Rash • Pancreatitis • Bullous pemphigoid • (Livertox, 2018)	

TABLE 10.3 *(Continued)*

Classification	Mechanism of Action	Types	Administration	Adverse Effects	Contraindications
		Alogliptin	Oral tablets of 6.25 mg, 12.5 mg, and 25 mg of alogliptin can be purchased and taken once a day without meals. Patients with type 2 diabetes mellitus often take 25 mg orally once a day (Terrell and Jacobs, 2023)	• Stevens-Johnson syndrome • Hepatic failure • Heart failure • Tubulointerstitial nephritis • Pancreatitis • Severe arthralgia • Rhabdomyolysis • (Terrell and Jacobs, 2023)	
SGLT2 inhibitor	Unlike other oral antihyperglycemic medications, SGLT-2 inhibitors function without insulin. Through glycosuria and natriuresis brought on by the suppression of glucose reabsorption at the kidney's proximal tubule, they lower blood sugar (Simes and MacGregor, 2019)	Dapagliflozin	When taken orally, dapagliflozin is quickly absorbed with peak plasma conc. Typically achieved in 2 h (faster state). Dapagliflozin has an absolute oral bioavailability of 78% following a dosage of 10 mg (Dhillon, 2019)	• UTI • Cystitis • Genital infection • (Saleem, 2017)	Renal impairment End-stage renal disease History of hypersensitivity toward dapagliflozin (Cada et al., 2014)
		Canagliflozin	Started with a daily dose of 100 mg just before breakfast. If the 100 mg dosage was well tolerated and the eGFR was 60 mL/min/1.73 m2 higher. Patients who require more glycemic control can raise the dose to 300 mg once daily (Sarnoski-Brocavich and Hilas, 2013)	• Dry mouth • Dry throat • Urgency • Nocturia	Patients with end-stage renal disease, dialysis, or a GFR <45mL/min/1.73m2 who are compromised should not take canagliflozin
Cycloset	The primary way that closure operates is by lowering high postprandial glucose levels (Alatrach et al., 2018).	Bromocriptine	Up to a maximum dose of 4.80 mg/day, the starting dose of 0.8 mg/day will ↑ be 0.8 mg/week until the required glycemic control is obtained (Ozery and Wadhwa, 2022).	• Nausea • Vomiting • Dizziness • Hypotension • Headache • Fatigue • Psychosis • Fibrosis • Cardiovascular incidents • (Ozery and Wadhwa, 2022)	T1DM Syncope Psychosis Breastfeeding patient CYP3A4 inhibitor (Ozery and Wadhwa, 2022)

10.4.2.3 INJECTABLE NONINSULIN MEDICATIONS

Diabetes treatment often includes injectable noninsulin medications, which are crucial for type 2 patients. Liraglutide and Exenatide, binding to glucagon-like peptide (GLP)-1 receptors, are effective alternatives. They suppress glucagon, slow stomach emptying, and boost insulin secretion in response to glucose, mimicking incretin hormones. They aid in glucose regulation, promote weight loss, and have positive cardiac effects—GLP-1Ras impact glucose homeostasis through these mechanisms (Drucker and Nauck, 2006). Amylin analogues, exemplified by pramlintide, mimic the effects of amylin, a hormone secreted with insulin. Pramlintide lowers postprandial glucose levels and increases satiety. Due to their novelty, these injectable noninsulin drugs offer customizable treatment plans for optimal glycemic control (Buse et al., 2020).

10.4.3 INSULIN DELIVERY SYSTEMS

10.4.3.1 SYRINGES AND NEEDLES

The first syringe, developed in 1853, was followed by the Fergusson syringe. Subcutaneous drug administration emerged in the early 19th century, while the intravenous route was documented in the 17th century. Becton, Dickinson and Company (BD), Franklin Lakes, NJ, USA, produced an insulin injection syringe in 1924, 2 years after insulin's discovery (Shah et al., 2016). In 1970, BD pioneered the first one-piece insulin syringe with an integrated needle. By 1983, the British Diabetic Organization recommended a shift to a single insulin strength (100 units/mL) from varied strengths. However, the glass syringes introduced had a flaw with "dead space," causing dosing errors. In 2012, BD introduced the BD Veo insulin syringe with a 6 mm ultrafine needle, reducing discomfort and dosing errors. This syringe became widely preferred. In 2016, the FDA approved a BD insulin series designed for U-500 insulin, addressing dosing challenges with the U-100 series for U-500 vial doses (Kesavadev et al., 2020).

10.4.3.2 INSULIN PEN

The introduction of insulin pens in 1985 by Novo Nordisk transformed insulin delivery, eliminating the drawbacks of vial and syringe injections.

Over the years, pharmaceutical companies have improved insulin pens, making them more precise, reusable, and safer with features like audible dosage clicks. Despite offering greater accuracy, convenience, and painlessness than traditional methods, their adoption varies globally. European countries embrace them more widely (around 80%) than the USA (approximately 15%), reflecting differences in healthcare practices and patient preferences (Shah et al., 2016).

104.3.3 INSULIN PUMP

An insulin pump is a small device that delivers fast-acting insulin continuously through a catheter under the skin, kept in place by adhesive. It infuses insulin via tubing connected to a cannula. Patch pumps use wireless tech. Standard rapid-acting insulins like Lispro are used. Insulin can be delivered continuously (basal) or as discrete meals or correction (bolus) doses. Basal insulin replaces long-acting insulin in injections and is influenced by physiology and life-stage factors.

10.4.4 PREVENTION OF COMPLICATIONS

Various strategies are employed to prevent complications in diabetes, such as regular monitoring, promoting a healthy lifestyle, managing blood pressure and cholesterol, and controlling blood glucose and lipids. Glucose management is critical in reducing the risk of microvascular issues (American Diabetes Association, 2020b). Additionally, managing blood pressure and cholesterol levels to address cardiovascular risk factors is highlighted as a way to prevent macrovascular complications. Lifestyle changes like regular exercise, quitting smoking, and weight control can prevent diabetes complications. Medication, diet, eye examinations, and health checkups are vital for managing diabetes effectively (Cosentino et al., 2020).

10.4.4.1 CARDIOVASCULAR RISK MANAGEMENT

Diabetes-related cardiovascular risk management targets multiple factors, focusing on cholesterol and blood pressure control. For those with diabetes, these factors notably increase cardiovascular disease risk. Strict BP control, typically below 130/80 mmHg, is recommended to minimize cardiovascular events. Lowering LDL cholesterol levels is crucial for effective risk reduction. Diabetes patients often take statins to lower cardiovascular risk, but lifestyle changes like a balanced diet, exercise, quitting smoking, and weight control are crucial for better heart health (Cosentino et al., 2020).

10.4.4.2 NEPHROPATHY PREVENTION

Managing blood pressure and glucose levels effectively is crucial to preventing diabetic nephropathy. Maintaining optimal blood glucose levels significantly reduces the risk of diabetic kidney disease. Early glycemic control is critical in avoiding nephropathy in individuals with diabetes. Maintaining strict blood pressure control (aiming for less than 130/80 mmHg) is crucial to slow or halt the progression of diabetic kidney disease. This involves using medications like renin angiotensin aldosterone system (RAAS) inhibitors and adjusting diet to limit sodium intake and promote heart health. These measures lower albuminuria and preserve renal function, which prevents nephropathy (American Diabetes Association, 2020d).

10.4.4.3 RETINOPATHY SCREENING AND MANAGEMENT

Preventing vision loss in people with diabetes relies on regular screening and treatment for diabetic retinopathy. Early detection through routine eye examinations, including dilated retinal examinations, is crucial. Timely interventions like intravitreal injections, laser treatment, or surgery such as vitrectomy become feasible with early identification. Diabetic retinopathy, a complication of both type 1 and type 2 diabetes, correlates with diabetes duration and glycemic control. A pooled meta-analysis of 35 studies (1980–2008) found global prevalence rates of 7.5% for proliferative diabetic retinopathy and 35.4% for any diabetic retinopathy (American Diabetes Association, 2020b).

10.4.5 MULTIPLE DISCIPLINARY CARE TEAMS

A diverse team is vital for optimal diabetes care. This includes nurses, pharmacists, dietitians, endocrinologists, physicians, educators, and mental health professionals. Comprehensive care addresses glucose, medication, lifestyle, mental health, and education. The team tailors treatment, empowers patients, communicates regularly, and emphasizes education, a holistic approach, and self-care.

10.5 SPECIAL CONSIDERATIONS

10.5.1 DIABETES IN CHILDREN AND ADOLESCENTS

Managing diabetes in children and adolescents requires tailored approaches due to unique challenges. Specialized strategies are crucial to address their complex needs effectively, considering physiological, psychosocial, and developmental factors. Effective glycemic management is essential to avoid long-term consequences, but achieving balance often involves considering development, puberty, and lifestyle changes. The psychological impact on kids and teens emphasizes the importance of holistic care, impacting self-control, peer relationships, and family dynamics. Advancements in insulin delivery and continuous glucose monitoring have improved diabetes management (American Diabetes Association, 2020c). Type 1 diabetes reduces life by 10–20 years with complications like hypoglycemia and DKA. Managing it in kids is stressful and linked to sadness. Delayed diagnosis increases DKA risks, especially lethal in children. Genetics and modern lifestyle cause T2DM, with strong hereditary influence evident in twins and certain ethnic groups (Los and Wilt, 2023).

10.5.2 DIABETES IN PREGNANCY

Gestational diabetes mellitus (GDM) is glucose intolerance during pregnancy. Types: A1GDM is managed by diet, and A2GDM needs medication. GDM increases the risk of diabetes postpregnancy. Treatment includes glucose monitoring, insulin, and other measures. Normalizing BMI prepregnancy helps. Managing obesity during pregnancy is challenging. Limiting weight gain in pregnancy is difficult (Quintanilla and Mahdy, 2023). Preexisting diabetes exacerbates glucose metabolism issues and insulin resistance, raising the risk of maternal hyperglycemia. This condition passes to the fetus via the placenta, increasing the likelihood of fetal hyperglycemia. Consequently, there has been heightened nutritional deposition and fetal hyperinsulinemia, potentially leading to macrosomia due to increased fetal pancreatic insulin synthesis.

10.5.3 OLDER ADULTS WITH DIABETES

Older individuals with diabetes face higher risks of acute and long-term complications compared to other age groups. These include lower limb amputations, heart attacks, vision problems, and kidney failure. Additionally, older patients are more likely to experience complications from hyperglycemia crises, leading to increased mortality rates and more visits to the emergency department due to hypoglycemia (Leung et al., 2018).

10.5.4 DIABETES AND COMORBIDITIES

10.5.4.1 HYPERTENSION

In diabetes, cardiovascular disease is a significant cause of illness and death. Research indicates that hypertension (HTN) is a primary risk factor for cardiovascular issues associated with diabetes. Therefore, it is crucial to identify and manage elevated blood pressure as part of comprehensive diabetic care. The causes of hypertension in diabetes involve immune system issues, environmental factors, vascular dysfunction, heightened RAAS activity, and autonomic nervous system changes. Studies demonstrate that reducing high blood pressure in diabetes reduces complications. As people with diabetes are at higher risk of cardiovascular disease, individualized care is vital, aiming for blood pressure below 130/80 mmHg (Naseri et al., 2022).

10.5.4.2 DYSLIPIDEMIA

Managing risk factors like dyslipidemia and hypertension is vital as they play a significant role in triggering cardiovascular disease in individuals with both T1DM and T2DM. Effective glycemic control in T1DM patients leads to lipid profiles similar to those of the general population. Atherosclerotic cardiovascular disease and high cholesterol and triglyceride levels are linked to both type 1 and type 2 diabetes. Individuals with diabetes have a higher likelihood of developing coronary heart disease (CHD) for every given blood cholesterol level, with the risk being more closely tied to triglyceride levels than in the general population. Cholesterol-lowering medication significantly reduces the risk of CHD in both diabetic and nondiabetic individuals (Schofield et al., 2016).

10.5.4.3 OBESITY

Obesity, as per the World Health Organization (WHO), is characterized by abnormal or excessive fat accumulation, which poses health risks. Given its systemic nature, obesity affects multiple organ systems (Lim and Boster, 2023). One diabetes risk factor is linked to insulin resistance in obesity. Adipose tissue in obese individuals releases elevated levels of pro-inflammatory cytokines, glycerol, and nonesterified fatty acids, all contributing to insulin resistance. Factors such as lipodystrophy, oxidative stress, endoplasmic reticulum stress, hypoxia in adipose tissue, and genetic background also influence insulin resistance (Wondmkun, 2020).

10.6 CONCLUSION

The study on DM underscores its complexity and the intricate interplay between biological causes, clinical symptoms, diagnostics, and treatment options. It covers diabetes' introduction, pathophysiology, clinical manifestations, diagnosis, monitoring, treatment options, preventive measures, and considerations for diverse populations. It emphasizes the need to mitigate long-term microvascular and macrovascular effects and address hyperglycemic crises. Medication therapy, insulin delivery devices, lifestyle changes, and multidisciplinary care teams are pivotal for successful management. Specific issues in children, adolescents, pregnant women, and the elderly are addressed, along with comorbidities like obesity, dyslipidemia, and hypertension, necessitating comprehensive care paradigms. The report delves into cutting-edge treatments such as artificial pancreas, stem cell and gene therapy, immunotherapy, and prevention programs, highlighting the quest for better modalities and potential cures. It offers a comprehensive overview of the current DM status and promising future developments.

KEYWORDS

- **diabetes mellitus**
- **Type 1 diabetes**
- **Type 2 diabetes**
- **insulin resistance**
- **complications**
- **management**
- **diagnosis**
- **neuropathy**
- **retinopathy**

REFERENCES

Akmal, M., Wadhwa, R. (2022). Alpha glucosidase inhibitors. In: *StatPearls*. StatPearls Publishing. https://www.ncbi.nlm.nih.gov/books/NBK534825/

Alatrach, M., Agyin, C., Adams, J., Chilton, R., Triplitt, C., DeFronzo, R.A., Cersosimo, E. (2018). Glucose lowering and vascular protective effects of cycloset added to GLP-1 receptor agonists in patients with type 2 diabetes. Endocrinology, Diabetes & Metabolism, 1(4), e00034. https://doi.org/10.1002/edm2.34

American Diabetes Association. (2020a). 2. Classification and diagnosis of diabetes: Standards of medical care in diabetes—2020. Diabetes Care, 43(Suppl. 1), S14–S31. https://doi.org/10.2337/dc20-S002

American Diabetes Association. (2020b). 9. Pharmacologic approaches to glycemic treatment: Standards of medical care in diabetes-2020. Diabetes Care, 43(Suppl. 1), S98–S110. https://doi.org/10.2337/dc20-S009

American Diabetes Association. (2020c). 13. Children and adolescents: Standards of medical care in diabetes-2020. Diabetes Care, 43(Suppl. 1), S163–S182. https://doi.org/10.2337/dc20-S013

American Diabetes Association. (2020d). 6. Glycemic targets: Standards of medical care in diabetes—2020. Diabetes Care, 43(Suppl. 1), S66–S76. https://doi.org/10.2337/dc20-S006

Azimova, K., San Juan, Z., Mukherjee, D. (2014). The cardiovascular safety profile of currently available diabetic drugs. Ochsner Journal, 14(4), 616–632.

Burrack, A.L., Martinov, T., Fife, B.T. (2017). T cell-mediated beta cell destruction: Autoimmunity and alloimmunity in the context of type 1 diabetes. Frontiers in Endocrinology, 8, 343. https://doi.org/10.3389/fendo.2017.00343

Buse, J.B., Wexler, D.J., Tsapas, A., Rossing, P., Mingrone, G., Mathieu, C., D'Alessio, D.A., Davies, M.J. (2020). 2019 update to: Management of hyperglycemia in type 2 diabetes, 2018. A consensus report by the American Diabetes Association (ADA) and the European Association for the Study of Diabetes (EASD). Diabetes Care, 43(2), 487–493. https://doi.org/10.2337/dci19-0066

Cada, D.J., Levien, T.L., Baker, D.E. (2014). Dapagliflozin. Hospital Pharmacy, 49(7), 647–662. https://doi.org/10.1310/hpj4907-647

Chae, H.W., Seo, G.H., Song, K., Choi, H.S., Suh, J., Kwon, A., Ha, S., Kim, H.S. (2020). Incidence and prevalence of type 1 diabetes mellitus among Korean children and adolescents between 2007 and 2017: An epidemiologic study based on a national database. Diabetes & Metabolism Journal, 44(6), 866–874. https://doi.org/10.4093/dmj.2020.0212

Chaitanya, M.V.N.L., Ramanunny, A.K., Babu, M.R., Gulati, M., Vishwas, S., Singh, T.G., Chellappan, D.K., Adams, J., Dua, K., Singh, S.K. (2022). Journey of rosmarinic acid as biomedicine to nano-biomedicine for treating cancer: Current strategies and future perspectives. Pharmaceutics, 14(11), 2401. https://doi.org/10.3390/pharmaceutics14112401

Chen, C., Cohrs, C.M., Stertmann, J., Bozsak, R., Speier, S. (2017). Human beta cell mass and function in diabetes: Recent advances in knowledge and technologies to understand disease pathogenesis. Molecular Metabolism, 6(9), 943–957. https://doi.org/10.1016/j.molmet.2017.06.019

Corcoran, C., Jacobs, T.F. (2023). Metformin. In: *StatPearls*. StatPearls Publishing. https://www.ncbi.nlm.nih.gov/books/NBK470150/

Correa, R., Quintanilla Rodriguez, B.S., Nappe, T.M. (2023). Glipizide. In: *StatPearls*. StatPearls Publishing. https://www.ncbi.nlm.nih.gov/books/NBK519556/

Cosentino, F., Grant, P.J., Aboyans, V., Bailey, C.J., Ceriello, A., Delgado, V., Federici, M., Filippatos, G., Grobbee, D.E., Hansen, T.B., Huikuri, H.V., Johansson, I., Jüni, P., Lettino, M., Marx, N., Mellbin, L.G., Östgren, C.J., Rocca, B., Roffi, M., Sattar, N., Seferović, P.M., Sousa-Uva, M., Valensi, P., Wheeler, D.C., ESC Scientific Document Group (2020). 2019 ESC guidelines on diabetes, pre-diabetes, and cardiovascular diseases developed in collaboration with the EASD. European Heart Journal, 41(2), 255–323. https://doi.org/10.1093/eurheartj/ehz486

Costello, R.A., Nicolas, S., Shivkumar, A. (2023). Sulfonylureas. In: *StatPearls*. StatPearls Publishing. https://www.ncbi.nlm.nih.gov/books/NBK551661/

Cunningham, A.M., Freeman, A.M. (2022). Glargine insulin. In: *StatPearls*. StatPearls Publishing. https://www.ncbi.nlm.nih.gov/books/NBK493213/

Dabhi, A.S., Bhatt, N.R., Shah, M.J. (2013). Voglibose: An alpha glucosidase inhibitor. Journal of Clinical and Diagnostic Research, 7(12), 3023–3027. https://doi.org/10.7860/JCDR/2013/6373.3838

Defronzo, R.A. (2009). Banting lecture. From the triumvirate to the ominous octet: A new paradigm for the treatment of type 2 diabetes mellitus. Diabetes, 58(4), 773–795. https://doi.org/10.2337/db09-9028

Dhillon, S. (2019). Dapagliflozin: A review in type 2 diabetes. Drugs, 79(10), 1135–1146. https://doi.org/10.1007/s40265-019-01148-3

Donnor, T., Sarkar, S. (2023). Insulin- pharmacology, therapeutic regimens and principles of intensive insulin therapy. In: Feingold, K.R. et al., Eds., Endotext. MDText.com, Inc. https://www.ncbi.nlm.nih.gov/books/NBK279083/

Driva, S., Korkontzelou, A., Tonstad, S., Tentolouris, N., Katsaounou, P. (2022). The effect of smoking cessation on body weight and other metabolic parameters with focus on people with type 2 diabetes mellitus. International Journal of Environmental Research and Public Health, 19(20), 13222. https://doi.org/10.3390/ijerph192013222

Drucker, D.J., Nauck, M.A. (2006). The incretin system: Glucagon-like peptide-1 receptor agonists and dipeptidyl peptidase-4 inhibitors in type 2 diabetes. Lancet, 368(9548), 1696–1705. https://doi.org/10.1016/S0140-6736(06)69705-5

Dutta, D., Mohindra, R., Mahajan, K., Sharma, M. (2023). Performance of fast-acting aspart insulin as compared to aspart insulin in insulin pump for managing type 1 diabetes mellitus: A meta-analysis. Diabetes & Metabolism Journal, 47(1), 72–81. https://doi.org/10.4093/dmj.2022.0035

Fletcher, B., Gulanick, M., Lamendola, C. (2002). Risk factors for type 2 diabetes mellitus. Journal of Cardiovascular Nursing, 16(2), 17–23. https://doi.org/10.1097/00005082-200201000-00003

Freeman, M.K. (2011). Efficacy and safety of linagliptin (Tradjenta) in adults with type-2 diabetes mellitus. P & T, 36(12), 807–842.

Fu, Z., Gilbert, E.R., Liu, D. (2013). Regulation of insulin synthesis and secretion and pancreatic Beta-cell dysfunction in diabetes. Current Diabetes Reviews, 9(1), 25–53. https://doi.org/10.2174/157339913804143703

Kasina, S.V.S.K., Baradhi, K.M. (2023). Dipeptidyl peptidase IV (DPP IV) inhibitors. In: *StatPearls*. StatPearls Publishing. https://www.ncbi.nlm.nih.gov/books/NBK554396/

Kesavadev, J., Murthy, L.S., Chaudhury, T., Yalamanchi, S.R., Giri, J., Gupta, S., Phatak, S., Modi, K.D., Chatterjee, S., Manjunath, A., Revanna, M., Bhattacharya, A. (2022). One-year safety and effectiveness of insulin degludec in patients with diabetes mellitus in routine clinical practice in India-TRUST (Tresiba real-world use study). Metabolism Open, 14, 100184. https://doi.org/10.1016/j.metop.2022.100184

Kesavadev, J., Saboo, B., Krishna, M.B., Krishnan, G. (2020). Evolution of insulin delivery devices: From syringes, pens, and pumps to DIY artificial pancreas. Diabetes Therapy, 11(6), 1251–1269. https://doi.org/10.1007/s13300-020-00832-2

Khan, H., Bangar, A., Grewal, A.K., Bansal, P., Singh, T.G. (2022). Caspase-mediated regulation of the distinct signaling pathways and mechanisms in neuronal survival. International Immunopharmacology, 110, 108951. https://doi.org/10.1016/j.intimp.2022.108951

Kimball, C. P., & Murlin, J. R. (1923). Aqueous extracts of pancreas: III. Some precipitation reactions of insulin. Journal of Biological Chemistry, 58(1), 337–346

Landman, G.W., de Bock, G.H., van Hateren, K.J., van Dijk, P.R., Groenier, K.H., Gans, R.O., Houweling, S.T., Bilo, H.J., Kleefstra, N. (2014). Safety and efficacy of gliclazide as treatment for type 2 diabetes: A systematic review and meta-analysis of randomized trials. PLoS One, 9(2), e82880. https://doi.org/10.1371/journal.pone.0082880

Lebovitz, H.E. (2019). Thiazolidinediones: The forgotten diabetes medications. Current Diabetes Reports, 19(12), 151. https://doi.org/10.1007/s11892-019-1270-x

Leung, E., Wongrakpanich, S., Munshi, M.N. (2018). Diabetes management in the elderly. Diabetes Spectrum, 31(3), 245–253. https://doi.org/10.2337/ds18-0033

Lim, Y., Boster, J. (2023). Obesity and comorbid conditions. In: *StatPearls*. StatPearls Publishing. https://www.ncbi.nlm.nih.gov/books/NBK574742/

LiverTox (2018). LiverTox: Clinical and Research Information on Drug-Induced Liver Injury [Internet]. Bethesda (MD): National Institute of Diabetes and Digestive and Kidney Diseases; 2012. Sitagliptin. [Updated 2018 January 3].

LiverTox (2021). LiverTox: Clinical and Research Information on Drug-Induced Liver Injury [Internet]. Bethesda (MD): National Institute of Diabetes and Digestive and Kidney Diseases; 2012. Acarbose. [Updated 2021 January 10]

Los, E., Wilt, A.S. (2023). Type 1 diabetes in children. In: *StatPearls*. StatPearls Publishing. https://www.ncbi.nlm.nih.gov/books/NBK507713/

Lucier, J., Weinstock, R.S. (2023). Type 1 diabetes. In: *StatPearls*. StatPearls Publishing. https://www.ncbi.nlm.nih.gov/books/NBK459237/

Maddatu, J., Anderson-Baucum, E., Evans-Molina, C. (2017). Smoking and the risk of type 2 diabetes. Translational Research, 184, 101–107. https://doi.org/10.1016/j.trsl.2017.02.004

Matschinsky, F.M., Wilson, D.F. (2019). The central role of glucokinase in glucose homeostasis: A perspective 50 years after demonstrating the presence of the enzyme in islets of Langerhans. Frontiers in Physiology, 10, 148. https://doi.org/10.3389/fphys.2019.00148

McIver, L.A., Preuss, C.V., Tripp, J. (2022). Acarbose. In: *StatPearls*. StatPearls Publishing. https://www.ncbi.nlm.nih.gov/books/NBK559242/

Meneghini, L.F. (2013). Insulin therapy for type 2 diabetes. Endocrine, 43(3), 529–534. https://doi.org/10.1007/s12020-013-9911-0

Milner, Z., Akhondi, H. (2023). Repaglinide. In: *StatPearls*. StatPearls Publishing. https://www.ncbi.nlm.nih.gov/books/NBK526098/

Miyagi, S., Takamura, T., Nguyen, T.T.T., Tsujiguchi, H., Hara, A., Nakamura, H., Suzuki, K., Tajima, A., Kannon, T., Toyama, T., Kambayashi, Y., Nakamura, H. (2021). Moderate alcohol consumption is associated with impaired insulin secretion and fasting glucose in non-obese, non-diabetic men. Journal of Diabetes Investigation, 12(5), 869–876. https://doi.org/10.1111/jdi.13411

Mohan, V., Saboo, B., Khader, J., Modi, K.D., Jindal, S., Wangnoo, S.K., Amarnath, S. (2022). Position of sulfonylureas in the current ERA: Review of national and international guidelines. Clinical Medicine Insights: Endocrinology and Diabetes, 15, 11795514221074663. https://doi.org/10.1177/11795514221074663

Munguia, C., Correa, R. (2023). Regular insulin. In: *StatPearls*. StatPearls Publishing. https://www.ncbi.nlm.nih.gov/books/NBK513346/

Nakrani, M.N., Wineland, R.H., Anjum, F. (2023). Physiology, glucose metabolism. In: *StatPearls*. StatPearls Publishing. https://www.ncbi.nlm.nih.gov/books/NBK541109/

Naseri, M.W., Esmat, H.A., Bahee, M.D. (2022). Prevalence of hypertension in type-2 diabetes mellitus. Annals of Medicine and Surgery, 78, 103758. https://doi.org/10.1016/j.amsu.2022.103758

National Center for Biotechnology Information. (2023). PubChem compound summary for insulin detemir. Retrieved December 6, 2023 from https://pubchem.ncbi.nlm.nih.gov/compound/Insulin-detemir

Noble, S.L., Johnston, E., Walton, B. (1998). Insulin lispro: A fast-acting insulin analog. American Family Physician, 57(2), 279–292.

Ozery, M., Wadhwa, R. (2022). Bromocriptine. In: *StatPearls*. StatPearls Publishing. https://www.ncbi.nlm.nih.gov/books/NBK557561/

Pociot, F., Lernmark, Å. (2016). Genetic risk factors for type 1 diabetes. Lancet, 387(10035), 2331–2339. https://doi.org/10.1016/S0140-6736(16)30582-7

Quintanilla Rodriguez, B.S., Mahdy, H. (2023). Gestational diabetes. In: *StatPearls*. StatPearls Publishing. https://www.ncbi.nlm.nih.gov/books/NBK544317/

Rewers, M., Stene, L.C., Norris, J.M. (2018). Risk factors for type 1 diabetes. 3rd edn. In: Cowie, C.C., et al., Eds., *Diabetes in America*. National Institute of Diabetes and Digestive and Kidney Diseases. https://www.ncbi.nlm.nih.gov/books/NBK567987/

Rix, I., Nexøe-Larsen, C., Bergmann, N.C., et al. (2019). Glucagon physiology. In: Feingold, K.R., et al., Eds., Endotext. MDText.com, Inc. https://www.ncbi.nlm.nih.gov/books/NBK279149/

Robertson, R.P., Harmon, J., Tran, P.O., Poitout, V. (2004). Beta-cell glucose toxicity, lipotoxicity, and chronic oxidative stress in type 2 diabetes. Diabetes, 53(Suppl 1), S119–S124. https://doi.org/10.2337/diabetes.53.2007.S119

Rohilla, M., Bansal, S., Garg, A., Dhiman, S., Dhankhar, S., Saini, M., Chauhan, S., Alsubaie, N., Batiha, G. E., Albezrah, N.K.A., Singh, T.G. (2023). Discussing pathologic mechanisms of diabetic retinopathy & therapeutic potentials of curcumin and β-glucogallin in the management of diabetic retinopathy. Biomedicine & Pharmacotherapy, 169, 115881. https://doi.org/10.1016/j.biopha.2023.115881

Rubin, R., Khanna, N.R., McIver, L.A. (2022). Aspart insulin. In: *StatPearls*. StatPearls Publishing. https://www.ncbi.nlm.nih.gov/books/NBK559864/

Saleem, F. (2017). Dapagliflozin: Cardiovascular safety and benefits in type 2 diabetes mellitus. Cureus, 9(10), e1751. https://doi.org/10.7759/cureus.1751

Saleem, F., Sharma, A. (2023). NPH insulin. In: *StatPearls*. StatPearls Publishing. https://www.ncbi.nlm.nih.gov/books/NBK560648/

Sapra, A., Bhandari, P. (2023). Diabetes mellitus. In: *StatPearls*. StatPearls Publishing. https://www.ncbi.nlm.nih.gov/books/NBK553050/

Sarnoski-Brocavich, S., Hilas, O. (2013). Canagliflozin (Invokana) is a novel oral agent for type-2 diabetes. P & T, 38(11), 656–666.

Schofield, J.D., Liu, Y., Rao-Balakrishna, P., Malik, R.A., Soran, H. (2016). Diabetes dyslipidemia. Diabetes Therapy, 7(2), 203–219. https://doi.org/10.1007/s13300-016-0167-x

Shah, R.B., Patel, M., Maahs, D.M., Shah, V.N. (2016). Insulin delivery methods: Past, present and future. International Journal of Pharmaceutical Investigation, 6(1), 1–9. https://doi.org/10.4103/2230-973X.176456

Sharabi, K., Tavares, C.D., Rines, A.K., Puigserver, P. (2015). Molecular pathophysiology of hepatic glucose production. Molecular Aspects of Medicine, 46, 21–33. https://doi.org/10.1016/j.mam.2015.05.003

Sharma, V.K., Singh, T.G. (2020). Insulin resistance and bioenergetic manifestations: Targets and approaches in Alzheimer's disease. Life Sciences, 262, 118401. https://doi.org/10.1016/j.lfs.2020.118401

Shoelson, S.E., Lee, J., Goldfine, A.B. (2006). Inflammation and insulin resistance. The Journal of Clinical Investigation, 116(7), 1793–1801. https://doi.org/10.1172/JCI29069

Simes, B.C., MacGregor, G.G. (2019). Sodium-glucose cotransporter-2 (SGLT2) inhibitors: A clinician's guide. Diabetes, Metabolic Syndrome and Obesity, 12, 2125–2136. https://doi.org/10.2147/DMSO.S200915

Singh, G., Can, A.S., Correa, R. (2023). Pioglitazone. In: *StatPearls*. StatPearls Publishing. https://www.ncbi.nlm.nih.gov/books/NBK519562/

Singh, R., Chandel, S., Dey, D., Ghosh, A., Roy, S., Ravichandran, V., Ghosh, D. (2020a). Epigenetic modification and therapeutic targets of diabetes mellitus. Bioscience Reports, 40(9), BSR20202160. https://doi.org/10.1042/BSR20202160

Singh, R., Farooq, S.A., Mannan, A., Singh, T.G., Najda, A., Grażyna, Z., Albadrani, G.M., Sayed, A.A., Abdel-Daim, M.M. (2022). Animal models of diabetic microvascular complications: Relevance to clinical features. Biomedicine & Pharmacotherapy, 145, 112305. https://doi.org/10.1016/j.biopha.2021.112305

Singh, R., Rao, H.K., Singh, T.G. (2020b). Advanced glycated end products (ages) in diabetes and its complications: An insight. Plant Archives, 20(1), 3838–3841.

Singh, R., Rao, H.K., Singh, T.G. (2020c). Neuropathic pain in diabetes mellitus: Challenges and future trends. Obesity Medicine, 18, 100215. https://doi.org/10.1016/j.obmed.2020.100215

Solis-Herrera, C., Triplitt, C., Reasner, C., et al., (2018). Classification of diabetes mellitus. In: Feingold, K.R., et al., Eds., Endotext. MDText.com, Inc. https://www.ncbi.nlm.nih.gov/books/NBK513830/

Terrell, J.M., Jacobs, T.F. (2023). Alogliptin. In: *StatPearls*. StatPearls Publishing. https://www.ncbi.nlm.nih.gov/books/NBK534804/

Thota, S., Akbar, A. (2023). Insulin. In: *StatPearls*. StatPearls Publishing. https://www.ncbi.nlm.nih.gov/books/NBK559381/

Trerattanavong, K., Tadi, P. (2023). Glimepiride. In: *StatPearls*. StatPearls Publishing. https://www.ncbi.nlm.nih.gov/books/NBK551549/

Vargas, E., Joy, N.V., Carrillo Sepulveda, M.A. (2022). Biochemistry, insulin metabolic effects. In: *StatPearls*. StatPearls Publishing. https://www.ncbi.nlm.nih.gov/books/NBK554537/

Weiss, M.A. (2009). The structure and function of insulin: Decoding the TR transition. Vitamins and Hormones, 80, 33–49. https://doi.org/10.1016/S0083-6729(08)00602-9

Wondmkun, Y.T. (2020). Obesity, insulin resistance, and type 2 diabetes: Associations and therapeutic implications. Diabetes, Metabolic Syndrome and Obesity, 13, 3611–3616. https://doi.org/10.2147/DMSO.S292539

World Health Organization. (2019). Classification of diabetes mellitus. https://www.who.int/publications/m/item/classification-of-diabetes-mellitus

Xu, G., Liu, B., Sun, Y., Du, Y., Snetselaar, L.G., Hu, F.B., Bao, W. (2018). Prevalence of diagnosed type 1 and type 2 diabetes among US adults in 2016 and 2017: Population-based study. BMJ, 362, k1497. https://doi.org/10.1136/bmj.k1497

Yoon, J.W., Jun, H.S. (2001). Cellular and molecular pathogenic mechanisms of insulin-dependent diabetes mellitus. Annals of the New York Academy of Sciences, 928, 200–211. https://doi.org/10.1111/j.1749-6632.2001.tb05651.x

Zhou, W., Tao, J., Zhou, X., Chen, H. (2019). Insulin degludec, a novel ultra-long-acting basal insulin versus insulin glargine for managing type 2 diabetes: A systematic review and meta-analysis. Diabetes Therapy, 10(3), 835–852. https://doi.org/10.1007/s13300-019-0608-x

CHAPTER 11

Challenges and Approaches for the Treatment of Metabolic Epilepsy

HIMANSHI RAHEJA[1*], SHUSHANK MAHAJAN[2], BHAVESH DHARMANI[2*], DIVYA KANWAR[2], SANJANA MEHTA[2], THAKUR GURJEET SINGH[2], PARMINDER NAIN[3], JASPREET KAUR[3], and RANIYA MALIK[4,5]

[1]Drug Safety Department, Mumbai, Maharashtra, India

[2]Chitkara College of Pharmacy, Chitkara University, Rajpura, Punjab, India

[3]School of Pharmaceutical Sciences, RIMT University, Mandi Gobindgarh, Punjab, India

[4]Discipline of Pharmacy, Graduate School of Health, University of Technology Sydney, Sydney, NSW, Australia

[5]Faculty of Health, Australian Research Centre in Complementary and Integrative Medicine, University of Technology Sydney, Sydney, NSW, Australia

*Corresponding author

ABSTRACT

Epilepsy is a widespread neurological disorder that affects individuals regardless of age, race, or social class. It arises from pathophysiological and metabolic disturbances, resulting in recurrent seizures due to abnormal electrical activity in the brain. These seizures may cause involuntary movements and altered behavior, often occurring

Pharmacotherapy Approaches Toward Endocrine and Metabolic Diseases.
Thakur Gurjeet Singh and Sanjana Mehta (Eds.)

DOI: 10.1201/9781779640154-11

subconsciously or unconsciously. Epilepsy is a chronic, noncontagious condition influenced by both genetic and environmental factors, with seizures classified into generalized, focal, and epileptic spasms. Despite ongoing scientific efforts, a complete cure remains elusive, and current treatments are still evolving. The disorder significantly impacts a patient's quality of life, requiring medical professionals to approach diagnosis and management with great attention to detail. Comprehensive care involves understanding seizure types, clinical manifestations, underlying physiology, and appropriate therapeutic strategies. Although epilepsy cannot always be entirely cured, it can often be effectively managed through strict adherence to medication regimens and quality primary care. However, the use of multiple antiepileptic drugs increases the risk of adverse effects. Thus, a deeper and more informed understanding of the disease is essential for improving treatment outcomes and enhancing the quality of life for individuals living with epilepsy.

11.1 INTRODUCTION

The description of epilepsy has been known to humankind for ages, but understanding its dynamics wholly is still challenging for all of us. It was accounted for in the Akkadian language for the first time in 2000 BC. Various signs and symptoms were described, but the etiology was very unclear; thus, it was superstitiously assumed that some unearthly powers were involved in causing such symptoms as turning hands and neck, eyes popping out, and jaw tightening (Singh and Singh, 2021). So, it was deduced that some evil power possessed the patient; thus, they tried to cure the patient with mythological methods. The patient with such symptoms was prohibited from being social or getting married. Later, as science advanced, many aspects of this disease were revealed. It was realized that there was no divine concept but the disturbances in the brain that were causing the disease. The understanding got better with the study of the neurophysiology of the brain (Moshé, 2020; Singh et al., 2020).

11.1.1 UNDERSTANDING CLINICAL DETAILS OF EPILEPTOGENESIS

11.1.1.1 NEUROTRANSMITTERS

As the name suggests, neurotransmitters carry messages from one nerve cell to another, which can also be called synaptic transmission. Neurotransmission is a very organized act, but it can be disturbed by many external factors, such as drugs, trauma, diseases, and so on.

11.1.1.2 EXCITATORY TRANSMISSION

In such transmission, the neuron fires off the message further to other neurons. Some common excitatory neurotransmitters are glutamate, histamine, epinephrine, and acetylcholine. Glutamate is the most common excitatory neurotransmitter, abundant in our nervous system (Teleanu et al., 2022; Khan et al., 2022).

11.1.1.3 INHIBITORY TRANSMISSION

Just opposite to the excitatory, it prevents generating any signal and does not let the message pass from one neuron to another. A few examples of inhibitory neurotransmitters are gamma-aminobutyric acid (GABA) and serotonin(Teleanu et al., 2022; Thapa et al, .2023).

GABA is one of the most prominent inhibitory neurotransmitters that stops our nervous system's excitability. It is broadly found in the brain, and when the inhibition crosses more than the required, it may cause seizures and many other issues. It is a push button for our mood and helps brain development, too. People have epilepsy either because of the lack of inhibitory neurotransmitters like GABA or due to the presence of excessive excitatory neurotransmitters like glutamate (Haas et al., 2024; Singh et al., 2021).

11.1.1.4 MODULATORY NEUROTRANSMITTERS

Neuromodulators can affect large numbers of neurons simultaneously. They can make connections with other neurotransmitters and influence their effects. Examples of neuromodulators are acetylcholine, dopamine, cannabinoids, serotonin, and histamine (Teleanu et al., 2022; Sharma et al., 2023) (Figure 11.1).

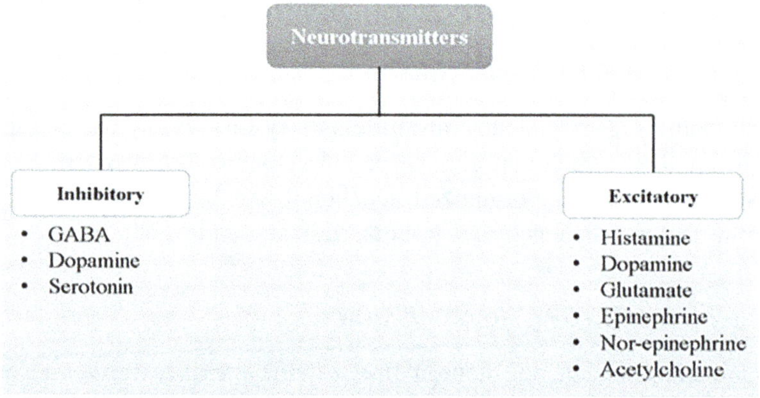

FIGURE 11.1 Examples of inhibitory and excitatory neurotransmitters.

11.2 EPILEPTIC DISORDERS

A class of neurological conditions referred to as epileptic disorders is defined by epileptic seizures. Episodes of epileptic seizures can range in duration from extended durations of intense shaking to short, essentially unnoticeable moments. Most epilepsy cases have an enigmatic etiology. Certain cases arise from birth abnormalities through a process called epileptogenesis, and some by brain injury, stroke, brain tumors, and brain infections (Sirven, 2015; Vishwakarma et al., 2022).

Two main categorization methods for seizures and epilepsies have been developed by the International League Against Epilepsy (ILAE): The International Categorization of Epileptic Seizures and the International Categorization of Epileptic Conditions and Epileptic Syndromes (Figures 11.2 and 11.3; Table 11.1).

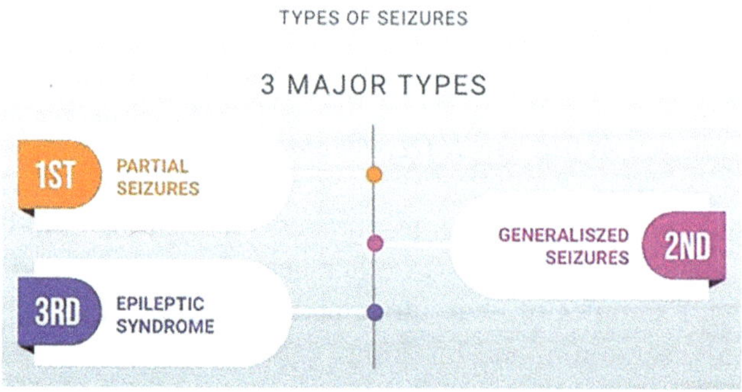

FIGURE 11.2 Types of seizures.

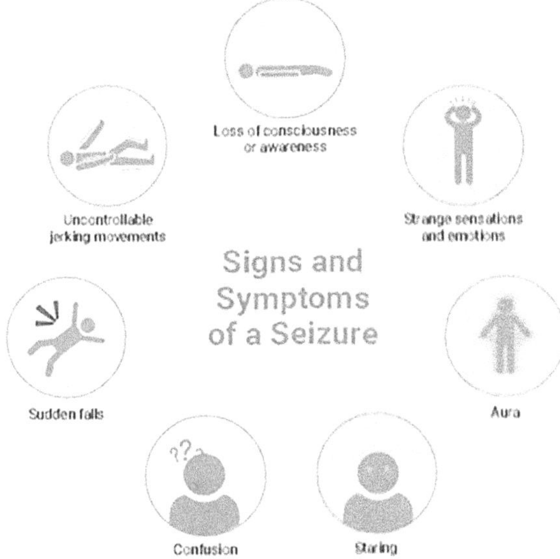

FIGURE 11.3 Symptoms of epilepsy.

TABLE 11.1 Various Types and Subtypes of Seizure Disorders

S. No.	Type of Seizure	Subtype
1.	Partial seizure/focal seizure	Simple partial seizure
		Complex partial seizure
		Secondarily generalized seizures
2.	Generalized seizure	Absence seizure
		Tonic seizure
		Clonic seizure
		Tonic–clonic seizure (GTC)
		Myoclonic seizure
		Atonic seizure
		Infantile spasms/hypsarrhythmia

11.2.1 CATEGORIZATION OF EPILEPTIC CONDITIONS AND EPILEPTIC SYNDROMES

11.2.1.1 PARTIAL SEIZURES

It is present in a single, localized brain region and can extend to a larger or smaller area or even the entire brain. Clinically, the focal origin may be obvious, or an ECG may show it.

- **Simple seizures (SPS):** SPS is defined as partial seizures that do not result in unconsciousness. Sometimes, patients describe somatosensory sensations as a "warning" sign before a generalized tonic–clonic seizure occurs. These alerts, sometimes called auras, are just primary partial seizures.
- **Complex partial seizures (CPS)/complicated partial seizures:** CPS are defined as partial seizures accompanied by altered awareness. The patient may have behavioral abnormalities, periods of memory loss, or automatisms when they have CPS. It has been wrongly determined that specific individuals with complicated partial epilepsy are experiencing psychotic episodes. Generalized tonic–clonic seizures can also develop from complex partial seizures. Individuals who suffer from complicated partial seizures usually lose memory of these incidents (Bench and Bedside, n.d.).

11.2.1.2 GENERALIZED SEIZURES

According to their behavioral impacts, generalized seizures can be categorized into many groups.

- **Absence seizures:** Absence seizures, also known as petit mal seizures, are characterized by a brief stoppage of consciousness during which the seizure victim seems empty and unresponsive (typically lasting up to 30 s). Muscle spasms might happen.
- **Myoclonic seizures:** Myoclonic seizures cause jerky movements of individual muscles or muscle groups and include very short (less than 0.1 s) muscular contractions.
- **Tonic seizures:** During a tonic seizure, the arms, legs, or trunk muscles suddenly stiffen or tense. The stiffness typically occurs during sleep and lasts for around 20 s. When someone has a tonic seizure while standing, they might trip and fall.
- **Clonic seizures:** Clonic seizures are characterized by periodic myoclonus, usually occurring at a frequency of two to three per second.
- **Tonic–clonic seizures (grand mal):** Tonic–clonic seizures involve an initial muscle contraction (tonic phase) that may include tongue biting, urinary incontinence, and the absence of breathing. This is followed by rhythmic muscle contractions (clonic phase).

- **Atonic seizures:** Atonic seizures result in a loss of muscular tone that sends the sufferer to the ground. These are commonly referred to as "drop attacks," although they should be differentiated from episodes that resemble those that may happen in cataplexy or narcolepsy (von der Brelie et al., 2013; Rehni et al., 2009).

11.3 ETIOLOGY

Epilepsy is brought on by any mechanism that modifies the structure (microscopic or macroscopic) or function of brain neurons. The structural alteration may be due to vascular processes, tumors, trauma, inborn errors, degenerative diseases, and so on. The exact cause is only sometimes found, so it is proposed. For example, compared to the younger generation, the most common cause of the condition in older people isvascular degenerative or neoplastic reasons (Bezabeh et al., 2004).

Some cases have shown this condition as the cause of genetic influence, the result of any kind of infection (human immunodeficiency viruses, meningitis, viral encephalitis, etc.), and developmental conditions (attention deficit hyperactivity disorder, autism, etc.).

11.4 INCIDENCE AND PREVALENCE OF EPILEPSY

Outcomes of various studies have shown that the prevalence of this condition is due to certain factors that include the age of the patient, family history of epilepsy or fever-related seizures, prenatal injury, traumatic head injury in early ages, brain infection, seizures in early ages, stroke and vascular diseases, dementia, and abuse of illegal drugs such as cocaine (Minardi et al., 2019; Rehni and Singh, 2010).

As per the World Health Organization report, produced on February 9, 2023, epilepsy affects over 50 million individuals worldwide, making it one of the most prevalent neurological conditions. Almost 80% of people with epilepsy reside in low- and middle-income nations. If given the correct diagnosis and care, up to 70% of people with epilepsy are thought to be able to enjoy seizure-free lives. Individuals with epilepsy have a threefold increased chance of dying young compared to the general population. In low-income nations, 75% of people with epilepsydo not receive the necessary therapy. People who have epilepsy and their families face stigma and prejudice in many areas of the world (Liu et al., 2023).

11.5 CLINICAL ASPECT OF EPILEPSY

Epilepsy syndrome: The ILAE defines an epilepsy syndrome as "a characteristic cluster of clinical and electroencephalogram (EEG) features, often supported by specific etiological findings (structural, genetic, metabolic, immune, and infectious)."

Signs are the indications the doctor will observe, and symptoms are the manifestations experienced by the patients (Table 11.2).

TABLE 11.2 Multiple Kinds of Epileptic Syndrome

Epileptic Syndrome	Onset	Causes	Signs and Symptoms
West syndrome/ Infantile spasms	The first year of a child's life is usually between 4 and 8 months	Genetical history Brain disorder or injury Idiopathic	Involuntary movements of hands, legs, and head Developmental delays Seizures mainly occur in clusters Hypsarrhythmia
Dravet syndrome	Early infancy	Defect in gene SCN1A	Stiffening and jerking of the whole body or some part of it Mainly focal or generalized seizure Developmental delays
Lennox-Gastaut syndrome	Early childhood, usually before four years	Genetic defects Tuberculosis Less blood flow in the brain Brain infection Idiopathic cause	Cognitive dysfunction and mental retardation Typically occur during sleep, myoclonic seizures, and generalized tonic–clonic seizures Life-threatening
Childhood absence epilepsy	Mostly between 4 and 8 years	Genetic and environmental components May have mutations in the gene GABRA1	Absence seizures Unresponsiveness for 10–20 s Absence seizures

Epilepsy syndrome can be featured based on the following parameters:

- Types of seizure
- Age of onset
- EEG pattern
- Severity and chronicity
- Patient history and family history

11.5.1 SIGNS AND SYMPTOMS

Epilepsy may strike anyone of any age, gender, color, or ethnicity. Individual differences can exist in seizure events. Throughout the episode, some people move their arms and legs, some have full-blown convulsions, and others look blankly. People with epilepsy may require emergency medical assistance if they experience two seizures a day or more (Stafstrom and Carmant, 2015) (Figure 11.3).

11.5.2 PATHOPHYSIOLOGY

The pathophysiology of epilepsy and seizures can explain the wide range of seizure disorders. A common feature of all epilepsies, though, is a dysregulated synaptic balance between excitatory (via glutamatergic signaling) and inhibitory (by GABAergic signaling) driving, which can cause seizures. The clinical manifestation of epilepsy is seizures, which are caused by disturbances in the neurotransmitters (Barker-haliski and White, 2015) (Figure 11.4).

11.5.3 EPILEPSY AND OTHER NEUROLOGICAL DISORDERS

Epilepsy, being a brain disorder, can lead to other comorbidities as it alters the functions of the brain. Patients with seizures face difficulties with their memories, which may eventually lead to dementia or Alzheimer's. Though there is no prominent evidence of such issues, possibilities are no less. Anxiety is also one of the common conditions among people with epilepsy. Comorbidities mean the occurrence of one disease with another simultaneously. In epilepsy, no age factor increases the risk of epilepsy; it may occur at any age in epilepsy patients. Adults may face anxiety and depression, whereas elders may face dementia. Almost all the patients with epilepsy face more than one issue (Sen et al., 2018) (Table 11.3).

11.6 DIAGNOSTIC EVALUATION OF DISEASE

Diagnosing epilepsy has always been a challenging task for doctors, as there are broad categories of brain disorders. The whole medical history,

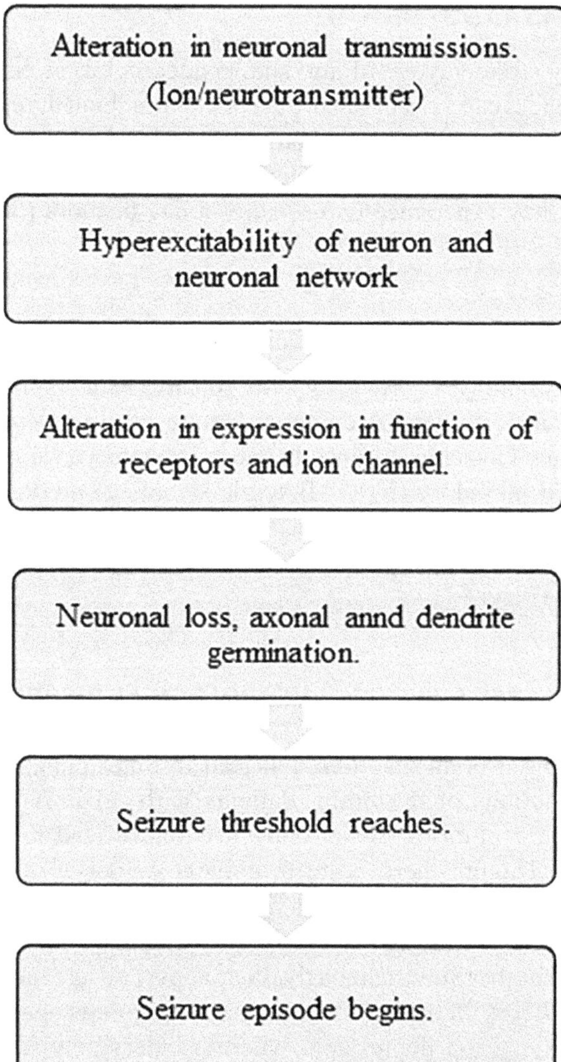

FIGURE 11.4 Flowchart showing the pathophysiology of epilepsy.

family, and genetic history must be tracked to know the correct type of epilepsy. Comorbidities always make the diagnosis a strenuous task for care providers. Correctly classifying and identifying seizure types is necessary to diagnose the disease. There is more than one way to diagnose epilepsy (van Donselaar et al., 2006; Kotsopoulos et al., 2003).

TABLE 11.3 Comorbid Conditions with Significantly Higher Rates of Epilepsy Than in the General Population

Medical	Psychiatric	Cognitive
Musculoskeletal system disorders	Depression	Attention-deficit hyperactivity disorder
Gastrointestinal and digestive disorders	Anxiety	Learning disability
Respiratory system disorders	Autism spectrum disorders	Mental retardation
Chronic pain disorders	Interictal dysphoric disorder	Alzheimer's disease/ dementia
Cerebrovascular accidents	Interictal behavior syndrome	
Migraine	Psychosis of epilepsy	
Neoplasia		
Arthritis/rheumatism		
Obesity		
Diabetes		
Infections		
Fractures		
Allergies		

A few are explained below.

- **Neurological exam:** This exam checks whether the neurological system works well. The doctor will test speech, behavior, body movements, concentration power, balance, and other neurological aspects.
- **Electroencephalogram (EEG)** is a commonly used test to diagnose epilepsy. Electrode sensors record brain activity, placing the electrodes on the scalp. If there is a suspicion of epilepsy, the pattern of waves in the brain will change. EEG can be done for a few minutes to a few hours, awake or asleep, to determine the type of seizure correctly. It is a safe and painless procedure.
- **Radiological testing:** The cause of epilepsy may be lesions, tumors, and injuries in the brain, which can be detected by radiological testing. Magnetic resonance imaging is used to check the magnetic field caused by the nerve cells. They will be altered from

regular activity in case of the disease. It is one of the best diagnostic tests for epilepsy. Functional magnetic resonance imaging tests the area responsible for specific brain functions like speech, memory, and movement.

- **Computerized tomography (CT):** X-rays detect abnormalities in the brain. A CT scan can show lesions, bleeding, and structural issues.
- **Positron emission tomography:** Radioactive glucose is injected into the brain to produce an image with minute details, which helps to notice brain cells' blood flow and activities.
- **Blood tests:** A complete blood test is done to check for specific markers and to determine whether an infection is suspected. It also examines the lipid and renal profiles.
- **Neuropsychological tests:** Patients with epilepsy face memory issues or other cognitive hardships. They sometimes have difficulty in speech and framing sentences, which multiple episodes of seizures can cause.

Psychological assessments can help care providers identify the severity of the disease. Often, simple puzzles and questions are given to the patient, and the ability of their responses is assessed, which helps in deciding on accurate therapy (Kotsopoulos et al., 2003).

11.7 TREATMENT PERSPECTIVES

As already discussed, epilepsy is a complicated disease and should be handled very vigilantly. A minor delay in identifying and solving the issue can lead to significant complications. Also, early detection of the signs of epilepsy can help in controlling the recurrence of seizures. There are various antiseizure drug therapies mentioned for curing the disease. Each kind of seizure is to be rightly identified and cured accordingly. However, the ideal cause of the disease is not yet known. The antiseizure drugs (ASDs) are used to cure the patient symptomatically (Stafstrom and Carmant, 2015) (Figure 11.5).

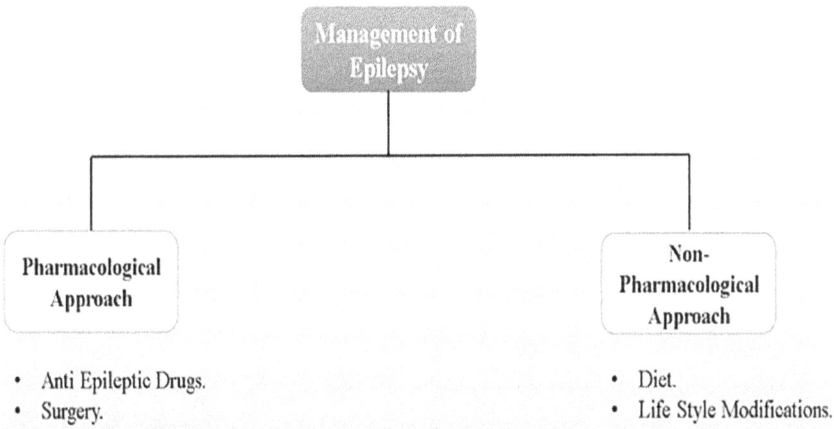

FIGURE 11.5 Approaches used in the management of epilepsy.

- **General approach to the treatment:** Not every seizure is epilepsy. A medical healthcare provider must be watchful for the signs and symptoms. There should be a specific approach when the patient complains of a seizure. Three steps can be followed to form a conclusion. First, patiently listen and observe the signs and symptoms of the patient and measure the severity according to the information presented. Second, if the issue is detected and the seizure turns out to be epileptic, then attentively categorize the type of epilepsy and note down the possible complications that occurred or may occur with that type of epilepsy. Third, a rational therapy for the patient should be created, and the patient should understand the situation's intensity (Ghosh et al., 2021) (Figure 11.6).

11.7.1 PHARMACOLOGICAL APPROACH TOWARD MANAGEMENT OF EPILEPSY

Epileptic drug helps in managing the signs and symptoms of the disease, but cannot cure it completely. They may help in improving the quality of life (Figure 11.7; Table 11.4).

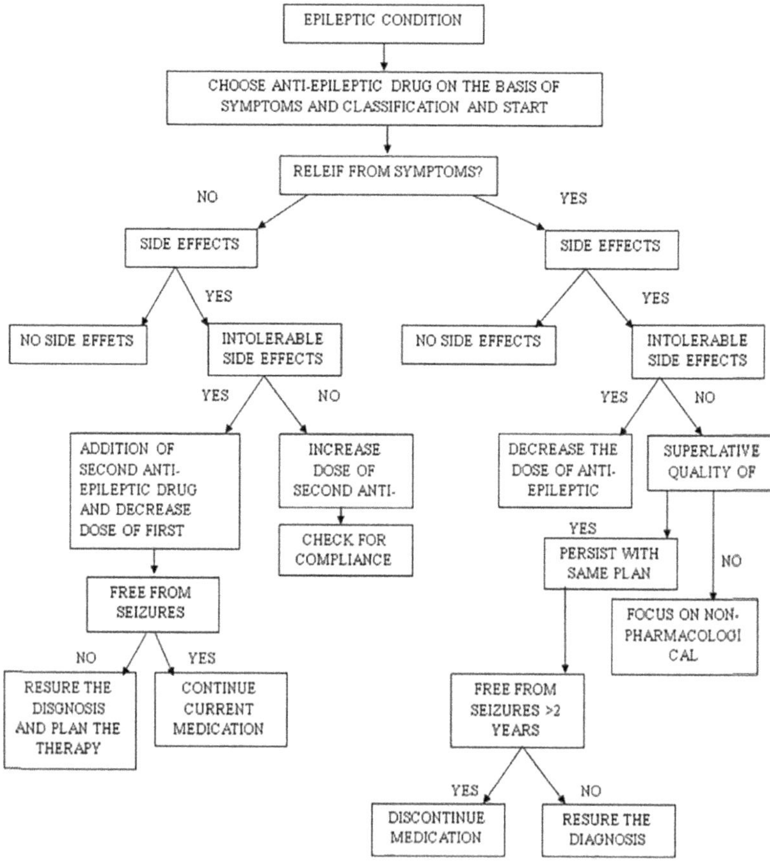

FIGURE 11.6 Algorithm for the management of epileptic condition.

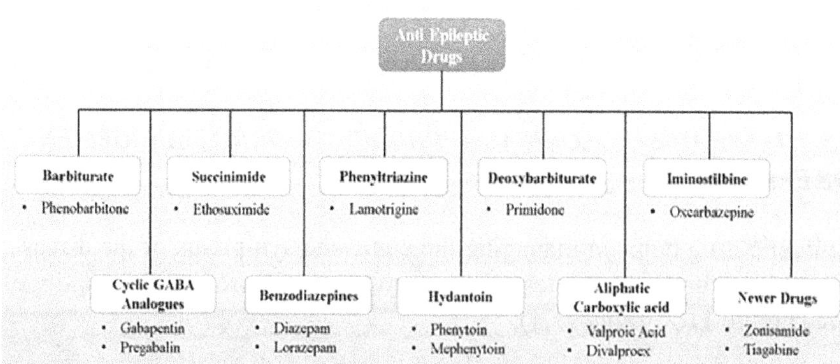

FIGURE 11.7 Classification of antiepileptic drugs.

TABLE 11.4 Choice of Antiepileptic Drugs

S. No.	Type of Seizure	First-Choice Drug	Second-Choice Drug	Alternative/Add-On Drugs
1	Generalized tonic clonic seizure/simple partial with or without generalization	Carbamazepine, phenytoin	Phenobarbitone, valproate	Primidone, gabapentin, lamotrigine, topiramate
	Complex partial with or without generalization	Phenytoin, valproate, carbamazepine	Lamotrigine, gabapentin	Topiramate, clobazam, zonisamide, tiagabine
2	Absence seizures	Valproate	Lamotrigine, ethosuximide	Clonazepam, clobazam
3	Myoclonic seizures	Valproate	Topiramate, lamotrigine	Clonazepam, primidone
4	Febrile seizures	Diazepam (rectal)	–	–
5	Atonic seizure	Valproate	Clobazam, clonazepam	Lamotrigine
6	Status epilepticus	Lorazepam (IV), Diazepam (IV)	Phenobarbitone (IV/IM), fosphenytoin (IV)	Gen. anesthetics

11.7.1.1 MANAGEMENT OF EPILEPSY

Epilepsy is a complicated disease and is not easy to comprehend, and as a result, it needs to be managed very carefully and patiently. Every detail should be very much understood before providing therapy to the patient. Every type of epilepsy requires a different approach, thus making it a more cumbersome process. There are various kinds of management for various age groups. Patient demographics are to be considered significantly before preparing a treatment chart.

There are many parameters to be considered before starting a treatment for epilepsy, like age, gender, frequency of seizure, mental status, comorbidities, family history, and medical history. After assessing all the major parameters, a plan is made to curtail the symptoms of epilepsy. Polytherapy may lead to drug-resistant epilepsy; thus, it is essential to consider monotherapy as a first choice. The ASD should be tolerable to the patient so that it does not hinder the quality of life. With comorbidities, it becomes more difficult to manage epilepsy as multiple drugs are administered. Therefore, drug–drug interactions should be well-studied before making a treatment chart (Galizia and Faulkner, 2018).

After administering the drug, adherence is the most significant part. Medical care providers should be very vigilant about adherence to the medication for the best results. Any negligence may result in drug-resistant epilepsy, and it may further complicate the treatment. Regular monitoring and evaluation of the disease and recovery are a must. Medical care providers should continually be updated with state-of-the-art technologies and should be curious to keep up with advancements (Cravo et al., 2020) (Figure 11.8; Table 11.5).

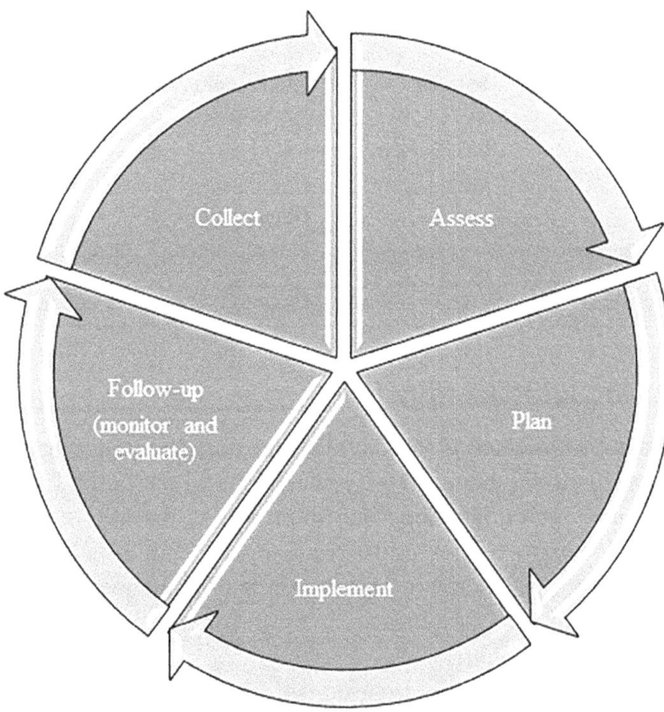

FIGURE 11.8 Patient-centered care cycle.

11.7.1.2 SURGICAL TREATMENT FOR EPILEPSY

Most of the time, some medications help in curtailing the signs and symptoms of epilepsy, but at times, surgical intervention becomes a must to understand and treat the disease. Epilepsy is usually convenient when the seizures that originate from a single location. Surgery is never to be counted as first-line treatment, but it should only be an option when the

TABLE 11.5 Approach to Antiseizure Medication (Pseudoresistance)

Incorrect Diagnosis	Unsuitable Antiseizure Drug	Incorrect Doses of Antiseizure Drugs		Lifestyle Factors and Medication Adherence
Examine the diagnosis of epilepsy (avoid mimicking epileptic seizures; examples include syncope, migraines, and movement abnormalities)	Review epilepsy type/ syndrome classification along with seizure type	Ensure you have trailed ideal dosages and titrated to the highest dose that can be tolerated	Review of concomitant drugs, including over-the-counter medications and antiseizure medications Medication interactions that impact antiseizure drugs	Nonadherence of antiseizure medication Recreational drug use Excessive alcohol use Sleep deprivation

seizures are uncontrollable, that too under many specific circumstances. Surgery is sometimes also considered when the patient is not able to tolerate the side effects of the drugs, and consequently, the quality of life is degrading.

Some surgeries are resective surgery, corpus callosotomy, hemispherectomy, and so on.

As already said, surgery is not the first option in the treatment of epilepsy, as there are multiple complications involved in and after such procedures. There may come multiple issues like language and speech problems, memory issues, headaches, anxiety, depression, lack of expressiveness, and many other severe effects on vital functions. To minimize these risks, presurgery testing and brain mapping are performed extensively (Shenoy et al., 2023).

11.7.2 NONPHARMACOLOGICAL APPROACH IN THE MANAGEMENT OF EPILEPSY

11.7.2.1 DIET AND LIFESTYLE MODIFICATIONS

Multiple food and daily habits may trigger seizures or make them worse, like a high intake of caffeine, which may result in restlessness and may also interfere with drug efficacy. It may make the patient more susceptible to seizures. Intake of alcohol and other addictive substances is especially to be avoided as they may become a severe hurdle in the treatment of the disease.

Sleeping habits play an essential role in curing the symptoms as good sleep provides relaxation to the brain, leading to fewer triggers of the seizures. An exercise routine may be set to minimize the stress hormones, which are a significant trigger of seizures. Making distance from the digital world may also help, like avoiding mobile phones one or two hours before sleeping and reducing screen time. A few minor changes in daily routine may significantly impact the treatment of the disease (Alqahtani et al., 2020).

11.8 PHARMACOLOGY OF ANTIEPILEPTIC DRUGS (AEDS)

- **Pharmacokinetics of antiepileptic drugs:** The use of AEDs has always been controversial because of their mechanism of action. These drugs usually work on the neurotransmitters by inhibiting or exciting them (Table 11.6).

TABLE 11.6 Pharmacokinetics of Antiepileptic Drugs

S. No.	Drug	Half-Life	Unchanged Percentage	Time to Steady State (Days)	Volume of Distribution	Percentage of Protein Binding	Metabolite (Clinically Important)
1.	Valproic acid	A = 8–20 C = 7–14	<5%	1–3	0.1–0.5	90-95 (binding saturates)	Can cause toxicity
2.	Zonisamide	24–60	–	5–15	0.8–1.6	40–60%	–
3.	Levetiracetam	7–10	–	2	0.7	<10%	–
4.	Felbamate	16–22	50%	5–7	0.73–0.82	Near around 25	–
5.	Carbamazepine	12 MT; 5–14 CT	<1%	21–28 for auto-induction completion	1–2	40–90	10,11-epoxide
6.	Primidone	A = 3.3–19 C = 4.5–11	40%	1–4	0.43–1.1	80	PB[c] PEMA[c]
7.	Phenobarbital	A = 46–136 C = 37–73	20–40%	14–21	0.6	50	–
8.	Ethosuximide	A = 60 C = 30	10–20%	6–12	0.67	0	–
9.	Tiagabine	5–13	Negligible	–	–	95	–
10.	Gabapentin[b]	5–40[d]	100%	1–2	0.65–1.04	0	–
	Topiramate	18–21	50–70%	4–5	Male: 0.55–0.8 Female: 0.23–0.4	15	–
	Lamotrigine	25.4 MT	0	3–15	1.28	40–50	–
	Phenytoin	A = 10–34 C = 5–14	<5%	7–28	0.6–8.0	90	–
	Oxcarbazepine	3–13	–	2	0.7	40%	10-Hydroxy-carbazepine

[a]A = adult, C = child, MT = monotherapy, CT = combination therapy; [b]the bioavailability of gabapentin is dependent upon its dose; [c]PB = phenobarbital, PEMA= phenylethylmalonamide; [d]renal functions are responsible for half-life.

- **First generation of antiepileptic drugs:** This generation of epileptic drugs, like clonazepam, carbamazepine, phenobarbital, phenytoin, and so on, plays a role in either inhibiting sodium ion channels or enhancing GABA receptor activity.
- Phenytoin blocks Na^+ channels in postsynaptic neurons and inhibits their action potential.
- **Second generation of antiepileptic drugs:** The drugs in the first generation had some drawbacks, resulting in the discovery of the second generation of ASDs, like gabapentin, felbamate, oxcarbazepine, topiramate, and so on. These drugs also block sodium channels and promote GABAergic activities but work beyond them. They further regulate excitatory neurotransmitters and work on calcium channels.
- **Third generation of antiepileptic drugs:** These generations of drugs are used for specific functions where other drugs are not effective. They also work on GABA receptors and sodium channels with more efficacy and specificity. Drugs like eslicarbazepine, lacosamide, rufinamide, and so on (Perucca, 2021).

11.9 DRUG-RESISTANT EPILEPSY

Though medication plays a massive part in curtailing the signs and symptoms of epilepsy, there are several impediments to the process of treatment. Sometimes, even with adequate therapy, a patient shows no improvement. When the patient is given at least two antiseizure medicines but does not show any recovery, then it can be said to be a case of drug-resistant epilepsy.

There are various factors involved in causing drug-resistant epilepsy:

- Seizures starting before one year of age can quickly become drug-resistant.
- Inaccurate choice of drugs according to the type of seizure may contribute to drug resistance.
- Administering multiple drugs may become an obstacle to drug efficacy.

- Poor medication adherence can become a severe cause of drug-resistant epilepsy.
- Poor diet and complicated lifestyle may reduce drug efficiency, thus causing drug-resistant epilepsy (Dalic and Cook, 2016).

11.9.1 CLINICAL MANAGEMENT

- Monotherapy can be considered instead of polytherapy.
- Seizure could be a promising option if the patient is facing drug resistance; in focal epilepsy, one part of the brain is responsible for triggering the seizures, and that part can be removed by surgery.
- Neuromodulators or neurostimulation devices, such as vagal nerve stimulation, deep brain stimulation, and responsive neurostimulation, can be used to control seizures.
- Genetic issues are also one of the causes; if there is a sodium voltage-gated channel alpha subunit 1 (SCN1A) pathogenic variant, a few medicines will not work, like carbamazepine and oxcarbazepine. Therefore, it is essential to know the correct type of epilepsy before starting the treatment.
- Patients should be able to tolerate the medicines; therefore, they should be regularly monitored. Medical care providers can usually check more frequently after administering the drug to look for intolerance or adverse effects.
- Comorbidities can play a big part in drug resistance; thus, a rational therapy should be prepared for the patient suffering from more than one disease.
- A ketogenic diet may be suitable for drug-resistant epilepsy (Guery and Rheims, 2021).

11.10 CONCLUSION

Frequent, spontaneous seizures characterize the neurological condition known as epilepsy. Its etiology is complex, encompassing aspects related to genetics, anatomy, metabolism, and infection. Antiepileptic medications are commonly used in pharmacological therapy to reduce seizures by modifying neuronal excitability. Nonpharmacological strategies include lifestyle changes, stress management, good sleep hygiene, and, in certain situations, surgical procedures. Cutting-edge medical technologies, such as precision medicine and neurostimulation, have benefits for individualized treatment planning, effectiveness optimization, and reduced adverse effects. Investigating aberrant neural activity and its impact on cognitive and affective processes is necessary to comprehend the physiological and pathological features of epilepsy. Technological and scientific developments keep improving our understanding of epilepsy and paving the way for more individualized and successful treatment plans.

KEYWORDS

- **epilepsy**
- **seizures**
- **neurological disorder**
- **therapy**
- **quality of life**

REFERENCES

Alqahtani, F., Imran, I., Pervaiz, H., Ashraf, W., Perveen, N., Rasool, M.F., Alasmari, A.F., Alharbi, M., Samad, N., Alqarni, S.A., Al-Rejaie, S.S., Alanazi, M.M. (2020). Non-pharmacological interventions for intractable epilepsy. Saudi Pharmaceutical Journal: SPJ: The Official Publication of the Saudi Pharmaceutical Society, 28(8), 951–962. https://doi.org/10.1016/j.jsps.2020.06.016

Barker-Haliski, M., White, H.S. (2015). Glutamatergic mechanisms associated with seizures and epilepsy. Cold Spring Harbor Perspectives in Medicine, 5(8), a022863. https://doi.org/10.1101/cshperspect.a022863

Bench, F., Bedside, T.O. (n.d.). *EPILEPSY 2019.*

Bezabeh, M., Tesfaye, A., Ergicho, B. (2004). *General Pathology.*

Cravo, T., Hashiguchi, O., Affairs, S., Affairs, S., Division, H. (2020). *OECD Health Working Papers. January.*

Dalic, L., Cook, M.J. (2016). Managing drug-resistant epilepsy: Challenges and solutions. Neuropsychiatric Disease and Treatment, 12, 2605–2616. https://doi.org/10.2147/NDT.S84852

Galizia, E.C., Faulkner, H.J. (2018). Seizures and epilepsy in the acute medical setting: Presentation and management. Clinical Medicine (London, England), 18(5), 409–413. https://doi.org/10.7861/clinmedicine.18-5-409

Ghosh, S., Sinha, J.K., Khan, T., Devaraju, K.S., Singh, P., Vaibhav, K., Gaur, P. (2021). Pharmacological and therapeutic approaches in the treatment of epilepsy. Biomedicines, 9(5), 470. https://doi.org/10.3390/biomedicines9050470

Guery, D., Rheims, S. (2021). Clinical management of drug resistant epilepsy: A review on current strategies. Neuropsychiatric Disease and Treatment, 17, 2229–2242. https://doi.org/10.2147/NDT.S256699

Haas, H.L., Sergeeva, O.A., Selbach, O. (2024). Histamine in the nervous system. Physiological Reviews, 88(3), 1183–1241. https://doi.org/10.1152/physrev.00043.2007.

Khan, H., Garg, N., Singh, T.G., Kaur, A., Thapa, K. (2022). Calpain inhibitors as potential therapeutic modulators in neurodegenerative diseases. Neurochemical Research, 47(5), 1125–1149. https://doi.org/10.1007/s11064-021-03521-9

Kotsopoulos, I.A., de Krom, M.C., Kessels, F.G., Lodder, J., Troost, J., Twellaar, M., van Merode, T., Knottnerus, A.J. (2003). The diagnosis of epileptic and non-epileptic seizures. Epilepsy Research, 57(1), 59–67. https://doi.org/10.1016/j.eplepsyres.2003.10.014

Liu, J., Zhang, P., Zou, Q., Liang, J., Chen, Y., Cai, Y., Li, S., Li, J., Su, J., Li, Q. (2023). Status of epilepsy in the tropics: An overlooked perspective. Epilepsia Open, 8(1), 32–45. https://doi.org/10.1002/epi4.12686

Minardi, C., Minacapelli, R., Valastro, P., Vasile, F., Pitino, S., Pavone, P., Astuto, M., Murabito, P. (2019). Epilepsy in children: From diagnosis to treatment with focus on emergency. Journal of Clinical Medicine, 8(1), 39. https://doi.org/10.3390/jcm8010039

Moshé, S.L. (2020). The Evolution of the Concepts of Seizures and Epilepsy : What's in a Name ? 2019, pp. 22–35. https://doi.org/10.1002/epi4.12375

Perucca, E. (2021). *The Pharmacological Treatment of Epilepsy : Recent Advances and Future Perspectives.*

Rehni, A.K., Singh, T.G. (2010). Levamisole-induced reduction in seizure threshold: A possible role of nicotinic acetylcholine receptor-mediated pathway. Naunyn-Schmiedeberg's Archives of Pharmacology, 382(3), 279–285. https://doi.org/10.1007/s00210-010-0543-4

Rehni, A.K., Singh, T.G., Kalra, R., Singh, N. (2009). Pharmacological inhibition of inducible nitric oxide synthase attenuates the development of seizures in mice. Nitric Oxide: Biology and Chemistry, 21(2), 120–125. https://doi.org/10.1016/j.niox.2009.06.001

Sen, A., Capelli, V., Husain, M. (2018). Cognition and dementia in older patients with epilepsy. Brain: A Journal of Neurology, 141(6), 1592–1608. https://doi.org/10.1093/brain/awy022

Sharma, V., Singh, T.G., Kaur, A., Mannan, A., Dhiman, S. (2023). Brain-derived neurotrophic factor: A novel dynamically regulated therapeutic modulator in neurological disorders. Neurochemical Research, 48(2), 317–339. https://doi.org/10.1007/s11064-022-03755-1

Shenoy, N., Srinivasan, S., Menon, G., Kurupath, R. (2023). Surgical treatment of epilepsy - Initial experience from a comprehensive epilepsy program in coastal South India. Journal of Neurosciences in Rural Practice, 14(3), 488–494. https://doi.org/10.25259/JNRP_116_2023

Singh, S., Singh, T.G. (2021). Emerging perspectives on mitochondrial dysfunctioning and inflammation in epileptogenesis. Inflammation Research: Official Journal of the European Histamine Research Society ... [et al.], 70(10–12), 1027–1042. https://doi.org/10.1007/s00011-021-01511-9

Singh, S., Singh, T.G., Rehni, A.K. (2020). An insight into molecular mechanisms and novel therapeutic approaches in epileptogenesis. CNS & Neurological Disorders Drug Targets, 19(10), 750–779. https://doi.org/10.2174/1871527319666200910153827

Singh, S., Singh, T.G., Singh, M., Najda, A., Nurzyńska-Wierdak, R., Almeer, R., Kamel, M., Abdel-Daim, M.M. (2021). Anticonvulsive effects of chondroitin sulfate on pilocarpine and pentylenetetrazole induced epileptogenesis in mice. Molecules (Basel, Switzerland), 26(22), 6773. https://doi.org/10.3390/molecules26226773

Sirven, J.I. (2015). *Epilepsy : A Spectrum Disorder.*

Stafstrom, C.E., Carmant, L. (2015). Seizures and epilepsy: An overview for neuroscientists. Cold Spring Harbor Perspectives in Medicine, 5(6), a022426. https://doi.org/10.1101/cshperspect.a022426

Teleanu, R.I., Niculescu, A.G., Roza, E., Vladâcenco, O., Grumezescu, A.M., Teleanu, D.M. (2022). Neurotransmitters-key factors in neurological and neurodegenerative disorders of the central nervous system. International Journal of Molecular Sciences, 23(11), 5954. https://doi.org/10.3390/ijms23115954

Thapa, K., Shivam, K., Khan, H., Kaur, A., Dua, K., Singh, S., Singh, T.G. (2023). Emerging targets for modulation of immune response and inflammation in stroke. Neurochemical Research, 48(6), 1663–1690. https://doi.org/10.1007/s11064-023-03875-2

van Donselaar, C.A., Stroink, H., Arts, W.F., Dutch Study Group of Epilepsy in Childhood (2006). How confident are we of the diagnosis of epilepsy. Epilepsia, 47(Suppl 1), 9–13. https://doi.org/10.1111/j.1528-1167.2006.00653.x

Vishwakarma, S., Singh, S., Singh, T.G. (2022). Pharmacological modulation of cytokines correlating neuroinflammatory cascades in epileptogenesis. Molecular Biology Reports, 49(2), 1437–1452. https://doi.org/10.1007/s11033-021-06896-8

von der Brelie, C., Malter, M.P., Niehusmann, P., Elger, C.E., von Lehe, M., Schramm, J. (2013). Surgical management and long-term seizure outcome after epilepsy surgery for different types of epilepsy associated with cerebral cavernous malformations. Epilepsia, 54(9), 1699–1706. https://doi.org/10.1111/epi.12327

CHAPTER 12

Concept and Therapeutic Applications: The Endocrine Pancreas

LAVISH VAID[1], JASLEEN KAUR[1], MRIDUL SHARMA[1], LOVELEEN KAUR[1*], MADHUKAR GARG[1], SANJANA MEHTA[1], THAKUR GURJEET SINGH[1], DEEPIKA RAINA[2*], and KESHAV RAJ PAUDEL[3]

[1]*Chitkara College of Pharmacy, Chitkara University, Chandigarh, Punjab, India*

[2]*School of Pharmacy, Graphic Era Hill University, Dehradun, Uttarakhand, India*

[3]*Centre for Inflammation, Centenary Institute and University of Technology Sydney, Faculty of Science, School of Life Sciences, Sydney, NSW, Australia*

*Corresponding author

ABSTRACT

The endocrine pancreas is the part of the pancreas that makes and distributes hormones directly into the bloodstream. The organ known as the pancreatic islets, called initially islets of Langerhans, comprises a group of cells. The endocrine pancreas produces four hormones: insulin, glucagon, somatostatin, and pancreatic polypeptide (PP). The two primary hormones controlling blood sugar levels are insulin and glucagon. Blood sugar levels are lowered as insulin encourages the body's cells to absorb glucose from the blood. Glucagon stimulates the liver to release glucose and increases blood glucose levels. Glucagon and insulin are inhibited by somatostatin, which keeps blood sugar levels within a healthy range. PP are believed to

Pharmacotherapy Approaches Toward Endocrine and Metabolic Diseases.
Thakur Gurjeet Singh and Sanjana Mehta (Eds.)

DOI: 10.1201/9781779640154-12

play a role in regulating digestion and appetite. A significant portion of the therapeutic applications involving the endocrine pancreas are related to managing diabetes mellitus and related conditions. These applications include insulin replacement therapy, glucagon administration, artificial pancreas, pancreatic islet transplantation, glucose monitoring, somatostatin analogs, pancreatic hormone replacement therapy, and many more. Medical research and technological advancements continuously advance therapeutic approaches involving the endocrine pancreas.

12.1 INTRODUCTION

Multiple important large vessels are located adjacent to the pancreas, surrounding it with several organs. It occupies an upper retroperitoneal space intensely and transversely. There is continuity between the pancreatic ducts and the duodenum at the distal point of the common bile duct. In addition, the pancreas is exceptionally well supplied with lymphatics and arteries. The endocrine compartment secures hormones into the bloodstream, while the exocrine compartment secretes enzymes and digestive juices (Daniels and Allum, 2011; Singh et al., 2020a). Several different types of hormones are secreted by the islets of Langerhans in the endocrine system. Pancreatic acini (acinar and duct cells) are the digestion-associated pancreatic exocrine function. Two vital functions of the pancreas are aiding food digestion and producing hormones, primarily responsible for controlling blood energy levels. Metabolism homeostasis depends mainly on the functioning of the endocrine pancreas. Langerhans islets constitute 2–3% of the organ's weight and are distributed throughout. The islets contain at least four types of cells (to which glucagon, somatostatin, insulin, and pancreatic polypeptide (PP) are secreted, respectively). Beta- and gamma-cells comprise approximately 20% and 75% of the islets. A characteristic feature of most islets is their cells' distribution: most cells are in the periphery, while the remaining cells are in the center. A paracrine signaling process is a form of intercellular communication between different types of cells. Islets function as a unit rather than four separate cell types (Lee et al., 2024; Thapa et al., 2021).

An endocrine pancreas produces insulin and glucagon, which regulate blood glucose levels. Glucagon facilitates glycogenolysis and gluconeogenesis, while insulin facilitates glucose uptake by tissues. Deficiencies in insulin-secreting cells, which are characteristic of diabetes, result in hyperglycemia due to abnormal regulation of blood sugar. As a paracrine hormone, somatostatin is also activated by cells that are immediately adjacent to it. As a critical hormone in the pancreas, somatostatin regulates blood flow and digestion. It inhibits the release of digestive enzymes from the exocrine pancreas and reduces gastric acid secretion. In order to maintain normal blood glucose levels and digestion, somatostatin is essential. Health problems may result from disorders of somatostatin secretion, such as somatostatinoma. Furthermore, the endocrine pancreas produces and secretes PP, an amino-acid peptide hormone. After consuming food, it enters the bloodstream and peaks about 2 h later. Additionally, PP may regulate blood sugar levels and metabolism (Röder et al., 2016; Rihal et al., 2022).

12.2 ENDOCRINE PANCREAS

An endocrine pancreas is composed of endocrine cells that are distributed primarily in the islets of Langerhans (islets). However, they are also located in clusters or on individual cells within and adjacent to connective tissues, exocrine acini, or exocrine pancreatic ductules (Figure 12.1). An islet is a cluster of cells that varies in size from 100 to 200 mm and is easily distinguished from the exocrine pancreas by its well-defined appearance. Based on the species, islets are concentrated in different lobes of the pancreas rather than distributed randomly throughout the organ. There are several distinct endocrine cells in each islet, each with a distinct function, yet they interact paracrinally through gap junctions and electrically through synapses (Da and Xavier, 2018).

TABLE 12.1 Hormones of Particular Cell Types with Their Structure

Hormone	Cell Type	Structure
Glucagon	A	Amino acids—29
Insulin	B	Two chains are present: A—21 = amino acids B—30 = amino acids
Amylin		Amino acids—37
Somatostatin	Δ	Two forms are present: S = Amino acids—14 S = Amino acids—28
Pancreatic Polypeptide	F	36 amino acids

Each pancreatic islet has four cell types, as shown in Table 12.1. Approximately 20% of each islet comprises alpha cells that produce glucagon. In order to regulate blood glucose levels, glucagon is an essential hormone. It is released in response to low blood glucose levels. Approximately 75% of the cells in each islet produce the hormone insulin. When blood glucose levels are elevated, insulin is released into the body. Somatostatin is a peptide hormone secreted by delta cells. The hypothalamus, stomach, and intestines are also responsible for releasing somatostatin (growth hormone-inhibiting hormone). Glucagon and insulin are inhibited by pancreatic somatostatin as inhibitory hormones. About 1% of islet cells contain PP cells, which secrete PP hormone. This hormone is also known to regulate the secretion of exocrine and endocrine hormones from the pancreas and appetite. In addition to its effect on reducing food consumption after a meal, PP can also be produced during fasting (Moede et al., 2020).

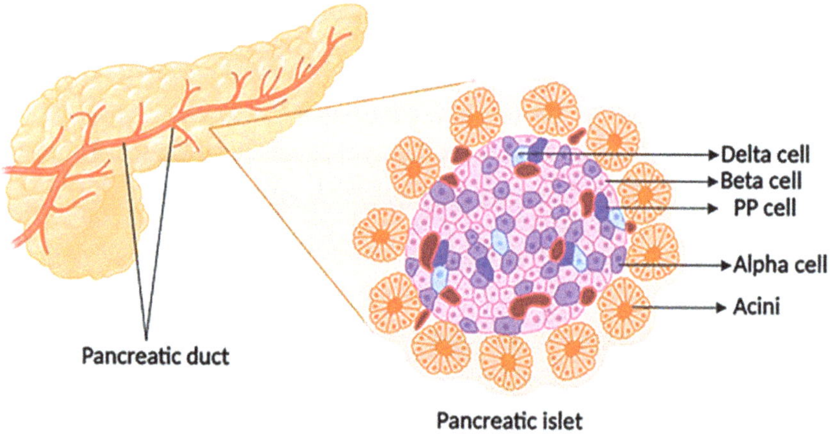

FIGURE 12.1 Pancreas (with pancreatic islet).

12.3 HORMONES OF THE ENDOCRINE PANCREAS

12.3.1 INSULIN

In 1928, insulin was first discovered to be a polypeptide, and it was determined that its amino acid sequence was in 1952. In terms of its molecular weight, it has a molecular mass of 5802 and consists of 51 amino acids linked by disulfide bridges. The isoelectric point of the protein is 5.5 pH.

In chain A, 21 amino acids are present, whereas 30 amino acids are in the B chain. A chain comprises two antiparallel helices at its N-terminus and a central helical segment at its C-terminus; the B chain has a central helical segment. A disulfide bond connects the A and C termini of the A chain with the central helix of the B chain (Figure 12.2). A connecting peptide connects Proinsulin to its B chain (Alyas et al., 2021; Rihal et al., 2023).

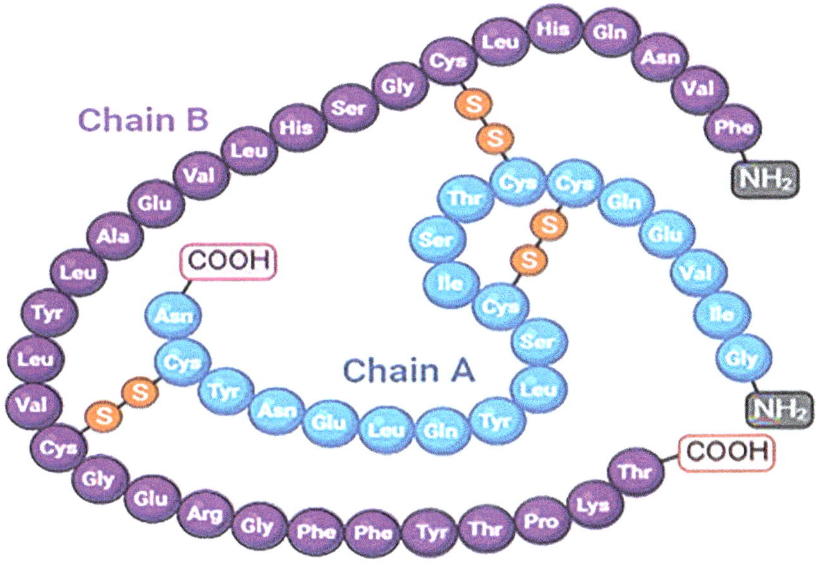

FIGURE 12.2 Structure of insulin.

As glucose levels rise, the cells release insulin from secretory granules, triggering the "first phase" of glucose-induced diabetic complications. Glucose-6-phosphate is formed when glucose enters the cell and is phosphorylated by glucokinase, generating adenosine triphosphate (ATP). A voltage-dependent calcium channel is activated upon closure of a K^+-ATP-dependent channel, thus increasing intracellular calcium levels and stimulating insulin secretion (Garg et al., 2022). The effect of glucose is enhanced by both a Ca^{2+}-dependent pathway and a Ca^{2+}-independent pathway, as well as by a K^+-ATP channel-independent pathway. The activity of protein kinase C and phospholipases is also increased (e.g., via acetylcholine), as is the activity of adenylyl cyclase and protein kinase A, which stimulates insulin secretion (Figure 12.3).

Several hormones may activate this mechanism, including capapeptide, glucagon-like peptide 1 (GLP-1), vasoactive intestinal peptide, and gastric inhibitory peptide. The second phase of glucose-mediated insulin secretion appears to be significantly affected by these factors following the refilling of secretory granules translocated from reserve pools (Sarmiento et al., 2019).

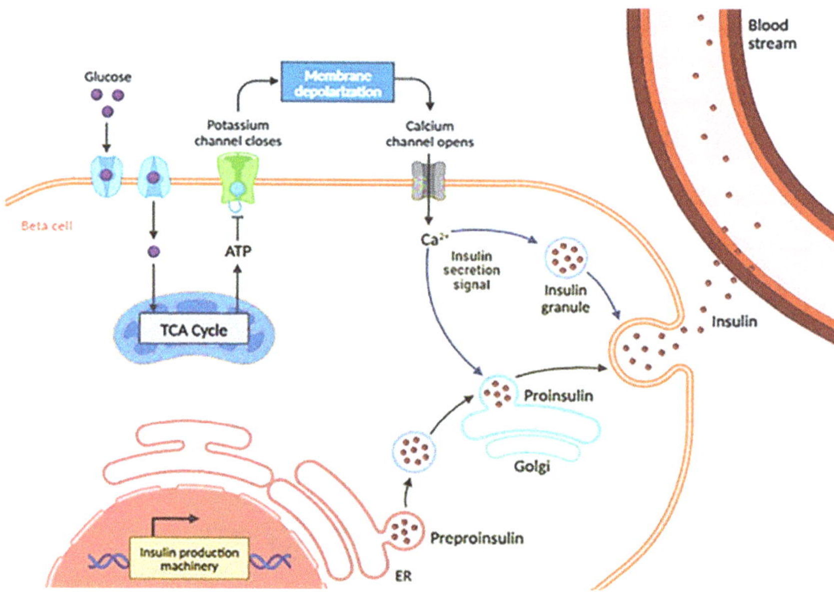

FIGURE 12.3 Insulin secretion through various cells.

12.3.2 SOMATOSTATIN

Somatostatin is a crucial cyclic peptide with strong regulatory properties throughout the body. In addition to the digestive tract, the hypothalamus, the pancreatic glands, and the central nervous system, this growth hormone inhibitor is produced in several locations. The peptide has two active forms, which differ in length at 14 and 28 amino acids, as shown in Figure 12.4. Regarding activity, both isoforms overlap considerably and differ primarily in the location at which they exert their effects. The short form (14 amino acids) is primarily found in the brain, while the longer form (28 amino acids) is found in the gastrointestinal tract. It has a half-life of 1–3 min (Rogoza et al., 2022).

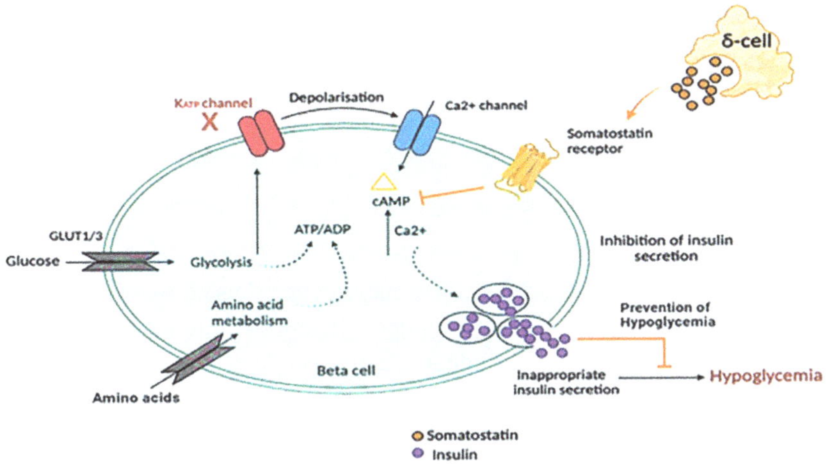

FIGURE 12.4 Illustration of the role of somatostatin in endocrine pancreas.

There are five subtypes of somatostatin receptors (SST1-5), which are expressed in several types of solid neoplasms, neuroendocrine tumors, and pituitary adenomas When agonists are released, g protein receptor kinases phosphorylate somatostatin receptor subtype 2 (SST2), which makes the receptor desensitized and internalized. As a result of these events and others, additional downstream signaling and antiproliferative effects are induced. However, the primary mechanism by which it inhibits secretion is by inhibiting cAMP, the second messenger (Neisig et al., 2003; Singh et al., 2022). Islet SST2 suppresses glucagon production, whereas SST2 and somatostatin receptor subtype 5 suppress insulin production. According to research, cAMP is hypothesized to act as an amplifier of insulin secretion in cells exposed to increased Ca^{2+} levels; somatostatin receptor ligands (SRLs) are thought to target this process to block insulin release. In addition to differences in receptor expression between congenital hyperinsulinism (CHI) patients and those with normal SST receptor distributions, the effects of somatostatin may differ based on the density and distribution of SST receptor subtypes in each tissue (van Albada et al., 2022; Rohilla et al., 2023).

During CHI, the pancreatic β-cell exhibits somatostatin receptors coupled to a G-protein. As intracellular ATP levels increase, K-ATP channels close, membranes depolarize, and Ca^{2+} ions are displaced from the cells. Insulin is released as a result of increased intracellular Ca^{2+} and cAMP levels. The somatostatin receptor activation produces inhibitory G-protein alpha subunit-guanosine triphosphate, inhibiting adenylate cyclase, preventing cAMP synthesis, and reducing insulin production (Prentki et al., 2013).

12.3.3 GLUCAGON

Glucagon is a hormone produced by pancreatic islets. A neuroendocrine convertase-2 synthesizes the native glucagon peptide from the proglucagon peptide encoded by the proglucagon gene. Aside from GLP-1, GLP-2, oxyntomodulin, and glicentin, proglucagon also encodes GLP-1, GLP-2, and oxyntomodulin. Proglucagon peptide is converted from proglucagon by neuroendocrine convertase-1-mediated cleavage in the brain and intestinal L cells (Singh et al., 2020b). A minimal promoter region and four enhancer elements have been identified in studies on proglucagon transcription. Several factors have been linked to transcription regulation, including amino acids, homeodomain transcription factors, cAMP in pancreatic and intestinal cells, and intestinal signaling. It is also known that insulin inhibits proglucagon expression in α-cells. Interestingly, this effect reverses in the intestine, where insulin pathological concentrations result in increased levels of GLP-1, resulting from the production of proglucagon (Holst, 2022).

Circulating glucose plays a vital role in regulating glucagon secretion. A hypoglycemic state results in glucagon release by pancreatic alpha cells, and a hyperglycemic state inhibits this release (Figure 12.5). ATP is generated in the mitochondria of alpha cells by glucose transporter 1 after glucose is absorbed by the membrane, followed by glycolysis. Therefore, ATP levels within alpha cells reflect glucose levels in the plasma. A low level of intracellular ATP and hypoglycemia in alpha cells reduces the efflux of potassium (K^+) through potassium channels sensitive to ATP. Consequently, the cell membrane is depolarized, which allows Ca^{2+} to enter the cell through voltage-dependent Ca^{2+} channels. As a result, intracellular Ca^{2+} levels increase, which triggers the exocytosis of glucagon granules from the alpha cells. In contrast, increased levels of circulating glucose lead to an increase in glucose influx into alpha cells, which triggers the release of intracellular ATP and opens KATP channels. Thus, establishing a membrane potential prevents glucagon secretion and Ca^{2+} influx.

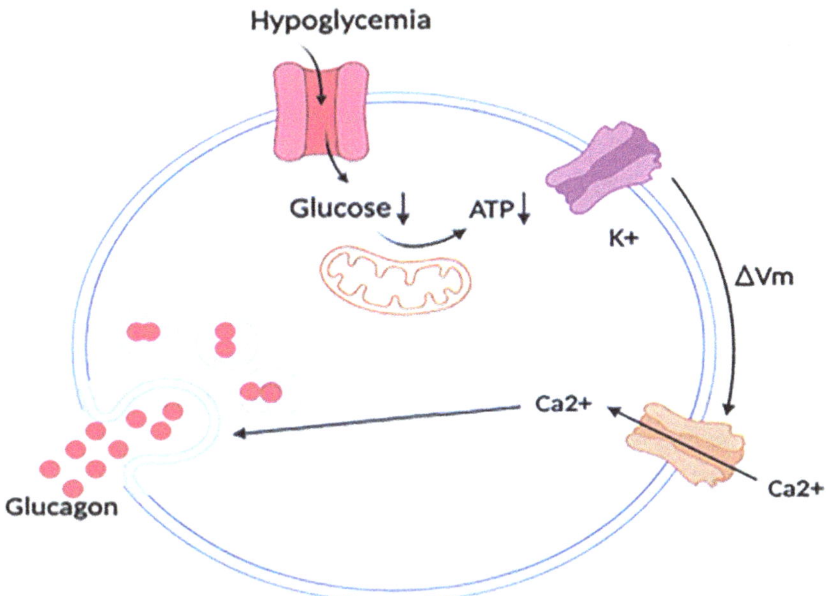

FIGURE 12.5 Illustration of the release of glucagon.

12.3.4 PANCREATIC POLYPEPTIDE

It is a hormone produced by the "F" or "PP" cells in the pancreas. The Langerhans islets originated from the ventral pancreatic bud and are components of the Langerhans islets. It has been proposed that the expression of PP immunoreactivity is a marker for the origin of the ventral pancreatic bud due to this unique embryonic derivation. In the pancreatic gland, PP cells are distributed inhomogeneously. They are located mainly on the periphery of the pancreatic islets. It has been reported that a minority of these cells are found in the acinar and the centroacinar-ductal segments of the pancreas unit (Dassaye et al., 2016).

Polypeptides produced by PP cells located in the head of the endocrine pancreas are known as PP. Approximately 4200 Da is this protein's molecular weight, consisting of 36 amino acids. This protein regulates the activity of the pancreatic secretory system (endocrine and exocrine); it also influences the level of glycogen in the liver and that of the gastrointestinal tract (Williams, 2014; Mehta et al., 2022). The human somatostatin level is significantly reduced by somatostatin and intravenous glucose when a protein meal is consumed, a fast is followed, exercise is performed, and acute hypoglycemia occurs. Studies have shown that plasma PP is reduced when food intake is increased and elevated when anorexia nervosa is present. Using PP pancreatic cells, Langerhans islets secrete PP. Drugs like this stimulate gastric secretion, while pentagastrine inhibits gastric secretion. Inhibiting pancreatic secretion stimulated by cholecystokinin, it acts as a cholecystokinin antagonist. Following a meal, the level of PP series is increased by 8–10 times compared to when fasting. In addition to blocking the PP's after-meal secretion, atropine is administered through the vagotomy. PP secretion is induced by gastrin, secretin, and cholecystokinin administration. The level of PP is also increased by glucose and fats, but when those substances are administered parenterally, the level of hormones does not change (Kumar and Singh, 2020; Mehta et al., 2022).

12.4 APPLICATIONS

The endocrine pancreas regulates blood sugar levels to maintain the body's energy balance and metabolism. As such, its applications are immense and far-reaching, impacting various aspects of health and well-being. Here is a breakdown of some critical applications.

12.4.1 *MAINTAINING BLOOD SUGAR LEVELS*

Insulin: This hormone helps cells absorb glucose from the bloodstream, lowering blood sugar after meals. Because of either insufficient insulin production or inefficient insulin use, its application is crucial to managing diabetes. Insulin injections or pumps have been used to control blood sugar levels and prevent further complications. Glucagon is another hormone used to maintain blood sugar levels, which acts opposite to insulin by raising blood sugar levels when they fall too low (Galicia-Garcia et al., 2020).

12.4.2 *METABOLIC REGULATION*

Other hormones produced by the endocrine pancreas include PP and somatostatin, which govern appetite, digestion, and the absorption of nutrients. Understanding these hormones and their interaction is essential to treating metabolic diseases like obesity and hypoglycemia (Prentki et al., 2013).

12.4.3 PANCREATIC TRANSPLANTATION

Transplantation of the pancreas (whole or partial) can be life-saving for a person suffering from severe pancreatic dysfunction in type 1 diabetes and chronic pancreatitis. The transplanted pancreas produces sufficient insulin and glucagon, reducing external injection requirements (Rickels and Robertson, 2019).

12.4.4 RESEARCH AND DEVELOPMENT

Ongoing research on the endocrine pancreas aims to understand better how its hormones interact with other systems, how disease states affect the organ's function, and to create novel therapeutic approaches for pancreatic illnesses like diabetes. This research may advance stem cell-based therapeutics, artificial pancreas systems, and customized medical techniques (Rožanc et al., 2021).

12.4.5 PUBLIC HEALTH AWARENESS

Public health initiatives can benefit from understanding the endocrine pancreas's significance and function in general health. Initiatives that support regular exercise, a good diet, and early diabetes identification can help prevent or treat pancreatic problems and enhance general health.

Understanding its critical function in controlling blood sugar and metabolism can help us create new treatments, encourage healthy living, and enhance the quality of life for those who suffer from pancreatic illnesses.

12.5 CONCLUSION

The pancreas is an exocrine and endocrine organ. Insufficient pancreatic exocrine secretion may result in malabsorption of several necessary digestive enzymes. Conversely, inappropriate activation of pancreatic enzymes results in pancreatitis. An endocrine pancreas is crucial in maintaining an average blood glucose level. The endocrine system tightly regulates pancreatic hormone secretion. An impaired glucose homeostasis and diabetes may result from damage to the endocrine pancreas and dysregulation of endocrine secretion.

Pancreatic islet cells produce glucagon, insulin, somatostatin, and PP, among other substances. There are several types of pancreatic islet cells. Insulin and glucagon are responsible for regulating glucose metabolism. It is the beta cells that produce insulin when there is a high level of blood glucose. As a result of the enzyme, glucose is better absorbed and metabolized by target cells and stored for future use. Almost all diabetics suffer from high blood glucose levels due to low insulin levels or resistance to insulin's effects. Diabetes mellitus is characterized by high blood glucose levels and insulin resistance. A decrease in blood glucose levels prompts the alpha cells of the pancreas to produce and secrete glucagon. Blood glucose levels are increased by glucagon, as it facilitates the stabilization of glycogen into glucose. Another hormone, somatostatin, is a true multitasker in the hormonal world and plays a crucial role in maintaining homeostasis in our bodies. Its primary function lies in inhibiting or suppressing the release of other hormones and secretions, acting like a conductor keeping the orchestra of our endocrine and digestive systems in harmony. In summary, the endocrine pancreas is a tiny miracle that controls much of our metabolism. New strategies for treating metabolic diseases and enhancing general health are made possible by our growing understanding of its complex mechanisms and therapeutic potential. Millions of people suffering from metabolic abnormalities could benefit significantly from endocrine pancreas-based medicines in the future with more study and development.

KEYWORDS

- **endocrine pancreas**
- **glucagon**
- **insulin**
- **somatostatin**
- **therapeutic applications**

REFERENCES

Alyas, J., Rafiq, A., Amir, H., Khan, S.U., Sultana, T., Ali, A., Hameed, A., Ahmad, I., Kazmi, A., Sajid, T., Ahmad, A. (2021). Human insulin : History, recent advances, and expression systems for mass production. Biomedical Research and Therapy, 8(9), 4540–4561.

Da, G., Xavier, S. (2018). The cells of the islets of langerhans. 1–17. https://doi.org/10.3390/jcm7030054

Daniels, I.R., Allum, W.H. (2011). The stomach. 17–37.

Dassaye, R., Naidoo, S., Cerf, M.E. (2016). Transcription factor regulation of pancreatic organogenesis, differentiation and maturation. Islets, 8(1), 13–34. https://doi.org/10.1080/19382014.2015.1075687

Galicia-Garcia, U., Benito-Vicente, A., Jebari, S., Larrea-Sebal, A., Siddiqi, H., Uribe, K.B., Ostolaza, H., Martín, C. (2020). Pathophysiology of type 2 diabetes mellitus. International Journal of Molecular Sciences, 21(17), 6275. https://doi.org/10.3390/ijms21176275

Garg, C., Khan, H., Kaur, A., Singh, T.G., Sharma, V.K., Singh, S.K. (2022). Therapeutic implications of sonic hedgehog pathway in metabolic disorders: Novel target for effective treatment. Pharmacological Research, 179, 106194. https://doi.org/10.1016/j.phrs.2022.106194

Holst, J.J. (2022). Glucagon and other proglucagon-derived peptides in the pathogenesis of obesity. Frontiers in Nutrition, 9, 964406. https://doi.org/10.3389/fnut.2022.964406

Kumar, U., Singh, S. (2020). Role of somatostatin in the regulation of central and peripheral factors of satiety and obesity. International Journal of Molecular Sciences, 21(7), 2568. https://doi.org/10.3390/ijms21072568

Lee, M.G., Ohana, E., Park, H.W., Yang, D., Muallem, S. (2024). Secretion general considerations. 39–74. https://doi.org/10.1152/physrev.00011.2011

Mehta, S., Nain, P., Agrawal, B.K., Singh, R.P. (2022). Vitamin D with calcium supplementation managing glycemic control with HbA1c and improve quality of life in patients with diabetes. Turkish Journal of Pharmaceutical Sciences, 19(2), 161–167. https://doi.org/10.4274/tjps.galenos.2021.62357

Moede, T., Leibiger, I.B., Berggren, P.O. (2020). Alpha cell regulation of beta cell function. Diabetologia, 63(10), 2064–2075. https://doi.org/10.1007/s00125-020-05196-3

Neisig, L., Enggaard, C., Hartmann, B., Juul, J. (2003). Somatostatin receptors. Biochimica et Biophysica Acta, 1616, 1–84. https://doi.org/10.1016/S0005-2736(03)00235-9

Prentki, M., Matschinsky, F.M., Madiraju, S.R. (2013). Metabolic signaling in fuel-induced insulin secretion. Cell Metabolism, 18(2), 162–185. https://doi.org/10.1016/j.cmet.2013.05.018

Rickels, M.R., Robertson, R.P. (2019). Pancreatic islet transplantation in humans: Recent progress and future directions. Endocrine Reviews, 40(2), 631–668. https://doi.org/10.1210/er.2018-00154

Rihal, V., Khan, H., Kaur, A., Singh, T.G. (2023). Vitamin D as therapeutic modulator in cerebrovascular diseases: A mechanistic perspectives. Critical Reviews in Food Science and Nutrition, 63(25), 7772–7794. https://doi.org/10.1080/10408398.2022.2050349

Rihal, V., Khan, H., Kaur, A., Singh, T.G., Abdel-Daim, M.M. (2022). Therapeutic and mechanistic intervention of vitamin D in neuropsychiatric disorders. Psychiatry Research, 317, 114782. https://doi.org/10.1016/j.psychres.2022.114782

Röder, P.V., Wu, B., Liu, Y., Han, W. (2016). Pancreatic regulation of glucose homeostasis. Experimental & Molecular Medicine, 48(3), e219. https://doi.org/10.1038/emm.2016.6

Rogoza, O., Megnis, K., Kudrjavceva, M., Gerina-Berzina, A., Rovite, V. (2022). Role of Somatostatin Signalling in Neuroendocrine Tumours. International Journal of Molecular Sciences, 23(3), 1447. https://doi.org/10.3390/ijms23031447

Rohilla, M., Rishabh, Bansal, S., Garg, A., Dhiman, S., Dhankhar, S., Saini, M., Chauhan, S., Alsubaie, N., Batiha, G.E., Albezrah, N.K.A., Singh, T.G. (2023). Discussing pathologic mechanisms of Diabetic retinopathy & therapeutic potentials of curcumin and β-glucogallin in the management of Diabetic retinopathy. Biomedicine & pharmacotherapy = Biomedecine & Pharmacotherapie, 169, 115881. https://doi.org/10.1016/j.biopha.2023.115881

Rožanc, J., Vajda, J., Cinˇ, L., Paradiž, E., Stožer, A. (2021). In vitro disease models of the endocrine pancreas. Biomedicines, *9*(10), 1415.

Sarmiento, B.E., Felipe, L., Menezes, S., Schwartz, E.F. (2019). Isolated from animal venoms : From basic research to drug development prospects. 1–31.

Singh, R., Farooq, S.A., Mannan, A., Singh, T.G., Najda, A., Grażyna, Z., Albadrani, G.M., Sayed, A.A., Abdel-Daim, M.M. (2022). Animal models of diabetic microvascular complications: Relevance to clinical features. Biomedicine & Pharmacotherapy = Biomedecine & Pharmacotherapie, 145, 112305. https://doi.org/10.1016/j.biopha.2021.112305

Singh, R., Rao, H.K., Singh, T.G. (2020a). Advanced glycated end products (ages) in diabetes and its complications: An insight. Plant Arch, 20(1), 3838–3841.

Singh, R., Rao, H.K., Singh, T.G. (2020b). Neuropathic pain in diabetes mellitus: Challenges and future trends. Obesity Medicine, 18, 100215

Thapa, K., Singh, T.G., Kaur, A. (2021). Cyclic nucleotide phosphodiesterase inhibition as a potential therapeutic target in renal ischemia reperfusion injury. Life Sciences, 282, 119843. https://doi.org/10.1016/j.lfs.2021.119843

van Albada, M.E., Mohnike, K., Dunne, M.J., Banerjee, I., Betz, S.F. (2022). Somatostatin receptors in congenital hyperinsulinism: Biology to bedside. Frontiers in Endocrinology, 13, 921357. https://doi.org/10.3389/fendo.2022.921357

Williams, J.A. (2014). Pancreatic polypeptide. 1–9. https://doi.org/10.3998/panc.2014.4

CHAPTER 13

MEN1 Syndrome, Diagnosis, and Its Pharmacotherapy

B. JEEVAN KUMAR[1], KONDAVEETI DEVAKI[1], KAVITA MUNJAL[2], KIRAN BHOPATE[3], HITESH CHOPRA[4], VINOD KUMAR GAUTTAM[5], MOHAMMAD AMJAD KAMAL[6,7,8,9,10*]

[1]*KL College of Pharmacy, Koneru Lakshmaiah Education Foundation, Vaddeswaram, Guntur, Andhra Pradesh, India*

[2]*Department of Pharmacy, Amity Institute of Pharmacy, Amity University, Noida, Uttar Pradesh, India*

[3]*IES Institute of Pharmacy, IES University, Bhopal, Madhya Pradesh, India*

[4]*Department of Biosciences, Saveetha School of Engineering, Saveetha Institute of Medical and Technical Sciences, Chennai, Tamil Nadu, India*

[5]*Department of Pharmacognosy, Shiva Institute of Pharmacy, Bilaspur, Himachal Pradesh, India*

[6]*Institutes for Systems Genetics, Frontiers Science Center for Disease-Related Molecular Network/West China Nursing School, West China Hospital, Sichuan University, Sichuan, China*

[7]*King Fahd Medical Research Center, King Abdulaziz University, Jeddah, Saudi Arabia*

[8]*Department of Pharmacy, Faculty of Allied Health Sciences, Daffodil International University, Birulia, Bangladesh*

[9]*Enzymoics, Hebersham, NSW, Australia*

[10]*Novel Global Community Educational Foundation, Hebersham, NSW, Australia*

*Corresponding author

Pharmacotherapy Approaches Toward Endocrine and Metabolic Diseases.
Thakur Gurjeet Singh and Sanjana Mehta (Eds.)

DOI: 10.1201/9781779640154-13

ABSTRACT

Wermer syndrome is another name for the uncommon hereditary endocrine tumor known as MEN1 (multiple endocrine neoplasia). It occurs approximately 1 in 30,000 people with an equal sex distribution experienced it. This syndrome results from mutations in tumor suppression gene/*menin* gene on chromosome 11. About 90% of cases have mutations inherited from afflicted parents, with secondary mutations accounting for 10% of cases. This syndrome primarily causes the neoplasm of the endocrine glands such as anterior pituitary gland (15–90% of cases), parathyroid gland (95% of cases), and the tissue of neuroendocrine tissue of gastro-entero-pancreatic organ system (30–80% of cases), nonfunctional tumors are reportedly present approximately 55% of patients. The opportunity to identify MEN1-related conditions in people who do not have a hereditary MEN 1 mutation has been made possible by breakthroughs in genetic identification. Clinically significant symptoms often appear in pediatric age, and screening should begin in the second decade, however early diagnosis reduces the morbidity and mortality. The genetic basis for MEN1 means the surgery interventions like parathyroidectomy is rarely curative. This chapter gives the insight of pathophysiology of MEN1 and its diagnosis along with latest innovation in treatment and surgery intervention.

13.1 INTRODUCTION

MEN1 syndrome is multiple endocrine neoplasia. Type 1 is a heterogenous and hereditary genetic disorder, also known as the Wermer syndrome, that mainly causes tumors in the endocrine glands, including a combination of more than 20 endocrine and nonendocrine tumors. The most common endocrine tumors seen in MEN1 involve the pituitary gland, parathyroid gland, neuroendocrine tumors (NETs), and islet cells of the cortical tumors (Singh et al., 2020). The common nonendocrine tumors were breast foregut carcinoma, cutaneous lipomas, and central nervous system tumor. Endocrine tumors in patients differ from MEN1, with sporadic tumors, with the onset of signs/symptoms occurring at a younger age and the presence of tumors at a younger age. It is mainly caused by the presence of mutations in the MEN1 gene; MEN1 is considered a tumor suppressor gene, and its dominant function is known to be tumor suppressor gene (Barlier et al., 2023; Carolina and Rachel, 2021).

13.1.1 EPIDEMIOLOGY

With an estimated frequency of 0.02–0.2 per 1000 and an incidence of 0.25%, MEN1 syndrome is considered uncommon. It has no gender-predisposing ethnic group or racial preference as a risk factor. It can affect all age groups, from 5 to 82 years (Marini et al., 2008; Singh et al., 2023).

The first case of MEN1 was reported in 1903 during the autopsy of a patient with the condition acromegaly and had seen four enlarged parathyroid glands. Later, in 1953, the first review was published on MEN1 syndrome, describing 14 cases by Underdahl and others. It was named Wermer in 1954 and first describes the MEN1 phenotype. The original name Wermer's syndrome was replaced by MEN1 syndrome (Marini et al., 2008; Bangar et al., 2024).

Parathyroid multiple adenomas are the primary organs affected, representing up to all patients by the time they are 50 years old. These constitute the initial clinical manifestation, with a mean age of 20–25 years, and in rare instances, cases as early as eight years old have been reported. The prevalence of pancreatic neoplasm is high in men, with a common manifestation being gastrinoma; thymic tumors were only observed in men, while pituitary tumors were somewhat more common in women (Singh et al., 2023; Marini et al., 2018; Mehta et al., 2022).

13.1.2 ETIOLOGY

In 90% of instances, the mutant gene is inherited from an afflicted parent; *de novo* mutations cause the remaining 10% of instances. Mutations in the MEN1 gene that cause germline inactivation result in the condition known as MEN1 syndrome. The menin protein, which has 610 amino acids, is produced by the tumor suppressor gene and is expressed in several tissues such as the brain, testes, pancreas, and lymphocytes. Numerous germline mutations, including missense, nonsense, frameshift, deletion, and mRNA splicing errors, can affect the *MEN1* tumor suppressor gene. These mutations can affect the gene's coding and noncoding regions (Singh et al., 2023; Lairmore et al., 2004; Mehta et al., 2022).

13.2 CLINICAL MANIFESTATIONS

Classical endocrine tumors and their corresponding secretory products are mostly linked to the clinical symptoms of MEN1 or overproduction or due to local mass effects. Typically, MEN1 is identified by several endocrine tumors in the pituitary, parathyroid, and GET tract. The most common symptoms are connected to complications from hormone excess release, which might result in severe ulcer disease or hypoglycemia (Lairmore et al., 2004). The clinical manifestations differ from person to person due to the type of association between endocrine and nonendocrine neoplasm. The clinical features of the MEN1-associated tumor (Figure 13.1) and its clinical features are shown in Table 13.1.

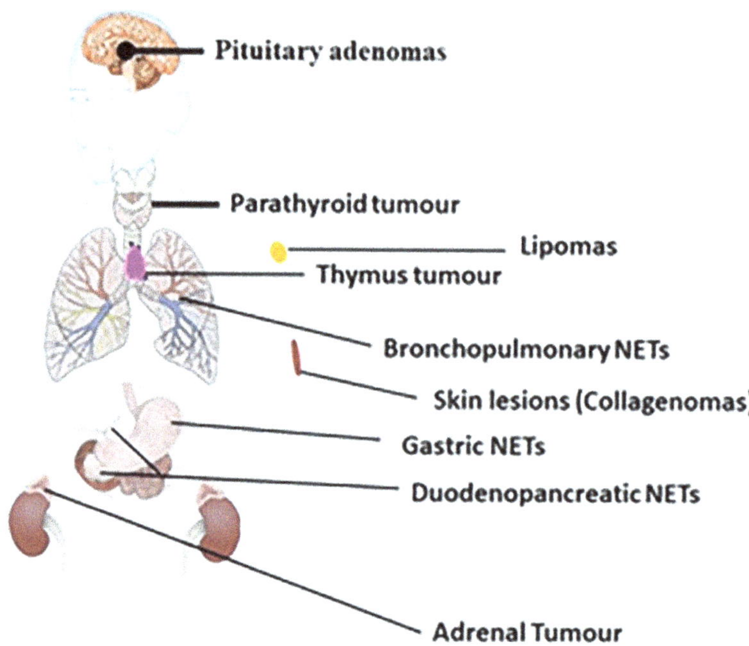

FIGURE 13.1 MEN1-associated tumors.

Source: Adapted from Carolina and Rachel, 2021.

13.2.1 PARATHYROID GLAND DISORDER

The most prevalent MEN1-associated endocrine condition is primary hyperparathyroidism (PHPT), in which 90% of individuals are affected by ages between 20 and 50. Morphologically, the parathyroid gland in MEN1 syndrome appears to be expected but differs in size, volume, and weight. The supernumerary glands (with multiple lesions) were reported in 20% of MEN1 syndrome individuals (Barlier et al., 2023; Giusti et al., 2012).

Interestingly, parathyroid hyperplasia is less frequent in MEN1 compared with PHPT. The MEN1 with PHPT has long-term asymptomatic hypercalcemia and low morbidity (Barlier et al., 2023; Sharma et al., 2021; Rihal et al., 2023).

13.2.2 PITUITARY GLAND DISORDER

Pituitary tumor prevalence might range greatly from 10% to 76% in MEN1 patients. Females are more likely than males to have pituitary adenoma. In these patients, mainly growth hormone and prolactin were producing tumors; pituitary adenomas larger than 10 mm are known as macroadenomas, and those less than 10 mm are known as microadenomas (Marini et al., 2018; John et al., 2022). Blurred vision, headaches, bitemporal hemianopia, and other visual field abnormalities can be caused by pituitary macroadenomas compressing the optic chiasm. Adrenocorticotropin (ACTH), which causes hypercortisolism, is secreted by 3% of MEN1-associated pituitary tumors, 25% of which release GH, and 60% of which secrete prolactin (prolactinomas) (Marini et al., 2008; Syro et al., 2012; Yao et al., 2011). The symptoms of prolactinomas in females include amenorrhea, galactorrhea, and infertility. In males, symptoms like hypogonadism, sexual dysfunction, gynecomastia, and impotence are common. The symptoms of GH-secreting tumors cause adults to develop acromegaly and gigantism in youngsters (Marini et al., 2018; Sharma et al., 2023a, 2023b; Khakha et al., 2023).

13.2.3 GASTROENTERIC PANCREATIC ORGAN SYSTEM DISORDER

Gastroenteropancreatic tumors occur in about 30–80% of cases and are the second most frequent clinical manifestations among MEN1, also known as NETs. NETs are categorized into nonfunctional NETs and functioning NETs. The most common cause of death was nonfunctional NET. They were delayed in diagnosis due to a lack of clinical findings or symptoms. The lesion size of nonfunctional NET was correlated with the risk of metastasis and death. Functional NETs can cause excess secretion of gastrin, insulin, and pancreatic polypeptide (Marini et al., 2008; Singh et al., 2023).

The most frequent clinical manifestations were gastrinoma, which can be pancreatic or duodenal. The pancreatic and duodenal gastrinoma were 45–95% associated with lymph node metastasis. Duodenal gastrinoma was due to neoplasm of islet cells; these patients have elevated gastrin levels (hypergastrinemia). Insulinoma is the second-most common among functional NETs; it represents about 30–40% of functional NETs; this tumor in the pancreas secretes a significant amount of insulin, which leads to hypoglycemia, including neuroglycopenic symptoms (Singh et al., 2023; Marini et al., 2008).

13.2.4 ASSOCIATED ENDOCRINE TUMOR

13.2.4.1 ADRENOCORTICAL TUMOR

The prevalence of bilateral adrenocortical tumors in MEN1 was about 9–40%. The majority of these tumors are nonfunctional. In this condition, the tumor secretes excess ACTH at an elevated level of cortical, causing primary hyperaldosteronism and primary hypercortisolism, leading to Cushing's syndrome. Marini et al., 2008; Wang et al., 2019).

13.2.4.2 PHEOCHROMOCYTOMA

It was a rare tumor, and its prevalence among the MEN1 was less than 1%. These tumors are usually characterized by excess catecholamine secretion, leading to headaches, palpitations, and sweating that lasts minutes to hours (Därr et al., 2012).

13.2.4.3 THYROID TUMORS

Although goiters were seen in over 25% of MEN1 patients, thyroid tumors are composed of adenoma. Thyroid disorders are common in the general population, so there is no significant association between thyroid cancer and MEN1 (Marini et al., 2008).

13.2.4.4 THYMUS TUMORS

The incidence of thymic tumor is infrequent, accounting for only 0.4% among MEN1; the typical clinical features of thymic tumor were found to be collagenoma of the skin, lipomas, and angiomyolipoma; symptoms were chest pain, dyspnea, and cough (Yliaska et al., 2022; Sadowski et al., 2017).

13.2.5 NONENDOCRINE TUMORS

13.2.5.1 CARCINOID TUMORS

Rare, slowly developing NETs called carcinoid tumors are caused by enterochromaffin cells that are spread throughout the thymus, pancreas, gastrointestinal tract, and bronchopulmonary system. Men are more likely than females to get thymic carcinomas, whereas females are more likely than men to develop bronchial carcinomas. Clinically, most carcinoids are quiet. Particularly among male smokers, thymic carcinoids can be deadly and aggressive. Less commonly, the carcinoid syndrome linked to dyspnea and flushing episodes is caused by the oversecretion of bronchial, gastric, and thymic carcinoids, growth-hormone-releasing hormone, calcitonin, serotonin, and ACTH (Marini et al., 2008; Scott and Holen, 2008).

13.2.5.2 FACIAL ANGIOFIBROMA'S AND COLLAGENOMAS

The prevalence of multiple angiofibroma in MEN1 is 40–90%. These benign tumors, composed of nonregressing acneiform papules, can expand over the lips' vermillion border and include connective tissue and blood vessels. Collagenomas, which are many hypopigmented, skin-colored cutaneous nodules distributed symmetrically throughout the upper limb, neck, and trunk, were seen in almost 70% of MEN1 patients (Marini et al., 2008; Khan et al., 2022; Sharma et al., 2023).

13.2.5.3 LIPOMAS

Lipomas are several fatty tissue tumors that primarily develop subcutaneously and are seldom visceral. The prevalence of lipomas among the MEN1 patients was 20–30% (Marini et al., 2008).

13.2.5.4 CNS SYSTEM TUMORS: MENINGIOMAS

The case of meningiomas was reported among 8% of MEN1 patients. Other CNS tumors like ependymomas (spinal cord) were less significantly associated with MEN1 syndrome (Marini et al., 2008).

TABLE 13.1 Clinical Features of MEN1-Associated Endocrine Neoplasia (Marini et al., 2008; Yliaska et al., 2022)

Endocrine Tumor	Prevalence	Hormone	Clinical Features/Symptoms
Primary hyperparathyroidism	90%	PTH	Hypertension, hypercalcemia, confusion anorexia
Pituitary gland	10–76%	GH FSH, LH ACTH PRL	Visual field defects, blurred vision, headaches, hypogonadism, sexual dysfunction, gynecomastia, and impotence
Gastroentero-pancreatic organ system	30–80%	Gastrin	Hypergastrinemia, insulinoma
Adreno-cortical tumor	9–40%	ACTH	Cushing's syndrome
Pheochromocytoma	<1%	VIP	Headache, palpitations, and sweating
Thyroid tumors	25%	TSH T3, T4	Adenoma, goiters
Carcinoid tumors	30%	GRF	Dyspnea, flushing attacks
Facial angiofibroma and collagenomas	40–90%	–	Diarrhea, skin rash
Lipomas	20–30%	–	Hypokalemia, skin rash
Meningiomas	8%	–	Headache, vomiting
Thymic tumor	>1%	–	Chest pain, dyspnea, and cough

PTH: parathormone; FSH: follicle-stimulating hormone; LH: luteinizing hormone; GRF: GH-releasing factor; TSH: thyroid-stimulating hormone

13.3 MOLECULAR GENETICS

The *MENI* gene is encoded by the protein menin, and its role is in the suppression of tumors and hyperplasia in endocrine organs and nonendocrine organs like the breast and lungs. Menin is the 610 amino acid nuclear protein and is less detectable in the cell membrane and cytoplasm; it is expressed ubiquitously and located on chromosome 11, identified in the year 1997. Menin has the potential to modify chromatin structure and draw a particular histone deacetylase aimed at a promoter to block JunD-mediated transcription so that the Menin may function as a negative regulator of DNA damage-induced cell growth. The level of expression of MEN1 varies from tissue to tissue. Based on the cellular role, transcription activators, transcription repressors, cell signaling proteins, and the other interaction partners are the four groups into which menin interacting proteins fall, the function ranging from structural integrity to DNA repair. The mutation in the *MEN1* gene leads to the loss of a functional role of the gene, leading to MEN1 syndrome. Ten percent of cases of MEN1 syndrome are the result of *de novo* mutations, whereas 90% of cases are inherited from afflicted parents. The *MEN1* gene has more than 1200 germline mutations known to exist; most germline mutations in MEN1 (69%) were predicted to be splicing problems, pathogenic premature truncation of frameshift mutations, nonsense mutations linked to extensive deletions, and other germline changes (25.5%) caused by missense mutations, and 5.5% by acid frame insertion or deletion (Marini et al., 2008; Kamilaris and Stratakis, 2019).

13.4 DIAGNOSIS METHODS

The basis for the MEN1 syndrome diagnosis is done through clinical, familial, and genetic criteria; the early diagnosis helps in the reduction of morbidity and mortality (Marini et al., 2008; Kamilaris and Stratakis, 2019).

- Clinical diagnosis was done by detecting lesions and MEN1-associated tumors and evaluating biochemical hormone levels, nuclear medicine, and imaging diagnostic tools (endoscopy, endoscopic ultrasonography, computed tomography, and magnetic resonance imaging). However, the biochemical and imaging diagnostic tools cannot distinguish sporadic with MEN1-associated tumors. For the correct diagnosis, an accurate medical history and solid clinical evidence are required (Marini et al., 2008).
- Familial MEN1 diagnosis: The detailed history of MEN1-associated tumor in the family or relative of first degree with MEN1 (Marini et al., 2008; de Laat et al., 2018).
- Genetic diagnosis aids in the early diagnosis even when there are no clinical or biochemical indications; however, by the most recent clinical practice guidelines, all patients who meet the diagnostic requirements for a clinical or familial MEN1 diagnosis should be provided DNA testing. Before DNA testing, pretest counseling is the most important aspect; they should be informed about all aspects of genetic counseling. MEN1 is diagnosed by proband, genetic counseling, and DNA testing (Marini et al., 2008).

- Screening of MEN1 syndrome: There are two screening services for identifying MEN1 syndrome: periodical screening or screening at the pediatric age. The main aim of these screenings was to reduce the morbidity of the MEN1 patients. Periodical screening was done by identifying gene mutations in patients. Family numbers were advised to undergo lifelong surveillance, and the clinic was visited annually for the physical examination, radiological screening, and biochemical screening at specific time intervals. The current guidelines from the recent endocrine society advise clinical and biochemical screening at five years, as shown in Table 13.2 (Carolina and Rachel, 2021; Kamilaris and Stratakis, 2019).

TABLE 13.2 Biochemical and Radiological Surveillance for MEN1 Mutation Carriers (Kamilaris and Stratakis, 2019).

Tumor	Starting Screening Age	Biochemical Test	Radiological Test
Insulinoma	5	Fasting glucose levels, insulin	Not necessary
Anterior pituitary	5	IGF-1, prolactin	MRI (at least once every three years)
Parathyroid	8	PTH, calcium	Not necessary
Pancreatic neuroendocrine tumor	Less than 10 years	PPP; CgA; glycogen; VIP	CT, MRI (annually)
Adrenal	Less than 10 years	None unless symptoms appear	CT/MRI (annually)
Thymic and bronchial carcinoid	15	None	MRI/CT (once in 1–2 years)
Gastrinoma	20	Gastrin (gastric pH)	Not necessary

IGF1: insulin-like growth factor-1; PTH: parathyroid hormone; PPP: pancreatic polypeptide; CgA: chromogranin A; VIP: vasoactive intestinal peptide; CT: computed tomography; MRI: magnetic resonance imaging

13.5 MANAGEMENT OF MEN1 SYNDROME

The patient's therapy depends on the clinical manifestations, severity, and diversity of MEN1 syndrome. Medicine and surgical interventions were used to manage MEN1-associated tumors; the possible medical interventions are explained below, such as pharmacotherapy management, surgical inventions, and radiation therapy.

13.5.1 PHARMACOTHERAPY/MEDICINE MANAGEMENT

The management of MEN1 syndrome-associated tumors is majorly done by surgery.

13.5.1.1 PHARMACOTHERAPY FOR INSULINOMA

A somatostatin analog drug known as octreotide prevents insulin release and controls glucose levels in the blood. This drug is initiated with short therapy with a dose of 20–30 mg taken 2–4 times/day. In addition to these, this drug may also have an antiproliferative effect (Okabayashi et al., 2013).

13.5.1.2 INTERVENTION STRATEGIES OF MEN1-ASSOCIATED GASTRINOMA

Therapy aims to treat acid secretion. Drugs of choice include Histamine H2 inhibitors (ranitidine, cimetidine, and famotidine) and H1-K1 ATPase inhibitors like lansoprazole, omeprazole, or pantoprazole to control acid hypersecretion. These drugs are well tolerated, and side effects are rare (Plöckinger, 2012; Khan et al., 2022).

13.5.1.3 PHARMACOTHERAPY OF PITUITARY TUMOR

To normalize cortisol levels in patients with Cushing's disease, medications like dopamine agonists (bromocriptine and cabergoline), somatostatin analogs (lanreotide, octreotide, and pasireotide), growth hormone receptor antagonists (pegvisomant), and ketoconazole were given. The choice of therapy depends upon the hypersecretion hormone levels and comorbidities of the patient's condition (Syro et al., 2012; John et al., 2022; Kaur et al., 2022).

13.5.1.4 PHARMACOTHERAPY FOR PARATHYROID TUMOR

Calcimimetics (cincalcet hydrochloride) are allosteric activators of CaR; they enhance the signaling and decrease parathyroid hormone (Liu et al., 2023).

13.5.1.5 PHARMACOTHERAPY FOR ADRENAL GLAND ADENOMA

For patients who are not suitable for surgery (advanced age, severe comorbidities), pharmacotherapy goals for alleviating the symptoms of patients by blocking the hormone receptors. For excess cortisol, drugs like mifepristone, glucocorticoid receptor antagonists, ketoconazole, and hyperaldosteronism, drugs like mineralocorticoid receptor antagonists like spironolactone or eplerenone were advised (Kapoor et al., 2011; Rajan and Giaccone, 2008).

13.5.1.6 PHARMACOTHERAPY OF THYMIC TUMOR

Chemotherapy is given for advanced thymic tumors. Combining cisplatin, cyclophosphamide, epirubicin, doxorubicin, and ifosfamide depends on drug severity and response (Rajan and Giaccone, 2008).

13.5.2 SURGERY INTERVENTIONS

13.5.2.1 SURGERY THERAPY FOR THE GASTRINOMA

The organs at the highest risk of developing tumors in MEN1 syndrome are the duodenum and pancreas; surgery is only curative and associated with high short pancreatic surgery (Carolina and Rachel, 2021).

13.5.2.1.1 Pancreas-Preserving Total Duodenectomy

PPTD requires an ultracareful surgical technique, which involves removing the whole duodenum while keeping the pancreatic head intact (Kamilaris and Stratakis, 2019).

13.5.2.1.2 Removal of Malignant Tumor

In asymptomatic patients, surgical removal of the malignant tumors before malignant transformation is an effort to reduce the death rate (Kamilaris and Stratakis, 2019).

13.5.2.2 SURGERY THERAPY FOR THE INSULINOMAS

Malignant insulinomas are extremely rare. The malignant tumor is unresectable, and medical therapy is limited to controlling the glucose levels in the blood (Okabayashi et al., 2013).

13.5.2.2.1 Partial Pancreatectomy

This surgery removes the tail alone or the tail with a portion of the body or often with the spleen depending upon the localization of the tumor mass and its malignancy effect and preserves the remaining pancreas parenchyma (Okabayashi et al., 2013).

13.5.2.2.2 Laparoscopic Resection and Radial Resection

The laparoscopy radial resection, a minimally invasive surgical procedure, is used when the lesions are not solitary, poorly encapsulated, more than 4 cm in diameter, and include or are close to the significant pancreatic duct (Okabayashi et al., 2013).

13.5.2.3 SURGERY INDICATION IN PITUITARY ADENOMAS

Surgery is the last resort for treating big, invasive, asymptomatic tumors, and symptomatic pituitary adenomas. It offers rapid relief from excess hormone production and mass impact (John et al., 2022).

13.5.2.3.1 Invasive Transsphenoidal Surgery

The minimally invasive transsphenoidal approach involves removing pituitary tumors using endonasal endoscopic surgery (computer-guided neuronavigational technique). It removes about 95% of pituitary tumors (John et al., 2022).

13.5.2.3.2 Submucosal Transseptal Surgery

The patient was put in the lawn chair posture, and an internal nasal incision was made for hemi-transfixation. The complete process of removing the osseous structure anterior to the pituitary gland was completed endonasally. The dude was opened, and the pituitary tumor was extracted in fragments or converted into subliminal for macroadenomas in children's cases (John et al., 2022).

13.5.2.3.3 Surgery by Pure Endoscopic Approach

This requires two surgeons and can be done in three or four hands (typically otolaryngologist and neurosurgeon with training in skull base surgery); one surgeon operates the endoscope while others have each hand free to remove the tumor using the microsurgical technique (John et al., 2022).

13.5.2.4 SURGERY INTERVENTION IN PARATHYROID

The optimal surgical approach in PHPT in MEN1 is under discussion between subtotal parathyroidectomy and total parathyroidectomy.

1. Subtotal parathyroidectomy is the elimination of three to half of the gland. This requires identifying all parathyroid glands, leaving a remnant of the parathyroid gland, approximately 20–30 mg. Careful dissection is necessary to preserve the fragile single end-artery and prevent ischemia and bleeding (Giusti et al., 2012).
2. Total thyroidectomy is resection of all four parathyroid glands followed by heterotopic auto implant (Giusti et al., 2012).

13.5.2.5 SURGERY INTERVENTION IN ADRENAL GLAND ADENOMA

Unilateral adrenalectomy is the preferred treatment for adenomas more significant than 4 cm, and for the surgical excision of adrenal masses, laparoscopic adrenalectomy ought to be the method of choice (Kapoor et al., 2011; Rajan and Giaccone, 2008).

13.5.3 RADIOLOGICAL THERAPY

Treatment with fractionated external beam radiation can lower the excess hormone production and the likelihood that a neoplasm will recur. Many consider cyberknife, gamma knife, linear accelerator stereotactic, or proton beam radiosurgery, an adjuvant treatment for pituitary tumors (John et al., 2022), for the pancreatic NETs. The radiation therapy for this indication was under the clinical trial phases I and II, in which 15.2% of patients had shown complete positive response, 30.3% of patients showed partial response, the remaining 42.4% and 12.2% were showing the stable disease and progress in the disease.

13.6 FUTURE PERSPECTIVE IN MANAGEMENT

There have been notable breakthroughs in the diagnosis of MEN1 and the early detection of malignancies through periodic screening programs that make use of sensitive radiography modalities. Unfortunately, there is a lack of scientific trials that evaluate the efficacy of specific treatments for MEN1-associated malignancies; therefore, the best way to treat these types of cancers is primarily unknown (Sherman, 2009). Although these studies have the potential to be fruitful, it may be challenging to recruit enough MEN1 patients to power them from a single national center. International and national MEN1 registries and partnerships should be established to address this. The effectiveness of this approach is demonstrated by clinical trials looking at the use of mTOR inhibitors for pancreatic NET and TRK inhibitors for MTC (Yao et al., 2011; Raymond and Dahan, 2011). Discovering crucial information on several elements, such as the necessity of surgery for nonfunctioning pancreatic NET and the natural course of adrenal lesions in MEN1 patients, has further proved the additional merits of such registries (Sakurai et al., 2012; Gatta-Cherifi et al., 2012). There must be a deeper molecular comprehension of MEN1 tumor biology to construct more solid foundational justifications for the proliferation of targeted and innovative therapies. This theory was reinforced by two recent investigations that identified therapeutic targets that disrupt the established relationship between menin and MLL1, an oncogenic cofactor that increases the transcription of genes. It has been demonstrated by crystal structures of both free and complexed human menin that this protein attaches to the short peptide of MLL1 through a deep pocket (Huang et al., 2012). Thienopyrimidine has been shown to have these activities in high-throughput screening tests that were looking for molecules that aim to inhibit menin's interaction with MLL. Two thienopyrimidine analogs were generated as a result of further structural and activity investigations; these bind to wild-type menin but not to mutant menins implicating the MLL interaction site (Grembecka et al., 2012). Future pharmacological therapies for MEN1 malignancies may be found in other analogs, which might be the subject of further research. For instance, molecular phenotyping of pancreatic NET might detect tumors linked to a bad prognosis and those with an active mTOR pathway. This would allow the evaluation of the impact of prior mTOR inhibitor therapy on clinical outcomes, as this approach could offer crucial information that might direct therapy. Furthermore, a future assessment in individuals with MEN1 is necessary to confirm the conclusion that individuals without MEN1 mutations, but with patients with mutations in the mTOR signaling pathway had a worse prognosis than those with pancreatic NET (MEN1 or DAXX/ATRX) (Jiao et al., 2011).

13.7 CONCLUSION

MEN1 mutant carriers may be mostly asymptomatic; early detection or diagnosis decreases the morbidity and mortality of the patients. Research activities, such as creating tumor biobanks related to MEN1, should thus be strongly supported. Lastly, in line to offer tailored medicines, patients should be informed about the significance of ongoing research and motivated to participate in these trials. Advances in medical treatment approaches, such as radiation therapy, medicine therapy, surgery interventions, and surveillance, improve the outcome of treatment.

KEYWORDS

- **multiple endocrine neoplasia1**
- **neuroendocrine neoplasm**
- **parathyroid**
- **pituitary gland**
- **islet cells**

REFERENCES

Bangar, A., Khan, H., Kaur, A., Dua, K., Singh, T.G. (2024). Understanding mechanistic aspect of the therapeutic role of herbal agents on neuroplasticity in cerebral ischemic-reperfusion injury. Journal of Ethnopharmacology, 319(Pt 2), 117153. https://doi.org/10.1016/j.jep.2023.117153

Barlier, A., Romanet, P., Pellegata, N.S. (2023). Editorial: New insights into multiple endocrine neoplasia type 1. Frontiers in Endocrinology, 14, 1266148. https://doi.org/10.3389/fendo.2023.1266148

Carolina, R.C.P., Rachel, S. (2021) Multiple Endocrine Neoplasia Type 1 http://dx.doi.org/10.3322/caac.21673

Därr, R., Lenders, J.W., Hofbauer, L.C., Naumann, B., Bornstein, S.R., Eisenhofer, G. (2012). Pheochromocytoma - update on disease management. Therapeutic Advances in Endocrinology and Metabolism, 3(1), 11–26. https://doi.org/10.1177/2042018812437356

de Laat, J.M., van Leeuwaarde, R.S., Valk, G.D. (2018). The importance of an early and accurate MEN1 diagnosis. Frontiers in Endocrinology, 9, 533. https://doi.org/10.3389/fendo.2018.00533

Gatta-Cherifi, B., Chabre, O., Murat, A., Niccoli, P., Cardot-Bauters, C., Rohmer, V., Young, J., Delemer, B., Du Boullay, H., Verger, M.F., Kuhn, J.M., Sadoul, J.L., Ruszniewski, P., Beckers, A., Monsaingeon, M., Baudin, E., Goudet, P., Tabarin, A. (2012). Adrenal involvement in MEN1. Analysis of 715 cases from the Groupe d'etude des Tumeurs Endocrines database. European Journal of Endocrinology, 166(2), 269–279. https://doi.org/10.1530/EJE-11-0679

Giusti, F., Tonelli, F., Brandi, M.L. (2012). Primary hyperparathyroidism in multiple endocrine neoplasia type 1: When to perform surgery. Clinics (Sao Paulo, Brazil), 67(Suppl 1), 141–144. https://doi.org/10.6061/clinics/2012(sup01)23

Grembecka, J., He, S., Shi, A., Purohit, T., Muntean, A.G., Sorenson, R.J., Showalter, H.D., Murai, M.J., Belcher, A.M., Hartley, T., Hess, J.L., Cierpicki, T. (2012). Menin-MLL inhibitors reverse oncogenic activity of MLL fusion proteins in leukemia. Nature Chemical Biology, 8(3), 277–284. https://doi.org/10.1038/nchembio.773

Huang, J., Gurung, B., Wan, B., Matkar, S., Veniaminova, N.A., Wan, K., Merchant, J.L., Hua, X., Lei, M. (2012). The same pocket in menin binds both MLL and JUND but has opposite effects on transcription. Nature, 482(7386), 542–546. https://doi.org/10.1038/nature10806

Jiao, Y., Shi, C., Edil, B.H., de Wilde, R.F., Klimstra, D.S., Maitra, A., Schulick, R.D., Tang, L.H., Wolfgang, C.L., Choti, M.A., Velculescu, V.E., Diaz, L.A., Jr, Vogelstein, B., Kinzler, K.W., Hruban, R.H., Papadopoulos, N. (2011). DAXX/ATRX, MEN1, and mTOR pathway genes are frequently altered in pancreatic neuroendocrine tumors. Science (New York, N.Y.), 331(6021), 1199–1203. https://doi.org/10.1126/science.1200609

John, A.J., Jr, Michael, P.C., Edward, R.L. (2022). Surgical treatment of pituitary adenomas. Endotext. https://doi.org/10.3389/fsurg.2023.1129387

Kamilaris, C.D.C., Stratakis, C.A. (2019). Multiple endocrine neoplasia type 1 (MEN1): An update and the significance of early genetic and clinical diagnosis. Frontiers in Endocrinology, 10, 339. https://doi.org/10.3389/fendo.2019.00339

Kapoor, A., Morris, T., Rebello, R. (2011). Guidelines for the management of the incidentally discovered adrenal mass. Canadian Urological Association journal = Journal de l'Association des urologues du Canada, 5(4), 241–247. https://doi.org/10.5489/cuaj.11135

Kaur, A., Singh, T.G., Khan, H., Kumar, M., Singh, N., Abdel-Daim, M.M. (2022). Neuroprotective effect of piclamilast-induced post-ischemia pharmacological treatment in mice. Neurochemical Research, 47(8), 2230–2243. https://doi.org/10.1007/s11064-022-03609-w

Khakha, N., Khan, H., Kaur, A., Singh, T.G. (2023). Therapeutic implications of phosphorylation- and dephosphorylation-dependent factors of cAMP-response element-binding protein (CREB) in neurodegeneration. Pharmacological Reports: PR, 75(5), 1152–1165. https://doi.org/10.1007/s43440-023-00526-9

Khan, H., Kaur Grewal, A., Gurjeet Singh, T. (2022). Mitochondrial dynamics related neurovascular approaches in cerebral ischemic injury. Mitochondrion, 66, 54–66. https://doi.org/10.1016/j.mito.2022.08.001

Lairmore, T.C., Piersall, L.D., DeBenedetti, M.K., Dilley, W.G., Mutch, M.G., Whelan, A.J., Zehnbauer, B. (2004). Clinical genetic testing and early surgical intervention in patients with multiple endocrine neoplasia type 1 (MEN 1). Annals of Surgery, 239(5), 637–647. https://doi.org/10.1097/01.sla.0000124383.98416.8d

Liu, Z., Zhao, Y., Han, X., Hu, X., Zhang, Y., Xu, L., Chen, G., Liu, C., Xu, S. (2023). Ultrasound-guided microwave ablation in the treatment of recurrent primary hyperparathyroidism in a patient with MEN1: A case report. Frontiers in Endocrinology, 14, 1175377. https://doi.org/10.3389/fendo.2023.1175377

Marini, F., Falchetti, A., Luzi, E., Tonelli, F., Maria Luisa, B. (2008). Multiple endocrine neoplasia type 1 (MEN1) syndrome. In: Riegert-Johnson, D.L., Ed., et al., *Cancer Syndromes*. National Center for Biotechnology Information (US).

Marini, F., Giusti, F., Brandi, M.L. (2018). Multiple endocrine neoplasia type 1: Extensive analysis of a large database of Florentine patients. Orphanet Journal of Rare Diseases, 13(1), 205. https://doi.org/10.1186/s13023-018-0938-8

Mehta, S., Nain, P., Agrawal, B.K., Singh, R.P. (2022). Vitamin D with calcium supplementation managing glycemic control with HbA1c and improve quality of life in patients with diabetes. Turkish Journal of Pharmaceutical Sciences, 19(2), 161–167. https://doi.org/10.4274/tjps.galenos.2021.62357

Okabayashi, T., Shima, Y., Sumiyoshi, T., Kozuki, A., Ito, S., Ogawa, Y., Kobayashi, M., Hanazaki, K. (2013). Diagnosis and management of insulinoma. World Journal of Gastroenterology, 19(6), 829–837. https://doi.org/10.3748/wjg.v19.i6.829

Plöckinger, U. (2012). Diagnosis and treatment of gastrinomas in multiple endocrine neoplasia type 1 (MEN-1). Cancers, 4(1), 39–54. https://doi.org/10.3390/cancers4010039

Rajan, A., Giaccone, G. (2008). Treatment of advanced thymoma and thymic carcinoma. Current Treatment Options in Oncology, 9(4–6), 277–287. https://doi.org/10.1007/s11864-009-0083-7

Raymond, E., Dahan, L. (2011). Sunitinib malate for treating pancreatic neuroendocrine tumours. The New England Journal of Medicine, 364, 501–513. https://doi.org/10.1056/nejmoa1003825

Rihal, V., Khan, H., Kaur, A., Singh, T.G. (2023). Vitamin D as therapeutic modulator in cerebrovascular diseases: A mechanistic perspectives. Critical Reviews in Food Science and Nutrition, 63(25), 7772–7794. https://doi.org/10.1080/10408398.2022.2050349

Sadowski, S.M., Cadiot, G., Dansin, E., Goudet, P., Triponez, F. (2017). The future: Surgical advances in MEN1 therapeutic approaches and management strategies. Endocrine-related Cancer, 24(10), T243–T260. https://doi.org/10.1530/ERC-17-0285

Sakurai, A., Suzuki, S., Kosugi, S., Okamoto, T., Uchino, S., Miya, A., Imai, T., Kaji, H., Komoto, I., Miura, D., Yamada, M., Uruno, T., Horiuchi, K., Miyauchi, A., Imamura, M., MEN Consortium of Japan, Fukushima, T., Hanazaki, K., Hirakawa, S., Igarashi, T., … Yamazaki, M. (2012). Multiple endocrine neoplasia type 1 in Japan: Establishment and analysis of a multicentre database. Clinical Endocrinology, 76(4), 533–539. https://doi.org/10.1111/j.1365-2265.2011.04227.x

Scott, N.P., Holen, K. (2008). Carcinoid tumors. Oncologist, 13(12): 1255–1269. https://doi.org/10.1634/theoncologist.2008-0207

Sharma, T., Kaur, D., Grewal, A.K., Singh, T.G. (2021). Therapies modulating insulin resistance in Parkinson's disease: A cross talk. Neuroscience Letters, 749, 135754. https://doi.org/10.1016/j.neulet.2021.135754

Sharma, V.K., Singh, T.G., Mehta, V., Mannan, A. (2023a). Biomarkers: Role and scope in neurological disorders. Neurochemical Research, 48(7), 2029–2058. https://doi.org/10.1007/s11064-023-03873-4

Sharma, V., Chhabra, T., Singh, T.G. (2023b). Correlation of covid-19 and Guillain–Barré syndrome: A mechanistic perspective. Obesity Medicine, 40, 100493. https://doi.org/10.1016/j.obmed.2023.100493

Sherman, S.I. (2009). Advances in chemotherapy of differentiated epithelial and medullary thyroid cancers. The Journal of Clinical Endocrinology and Metabolism. 94, 1493–1499. https://doi.org/10.1210/jc.2008-0923

Singh, G., Mulji, N.J., Jialal, I. (2023). Multiple Endocrine Neoplasia Type 1. In: *National Institutes of Health*. http://dx.doi.org/10.1016/j.soc.2015.06.008

Singh, R., Rao, H.K., Singh, T.G. (2020). Advanced glycated end products (ages) in diabetes and its complications: An insight. Plant Arch, 20(1), 3838–3841

Syro, L.V., Scheithauer, B.W., Kovacs, K., Toledo, R.A., Londoño, F.J., Ortiz, L.D., Rotondo, F., Horvath, E., Uribe, H. (2012). Pituitary tumors in patients with MEN1 syndrome. Clinics (Sao Paulo, Brazil), 67(Suppl 1), 43–48. https://doi.org/10.6061/clinics/2012(sup01)09

Wang, W., Han, R., Ye, L., Xie, J., Tao, B., Sun, F., Zhuo, R., Chen, X., Deng, X., Ye, C., Zhao, H., Wang, S. (2019). Adrenocortical carcinoma in patients with MEN1: A kindred report and review of the literature. Endocrine Connections, 8(3), 230–238. https://doi.org/10.1530/EC-18-0526

Yao, J.C., Shah, M.H., Ito, T., Bohas, C.L., Wolin, E.M., Van Cutsem, E., Hobday, T.J., Okusaka, T., Capdevila, J., de Vries, E.G., Tomassetti, P., Pavel, M.E., Hoosen, S., Haas, T., Lincy, J., Lebwohl, D., Öberg, K., RAD001 in Advanced Neuroendocrine Tumors, Third Trial (RADIANT-3) Study Group (2011). Everolimus for advanced pancreatic neuroendocrine tumors. The New England Journal of Medicine, 364(6), 514–523. https://doi.org/10.1056/NEJMoa1009290

Yliaska, I., Tokola, H., Ebeling, T., Kuismin, O., Ukkola, O., Koivikko, M.L., Lesonen, T., Rimpiläinen, J., Felin, T., Ryhänen, E., Metso, S., Schalin-Jäntti, C., Salmela, P. (2022). Thymic neuroendocrine tumors in patients with multiple endocrine neoplasia type 1. Endocrine, 77(3), 527–537. https://doi.org/10.1007/s12020-022-03099-4

Index

D

S

T

U

V

W

X

Z

For Product Safety Concerns and Information please contact our EU
representative GPSR@taylorandfrancis.com
Taylor & Francis Verlag GmbH, Kaufingerstraße 24, 80331 München, Germany

www.ingramcontent.com/pod-product-compliance
Lightning Source LLC
LaVergne TN
LVHW020627300926
849161LV00004B/630
* 9 7 8 1 7 7 9 6 4 0 1 4 7 *